The Biological Basis of Mental Health Nursing

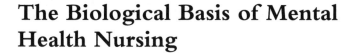

Written by an experienced nurse lecturer who also trained as a mental health nurse, this book explores the underlying biology associated with the pathology of mental health disorders and the related nervous system. Fully revised for this second edition, the text includes three new chapters on brain development, pharmacology and learning, behavioural and developmental disorders.

Integrating up-to-date pharmacological and genetic knowledge with an understanding of environmental factors that impact on human biology, *The Biological Basis of Mental Health Nursing* covers topics including:

*   the physiology of neurotransmission and receptors
*   hormones and mental health
*   the biology of emotions, stress, anxiety and phobic states
*   the biology of substance abuse
*   developmental disorders
*   brain development
*   the biology of behaviour
*   genetics and mental health
*   affective disorders: depression and suicide
*   schizophrenia
*   autism and other syndromes
*   the ageing brain and dementia
*   degenerative diseases of the brain
*   epilepsy and sleep disorders.

Accessibly laid out, with plenty of diagrams and overviews at the beginning of each chapter, this is an essential text for mental health nursing students, practitioners and educators.

William T. Blows, RMN, RGN, RNT, OStJ, BSc (Hons), PhD is currently Lecturer in Applied Biological Sciences at City University, London. He is also the author of *The Biological Basis of Nursing: Clinical Observations* and *The Biological Basis of Nursing: Cancer.*

The Biological Basis of Mental Health Nursing

Second edition
William T. Blows

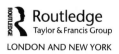

Routledge
Taylor & Francis Group

LONDON AND NEW YORK

First edition published 2003
by Routledge

This edition published 2011
by Routledge
2 Park Square, Milton Park, Abingdon, Oxon OX14 4RN

Simultaneously published in the USA and Canada
by Routledge
270 Madison Avenue, New York NY 10016

Routledge is an imprint of the Taylor & Francis Group, an informa business

Typeset in Bembo by Swales & Willis Ltd, Exeter, Devon
Printed and bound in Great Britain by TJ International Ltd, Padstow, Cornwall

British Library Cataloguing in Publication Data
A catalogue record for this book is available from the British Library

Library of Congress Cataloging in Publication Data
Blows, William T., 1947–
   The biological basis of mental health nursing / William Blows.—2nd ed.
   p. ; cm.
   Rev. ed. of: Biological basis of nursing. Mental health / William T. Blows. 2003.
   Includes bibliographical references and index.
   1. Biological psychiatry. 2. Mental illness—Physiological aspects.
   3. Brain—Diseases. 4. Psychiatric nursing.
   I. Blows, William T., 1947– Mental health. II. Title.
   [DNLM: 1. Biological Psychiatry—Nurses' Instruction.
   2. Mental Disorders—Nurses' Instruction.
   3. Brain—physiology—Nurses' Instruction. WM 140]
   RC455.4.B5B62 2011
   616.89—dc22
   2010027434

ISBN13: 978–0–415–57097–8 (hbk)
ISBN13: 978–0–415–57098–5 (pbk)
ISBN13: 978–0–203–83388–9 (ebk)

Contents

1 Introduction to the brain

- **Introduction**
- **The meninges and cerebrospinal fluid**
- **The cerebrum**
- **The limbic system**
- **The thalamus, hypothalamus and pituitary gland**
- **The basal ganglia and the cerebellum**
- **The brain stem**
- **The autonomic nervous system**
- **The pathways involved in mental health**
- **The basic principles of brain pathologies affecting mental health**
- **Key points**

Introduction

The human brain is one of Nature's greatest achievements. It is the development of the brain which has allowed humans to progress from their humble origins to putting a man on the moon. This chapter consists of an overview of the brain and contains many references to other pages where the area of the brain in question is explored further in more detail, usually in relation to a particular mental health pathology. At the simplest level the brain works something like a computer, but this is a computer like no other. It has been said that to build a computer to do everything the human brain does, the computer would have to be the size of Europe. Like a computer, the brain has an input (called a **sensory nervous system**) and an output (called a **motor nervous system**). Between these two systems, the brain carries out **cognitive functions**, i.e. mental processing such as thought, language, intellect, memory and interpretation of the world about us.

As with a computer, things can go wrong with the brain, and when they do, symptoms occur, just as with any other organ. The pathological conditions associated with the brain may be either **neurological** or **psychiatric**, depending on the degree of physical disturbance (neurological) or mental health disturbance (psychiatric) identified. These two types of brain dysfunction are becoming increasingly overlapped, with the distinction between them becoming blurred. This is because we are learning that neurological conditions often involve disturbance of the mind and that mental health disturbance has some degree of physical (or biological) basis.

The brain can be divided into several anatomical, developmental and functional areas as we move downwards from the top towards the base (Figure 1.1). The **cerebrum**, at the top, is the largest and most advanced region of the brain, carrying out all our cognitive and conscious processes. Beneath this is the **limbic cortex** (cortex = surface layer), the area concerned with preservation of both the individual and the species. This is the area involved in emotions, such as fear, and behavioural patterns, such as eating, which are designed to keep us alive. Beneath this are the **basal ganglia** and the **cerebellum**, areas involved in control of movement at a subconscious (automatic) level. Finally, at the very base of the brain, the **brain stem** is involved in keeping the individual alive at the physiological level, controlling the heart, the blood pressure and the lungs amongst other functions (Martini and Nath 2008).

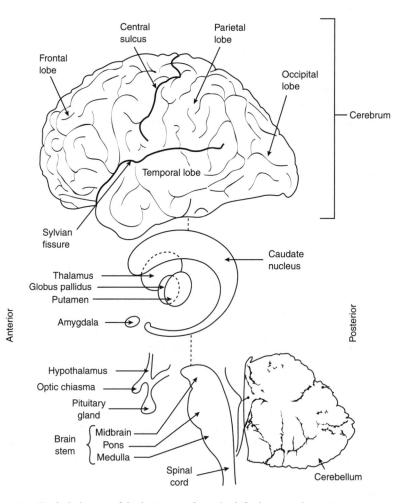

Figure 1.1 Exploded view of the brain seen from the left, showing the main components.

At tissue level, the areas of the brain are either **grey matter**, made from the cell bodies of **neurons** (brain cells), or **white matter**, made from the **axons** of neurons. Grey matter dominates the outer surfaces of the brain, known as a **cortex**, *See page 43* with white matter inside. The surfaces, or cortex, are folded into **gyri** (singular **gyrus**, i.e. the top of a fold), and **sulci** (singular **sulcus**, i.e. the bottom of a fold) in order to increase the surface area for the purpose of packing in more neurons. Cell bodies which are separate from the main outer surface, i.e. patches of grey matter deeper inside the white matter, are called **ganglia** (e.g. the basal ganglia). **Nuclei** are patches of grey matter which have a specific controlling function (e.g. the cranial nerve nuclei of the brain stem). Several areas of the brain, such as the **thalamus** and **hypothalamus**, are actually discrete collections of distinct nuclei which are linked together by one name because they are anatomically positioned together, and they have similar, related functions.

The meninges and cerebrospinal fluid

The brain and the cord are covered by membranes called the **meninges**, which form three layers (Figure 1.2). The innermost layer is the **pia mater** ('gentle mother'), the middle is the **arachnoid mater** ('spider mother') and the outermost is the **dura mater** ('tough mother'). Between the arachnoid mater and pia mater is the **subarachnoid space** containing a watery fluid called **cerebrospinal fluid** (**CSF**). This is formed from blood plasma inside the **ventricles** of the brain, i.e. the cavities within the brain substance (Martini and Nath 2008). CSF fills the two **lateral ventricles**, the **third ventricle** and the **fourth ventricle** before it flows out into

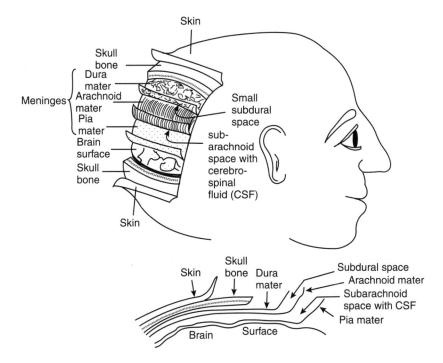

Figure 1.2 The meninges between the brain and the skull.

the subarachnoid space. From here it circulates over the brain and cord surface before being absorbed back into blood via small projections of the arachnoid mater called **villi**. CSF also flows from the fourth ventricle through the **central canal** of the cord. CSF has several important functions.

1   It protects the central nervous system by acting as a water jacket, giving a cushioning effect to the central nervous system. This is a very important function, helping to reduce brain injury in accidents involving the head.
2   It provides support and flotation for the brain, which would otherwise weigh 30 times heavier without it!
3   It delivers nutrition to some parts of the nervous system, since the CSF contains not just water but also some minerals and glucose.
4   It acts as part of an excretory pathway for the end products of neurotransmitter metabolism (known as **metabolites**) and some psychoactive drugs. These wastes pass from the brain into the CSF, then into the blood, which then goes on to the kidneys for filtering and the excretion of the wastes in urine.

CSF is often very important in mental health because of this role as an excretory pathway. One investigation, called **lumbar puncture**, is a method of collecting a sample of CSF in which the excretory products from brain chemicals or drugs can be measured (Blows 2002a). A needle is put into the spinal subarachnoid space below the level of lumbar vertebra 2 (L2) so as not to hit the solid spinal cord. The quantity of metabolite found in the CSF sample gives an indication of the amount of neurotransmitter that is active in the brain.

The cerebrum

The largest and uppermost area of the brain, the cerebrum (Figure 1.1), is divided into two **hemispheres**, left and right, each of which is further divided into four **lobes**: the frontal, parietal, temporal and occipital lobes. **Brodmann numbers** (Figure 1.3) form an internationally agreed numbering system to identify and map the major areas of the cerebral cortex (outer surface) according to their functions.

Frontal lobe

The **frontal lobes** contain the main **motor cortex** (motor = movement) (Brodmann 4) for each side of the body. Each cortex, left and right, controls skeletal muscles via long pathways descending into the spinal cord, then out to the muscles; these motor pathways are called the **pyramidal tracts** (Martini and Nath 2008). In addition, the **premotor cortex** (Brodmann 6), just anterior to the motor cortex, is involved in **motor planning**, a process that is vital for the swift and accurate execution of complex motor tasks. Speech motor areas (Brodmann 44 and 45), also known as **Brocha's area**, control the muscles of the speech.

The frontal lobe also has areas concerned with the following range of important higher intellectual activities:

1   Achieving and sustaining attention and concentration;
2   Carrying out language activities, both spoken and in thought;

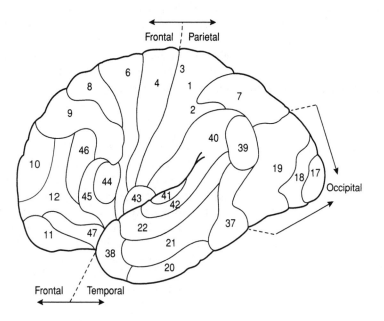

Figure 1.3 A functional map of the left cerebral cortex showing Brodmann numbers.

3   Maintaining memory;
4   Forming part of the pathways involved in emotions;
5   Carrying out complex skills involving visual space (i.e. **visuospatial tasks**) which require, for example, sequence planning or detailed copying of figures;
6   Performing **executive functions** such as monitoring one's own performance and making corrections as required, formulating and achieving goals, planning, judgement and reasoning.

The frontal lobes are the last part of the brain to mature, sometime after puberty, so teenagers function with reduced levels of emotional control and reasoning.

See page 34

The frontal lobes are the main centres of consciousness, particularly of self (i.e. self-awareness). Much of our **thought processes**, particularly **planning** (which requires forward thinking towards the future), reasoning and deduction, are carried out by the frontal lobe, and in particular the prefrontal cortex. It has the most neural connections, it makes the most complex integrations with other systems, and it requires more than twice the energy requirements of other brain areas such as the limbic system. Thought processes, unlike other brain functions, do not rely on sensory input directly; they are an 'internal' mental function. Thought does require, however, previous stored information and knowledge, in particular knowledge of language. Thought content and processing is strongly influenced by the hippocampus, and disruption of the hippocampus, as in **schizophrenia**, causes symptoms such as thought disorder.

Many components of what we regard as our **personality** are due to the activities of the frontal lobes. It should therefore not be surprising to learn that many psychiatric disorders and some specific mental health symptoms either manifest within or involve the frontal lobes of the brain. No wonder that one of the very few psychosurgical operations carried out in the past for mental health reasons was a **prefrontal leucotomy**, which involved severing pathways leading from the frontal lobe to the other parts of the brain. Three main pathways involved in mental health disturbance connect the frontal lobe to deeper structures in the brain. These are the **dorsolateral prefrontal circuit**, the **lateral orbitofrontal circuit** and the **anterior cingulate circuit** (McPherson and Cummings 1999).

See page 20

Parietal lobe

The **parietal lobe** involves the main **somatic** (i.e. soma = body, thus somatic = from the body) sensory cortex (Brodmann 1, 2 and 3), and the somatic sensory association area (Brodmann 7). **Association areas** are essential for the interpretation and memory of senses, and therefore the understanding of sensory stimuli. This is important because the brain is itself shut away from the world inside the skull. The only way the brain is going to know what is happening outside the skull is via the sensory nervous system, and by its ability to interpret those signals brought in by this sensory system. Association areas are therefore critical in the brain's understanding of the world around us. A language area, which is also part of the parietal lobe, is Brodmann 39 (also known as **Wernicke's area**) and is the main site for formulation of spoken sentences.

Temporal lobe

The **temporal lobe** houses the auditory area for the *conscious* sensation of hearing (Brodmann 41 and 42) and the auditory association area (Brodmann 22). What we actually hear is generated in the temporal lobe auditory area and not in the ears. Ears are organs necessary to convert sound waves into nerve impulses. The temporal lobe makes sense of these impulses as sound. This lobe is also involved in the creation of personality and in emotional responses to sensory stimuli.

Occipital lobe

The **occipital lobe** has the main visual cortex (Brodmann 17) and the visual association areas (Brodmann 18 and 19) (Blows 2000a). This is therefore the *conscious* area for vision; that is, as with the temporal lobe and hearing, we actually 'see' the world with the back of the brain. The eyes only convert light energy into nerve impulses; it is the occipital lobe that makes sense of these impulses as a visual picture that we are aware of.

Functions of the cerebrum

One of the most important functions of the cerebrum is the government of three important aspects of **consciousness**: awareness (sensory); cognition (e.g. thought); and response (motor). The entire cortex plays a role in consciousness, although for the most part the parietal, temporal and occipital lobes are involved with conscious interpretation of sensory stimuli, whilst the frontal lobe is concerned with cognition and consciousness of the 'self'. A discussion of consciousness and its relation to nursing observations can be found in *The Biological Basis of Nursing: Clinical Observations* (Blows 2001, Chapter 7) (see also Blows 2000b).

The left hemisphere of the cerebrum is dominant for several functions, notably fine motor control, logic, analytical work, language and verbal tasks. Fine motor control means digital and hand movements, an essential part of many activities. Since most of the motor (i.e. pyramidal) fibres cross in the medulla, the dominance of motor control in the left hemisphere makes most people right handed. However, we know that it is entirely normal for left-handed people to be an exception to this, although left-handed dominance has not always been accepted by society. In the past, left-handed children were sometimes forced to write right handed. The right hemisphere is dominant for non-language skills, spatial perception and artistic and musical endeavours. People who have a general dominance of left hemisphere function are sometimes called *thinkers*, whilst those with right hemisphere function dominance are sometimes referred to as *creators*. This image of hemisphere functions may give the impression that the two hemispheres work in isolation. This is not true; they work together, communicating with each other through a bridge connection that joins the left hemisphere with the right hemisphere known as the **corpus callosum** (Martini and Nath 2008).

Sleep is a vital function for the brain, and the cerebrum in particular. It was thought for many years that sleep was a state of rest for the brain as well as for the body. We now know, from modern imaging techniques and **electroencephalograms** (**EEG**), that sleep is a time when the brain is very active, and occasionally more active than when awake. The real reason for sleep is still unknown, but a significant amount of research is trying to establish why we spend about a third of our lives sleeping. This is important because sleep patterns are often disturbed in mental health disorders, such as in depression. The triggers for sleep are also unknown but it appears there are complex hormonal and neurological changes occurring as sleep approaches. These changes involve the reticular activating system of the brain stem and chemical changes within the brain. *See page 243*

There are two main phases of sleep: **REM** (**rapid eye movement**) and **NREM** (**non-rapid eye movement**). The terms come from observations made of the eye movements during sleep, movements which can distinguish these two phases, one from the other. When the eyes are still (NREM) the brain goes through four stages in order as follows:

Stage 1: A light sleep, recognised by brain waves called **theta waves** seen on an electroencephalogram (EEG) (for details of EEG see Blows 2002b).
Stage 2: A deeper sleep, recognised by a special form of brain waves called 'sleep spindles' seen on the EEG.
Stage 3: Even deeper sleep, recognised by the presence of delta waves on the EEG.
Stage 4: The deepest form of sleep, recognised by a change to a greater intensity of delta waves.

During a typical night's sleep, the brain moves through NREM stages 1 to 4, then reverses back through the stages 4 to 1. This NREM cycle takes from seventy to ninety minutes. There is then a move into REM sleep, when the EGG pattern is similar to that seen when awake (the brain, when awake, produces alpha waves). This lasts five to fifteen minutes, followed by a return to the NREM cycle. The rest of the night's sleep is composed of repeated cycles of NREM with REM, with each cycle seeing a shortening of NREM and a lengthening of the REM periods. We finally awake from REM. Apparently, it is during REM that people dream, and waking up from REM allows some people to remember their dreams. The function of dreams is not understood, despite the many attempts to interpret the meaning of dreams. What is known is that sleep is essential, and loss of sleep causes serious problems, including irritability, blurred vision, slurred speech, loss of concentration, memory loss, confusion, fatigue and even hallucinations. When sleep is restored, the effects of the sleep loss are quickly reversed without long-term effect.

Sleep patterns change with age as follows:

* Newborn babies require sixteen hours per day in sleep, approximately 50 per cent of the time in REM and 50 per cent in NREM. During the first year of life the total amount of sleep needed per day drops sharply. By the second year the child needs between nine and twelve hours of sleep per day.
* Adults require six to nine hours of sleep per day, 25 per cent in REM, 75 per cent in NREM.
* Elderly people require about six hours of sleep per day, mostly in NREM (REM is less than 20 per cent).

Recently, the concept of the restless brain came into sharper focus with the discovery of the **default mode network** (**DMN**). During waking hours, the brain is able to concentrate on the specific task at hand, but there are times when the brain is allowed to wander, and not concentrate on anything. During this time, it would be easy to suspect the brain is inactive, but this is far from the truth. The brain appears to be active on 'internal matters' rather than 'external matters', but these internal matters remain unknown to us, and this activity has therefore been called *dark energy*. The DMN is the system in the brain responsible for dark energy; it is a system which keeps active even when the brain is not doing anything. This is rather similar to a car engine 'ticking over' or 'running idle' when not involved in moving the car. In a way, the DMN is probably very much involved in establishing and maintaining consciousness, and it keeps the brain in a state of instant readiness for when that moment comes that focus on a specific activity is necessary. Prior to the discovery of the DMN, neurologists thought that the brain was cycling between moments of no activity and moderate activity; but now the new concept is that the brain is cycling between moderate activity and high activity. This, plus the notion that the brain is active during sleep, suggests that, from birth to death, the brain *never* rests. The main areas of the brain that make up the DMN are the **medial prefrontal cortex**, the **medial parietal cortex**, the **lateral temporal cortex** and the **lateral parietal cortex**. Other areas are also involved but these four regions appear to control the activity levels of the brain's idle state. This new discovery may be important for mental health because there is growing evidence that altered connections in the DMN are possibly linked to disorders such as autism, depression, Alzheimer's disease (AD) and even schizophrenia. In fact, some researchers are suggesting that one-day AD may be classified as a disorder of the DMN (Raichle 2010).

Learning and *memory* are also two vital functions for the brain. Learning is the process by which memory is formed. These are covered in more detail in Chapter 2.

See page 33

The limbic system

The limbic system provides the brain's emotional centres, and it is also important for learning and for maintaining the brain's role in relation to a sense of human needs and safety. The system consists of a ring of structures, notably the amygdala, the hippocampus, the cingulate gyrus, the mammillary bodies of the hypothalamus and the orbitofrontal cortex (see Chapter 9 and Figure 9.1).

The amygdala

The amygdala is a small pea-sized collection of nuclei situated at the tail end of the caudate nucleus (Figure 1.4). This tiny area is the emotional centre of the brain. It receives sensory input from several sources, particularly the cerebral cortex, the thalamus and the hippocampus (Figure 1.5) (Blows 2000c). All kinds of stimuli from the external environment, or from the internal environment of the body, pass through the amygdala. The amygdala may respond to these stimuli by initiating specific emotional responses. Any adverse stimuli are known as **stressors** – i.e. potential threats to which the brain must respond with either an emotional or physical change. Output from the amygdala, in response to good stimuli, or stressors, is to the brain stem (for emotional responses) and to the hypothalamus (for any physical response) (Figure 1.5). The amygdala is described in more detail in Chapter 9 in relation to emotions and phobic states.

See page 163

The hippocampus

The hippocampus is tucked up underneath the temporal lobe of the cerebrum (Figure 1.6). The main function of this area is that of short-term memory, i.e. memory of very recent events (within the last few hours), which is held temporarily until it is either committed to long-term memory or forgotten (Blows 2000c). It is also involved in learning, which should not be surprising since learning is

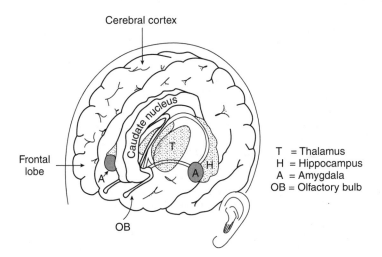

Figure 1.4 The components and location of the limbic system.

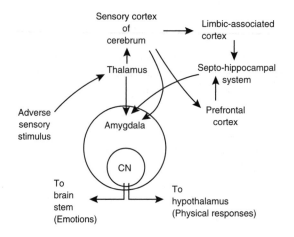

Figure 1.5 Simplified connections of the amygdala. CN = central nucleus.

See page 164
See page 89
interlinked with memory. Emotional behaviour and thinking are both influenced by hippocampal activity, notably aggression. The hippocampus is described in more detail in relation to schizophrenia.

The cingulate gyrus

This is the mass of neurons that overlies the upper surface of the corpus callosum, from front to back, and tucks beneath the corpus callosum anteriorly (Figure 9.1). The functions are becoming better understood. The anterior aspect is involved in mood, the central section controls response selection, and the posterior section is

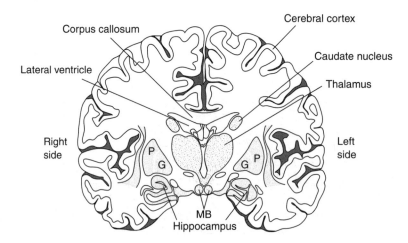

Figure 1.6 Coronal section through the brain showing the location of the cerebral cortex, the corpus callosum, the thalamus, the hippocampus, the mammillary bodies (MB) of the hypothalamus and parts of the basal ganglia. P = putamen; G = globus pallidus.

important in memory. This part of the brain has strong links with the rest of the limbic system.

The orbitofrontal cortex

Although strictly part of the cerebrum, the orbitofrontal cortex has strong links with the limbic system and is sometime considered to be part of what is called the *limbic associated cortex*. This part of the frontal lobe lies ventral to the prefrontal cortex, i.e. it is the brain area found immediately above the eyes. It is one of the most complex parts of the brain, and its functions are only just coming to light. All sensory stimuli (vision, hearing, and so on), are first processed by the relevant sensory areas, then pass into the posterior orbitofrontal cortex. The main function of the orbitofrontal cortex is to use this sensory input to guide behaviour, learning, memory and pleasure-seeking activity.

The thalamus, hypothalamus and pituitary gland

The thalamus

The thalamus is a collection of more than 30 nuclei situated underneath the cerebrum, close to the midline of the brain on each side (Figure 1.6) (Blows 2000c). The nuclei are set in four main groups: anterior, medial, midline and lateral. The thalamus is the *sensory relay station*; i.e. sensory impulses originating in the body (somatic) or the special senses (e.g. vision and hearing) pass into the thalamus, from where they are relayed to the appropriate part of the cerebrum. Visual nerve impulses from the retina must be relayed by the thalamus to the visual cortex of the occipital lobe (Brodmann 17, Figure 1.3), and nerve impulses generated from sound by the ear are relayed by the thalamus to the auditory cortex in the temporal lobe (Brodmann 41 and 42, Figure 1.3). Even somatic sensations from the body, e.g. touch or pain, are relayed to the appropriate part of the sensory cortex in the parietal lobe (Brodmann 1, 2 and 3, Figure 1.3). The sensory cortex has a cellular layout rather like a body plan, with cells in specific sites on the cortex accepting sensations from particular parts of the body. Impulses arising from the toes, for example, would be directed by the thalamus to the cortex occurring down the midline division, whilst impulses destined for the cells that accept sensations from the face would be directed to the lateral aspect of the cortex (Blows 2000b, p. 47). Pain is the only sensation that is 'conscious' at both thalamic and cerebral levels, whilst all other sensations must arrive at the cerebrum before we become aware of them.

The thalamus also focuses attention to specific sensations by making certain sensory areas of the cerebrum more receptive to sensory stimuli and other areas less receptive. Integration of some different sensory stimuli takes place inside the thalamus, a process essential for full appreciation of the information received by the sense organs.

The thalamus has a motor function as well. One particular thalamic nucleus links with the premotor cortex (Brodmann 6) of the frontal lobe, influencing motor function by increasing the focus of attention on the motor activity in progress. This influence is normally deactivated by the **basal ganglia motor loop** when no movement is happening, or activated when movement begins. *See page 262*

The hypothalamus

The hypothalamus occurs as a collection of nuclei at the base of the brain (Figure 1.6) (Blows 2000c). These nuclei are arranged in anterior, posterior, ventromedial, dorsomedial and lateral groups. The **mammillary body**, a bulbous part of the hypothalamus, is a member of the posterior group of nuclei and a useful landmark on the undersurface of the brain. The hypothalamus is connected to the **pituitary gland** by a narrow stalk, the **pituitary stalk** (or **infundibulum**) (Martini and Nath 2008).

The hypothalamus has a wide range of functions and controlling centres:

See page 17 1   It is part of the **reticular formation** (see brain stem) that controls the **sleep–wake cycle**; the role of the hypothalamus is that of the **alerting centre**; that is, it wakes the brain from sleep by sending impulses out to the cerebrum.

2   It controls the body's temperature; that is, it is the **temperature regulation centre** keeping the body at 37°C. By monitoring blood temperature and acting as a thermostat it corrects the temperature if it goes too high or too low. The *anterior* part of the hypothalamus controls heat loss if the body gets too hot (e.g. by promoting sweating) and the *posterior* part controls heat conservation if the body gets too cold.

3   It regulates eating by giving a feeling of fullness (**satiation**), which prevents further food intake. This is the function of the **satiety centre** within the ventromedial part of the hypothalamus. Hunger and the seeking of both food and drink, however, are controlled by the lateral part of the hypothalamus.

See page 18 4   It controls the functions of both the **sympathetic** and **parasympathetic** components of the **autonomic nervous system** (**ANS**).

5   It influences sexual activity in combination with other regions of the brain.

6   It plays a role in emotions.

7   It controls the hormonal output of the pituitary gland, both anterior and posterior lobes, by the following mechanisms.

Anterior pituitary lobe. **Releasing hormones** (**RH**) or **inhibiting hormones** (**IH**) (sometimes called releasing or inhibiting *factors*) pass down from the hypothalamus into the anterior lobe and either release, or inhibit the release of, the anterior lobe hormones. Anterior pituitary lobe hormones are:

- **growth hormone** – as the name suggests, it is important for growth;
See page 147 - **adrenocorticotropic hormone** (**ACTH**), which acts on the adrenal cortex to stimulate the production of **cortisol**;
See page 82 - **thyroid–stimulating hormone** (**TSH**), which acts on the thyroid gland and causes release of the thyroid hormones **T3** and **T4**;
- **prolactin**, which promotes breast milk production during breastfeeding;
- **follicle–stimulating hormone** (**FSH**), which stimulates the ovarian follicles to mature the ova (egg cells) in females and stimulates cells in the male testes to produce sperm;
- **luteinising hormone** (**LH**), which promotes ovulation in females and stimulates the production of **testosterone** from the male testes.

Posterior pituitary lobe. The hormones that are released from the posterior lobe are produced in the hypothalamus. They pass down into the pituitary gland, where they are stored and released by hypothalamic control. These hypothalamic hormones are:

- **antidiuretic hormone (ADH)**, from the **supraoptic nucleus** of the hypothalamus, a hormone which is released into the blood and acts on the **renal nephron** to conserve water;
- **oxytocin**, from the **paraventricular nucleus** of the hypothalamus, a hormone which is released into the blood and causes smooth-muscle contraction (for example, it contracts the uterus during labour), and also contraction of special breast cells which push milk towards the nipple during breastfeeding.

The basal ganglia and the cerebellum

These areas are part of what is called the **extrapyramidal tract** system; that is, they control the finer details of skeletal muscle movement at a subconscious level (Blows 2000c; 2001a, pp. 196–199). The extrapyramidal tract side-effects of drugs such as the antipsychotics are caused by disturbance to this system, particularly the basal ganglia.

The basal ganglia

The basal ganglia are made up of five main nuclei: the **putamen**, the **caudate nucleus**, the **globus pallidus**, the **substantia nigra** and the **subthalamus** (it is important not to muddle the thalamus with the hypothalamus and the subthalamus) (Figure 1.7). Several terms are used to describe the different ways in which some of these nuclei are grouped. The **corpus striatum** is the area involving the putamen and the caudate nucleus combined, with the main pyramidal motor pathways, called the **internal capsule**, passing between them. But the putamen is also part of the **lentiform nucleus**, which also includes the globus pallidus (Figure 1.7).

Collectively, the function of the basal ganglia is the fine control of muscle contraction (Martini and Nath 2008). The corpus striatum receives input from the main motor and sensory areas of the cerebrum, as well as inputs from the thalamus, subthalamus and the brain stem (particularly the substantia nigra). Degeneration of the caudate nucleus is seen in Huntington's disease where excessive uncontrollable movement is a major symptom.

Output from the corpus striatum passes via the globus pallidus to the motor areas of the frontal lobe. The globus pallidus has several vital functions, notably the control of trunk and limb movements, including the positioning of limbs just prior to the movements of the digits, a function of the main motor cortex.

The globus pallidus and the putamen are also involved in the **basal ganglia motor loop** (Figure 1.8; see also Blows 2001a, pp. 198–200). When the body is not moving, the globus pallidus inhibits a particular thalamic nucleus which, when active, influences movement. As movement starts, stimulation of the putamen causes a blocking of the globus pallidus, removing the inhibition on the thalamus. The thalamus then becomes free to influence the main motor areas of the frontal lobe.

The substantia nigra is particularly important as the area decreasing **muscle tone**, the state of tension within a muscle, which is essential for the muscle to achieve full

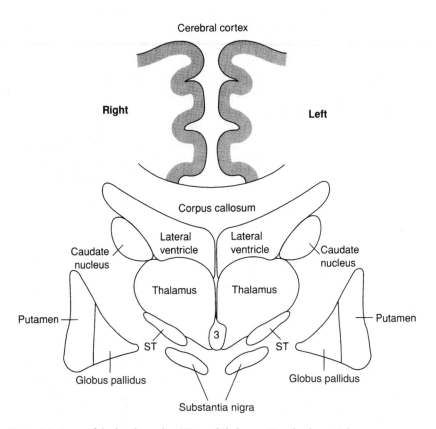

Cerebral cortex

Right   Left

Corpus callosum

Lateral
ventricle

Lateral
ventricle

Caudate
nucleus

Caudate
nucleus

Thalamus   Thalamus

Putamen   Putamen

ST   3   ST

Globus pallidus   Globus pallidus

Substantia nigra

Figure 1.7 Areas of the basal ganglia. ST = subthalamus, 3 = third ventricle.

contraction. The axonal tracts coming from the substantia nigra to go to the corpus striatum are the **nigrostriatal pathway**, and these neurons use the neurotransmitter dopamine. Degeneration of the substantia nigra causes Parkinson's disease, and *See page 236* Parkinsonian-like symptoms are a feature of some drug side-effects.

The subthalamus has the role of inhibiting excessive motor activity from the cerebral motor cortex (i.e. acting as a breaking system for the pyramidal tracts). Disturbance of this function can result in excessive pyramidal activity affecting skeletal muscle contraction.

Apart from Huntington's disease and Parkinson's disease, disturbance of basal ganglia function includes several other different movement disorders, which are *See page 204* described in relation to psychotropic drug side-effects.

The cerebellum

The cerebellum (Figure 1.9) is another part of the extrapyramidal tract system, controlling muscle function at a subconscious level (Blows 2000d). There are two hemispheres, as in the cerebrum, but just three main lobes: the **anterior, posterior** and **flocculonodular** lobes. Each lobe is further subdivided into smaller regions of surface area. This surface is made of grey matter, which is folded to increase the area to

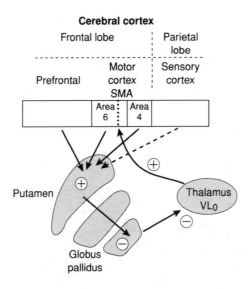

Figure 1.8 The basal ganglia motor loop. Input to the putamen comes from the frontal cortex, with less input coming from the parietal sensory cortex. This activates (+) neurons running from the putamen to the globus pallidus which, in turn, then deactivates (−) neurons linking the globus pallidus with the ventral lateral nucleus of the thalamus (VLo). These globus pallidus neurons were preventing (i.e. inhibiting, shown as −) any feedback from the VLo to the cerebral cortex. However, deactivation from the putamen has removed this inhibition, and the VLo then is free to feed back to the cortex (+) (more precisely, the supplementary motor area (SMA) of area 6 of the motor cortex).

about 75 per cent of the surface area of the cerebrum. There is white matter below the surface and at the core of this white matter are further patches of grey matter, the **cerebellar nuclei**. The routes for impulses to pass into and out from the cerebellum are through the brain stem via the **cerebellar peduncles**, foot-like connections between the cerebellum and the brain stem (Martini and Nath 2008).

The functions of the cerebellum are as follows:

1   To maintain the balance of the body. The cerebellum makes fine adjustments to muscle tensions to stabilise body position, especially when upright, to prevent falling over. Sensory feedback on balance, to the cerebellum, is from somatic **proprioception** (sensory information on body position from muscles, tendons and joints), and **vestibular** information from the semicircular canals of the inner ear. The proprioception impulses enter the anterior lobe of the cerebellum, whilst vestibular impulses pass into the flocculonodular lobe.

2   To smooth out muscle movement, preventing erratic movements and facilitating fine, well-controlled movements.

3   To increase muscle tone in opposition to the substantia nigra.

4   To effect *synergy*, i.e. a collection of different muscle movements made simultaneously to achieve a particular objective. The cerebellum creates a motor plan,

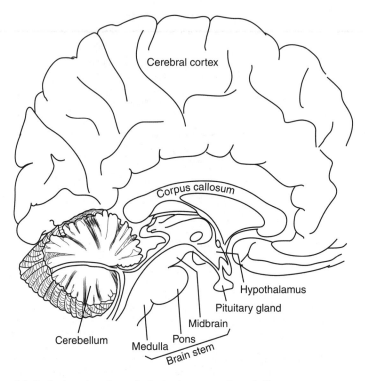

Figure 1.9 Sagittal section through the brain stem and cerebellum.

whereby multiple muscles function together in one activity. A good example is the coordination required to catch a ball which is moving towards you. Visual information on the nature of the object, its speed and direction, is flashed to the cerebellum. The entire muscle sequence needed to catch the ball is planned, slightly ahead of time (to allow for movement of the ball whilst planning and muscle movement takes place), and the activity is then executed.

These skills are not present in the newborn infant. The cerebellum has to learn, by trial and error, to balance the body, smooth and coordinate muscle activity and to interact with moving objects. Parents can often identify the moments in the development of a child when the cerebellum achieves a new skill, such as the first moment the infant stands unsupported, balancing on both legs. Repeated attempts at a skill, along with sensory feedback, improve the cerebellum's ability to learn and perfect that skill. *Practice makes perfect* could be rewritten to read *practice makes better cerebellar function*.

The brain stem

This part of the brain is the most primitive in that it carries out the basic functions of living (Blows 2000d). It is the lowest area of the brain (Figure 1.9) and is continuous with the spinal cord. The distinction between brain stem above and cord below is approximately at the level of the **foramen magnum**, the 'large window' at the base of the skull.

The brain stem is divided into three parts, the uppermost part being the **midbrain**. Below this and bulging anteriorly is the **pons**, and the lowest part is the **medulla** (Figure 1.9). The pons is often referred to as *bulbar*, meaning it is swollen like a bulb. The brain stem houses many nuclei, a number of which are those that control the functions of most of the 12 pairs of **cranial nerves** (numbers III to XII). Cranial nerves are the nerves that come direct from the brain. Cranial nerves I (olfactory) and II (optic) come from the brain at a higher level than the brain stem.

The midbrain is the smallest part of the brain stem, just above the pons. Here cranial nerve nuclei numbers III (oculomotor) and IV (trochlear) are found. These nerves and their nuclei are concerned with eye movements.

The pons has cranial nerve nuclei numbers V (trigeminal), VI (abducent), VII (facial) and VIII (vestibulocochlear). Two other nuclei are part of the respiratory control centres shared with the medulla.

The medulla is the lowest part of the brain stem. The remaining cranial nerve nuclei are found here with their associated nerves: IX (glossopharyngeal), X (Vagus), XI (accessory) and XII (hypoglossal). The medulla also contains the vital centres which keep the body alive: the **cardiac centre** essential for heart function, the **respiratory centres** (shared with the pons) which together keep the individual breathing, and the **vasomotor centre** (**VMC**), a diffuse set of nuclei which collectively influence peripheral vascular resistance, part of the mechanism for maintaining blood pressure. The medulla is also the location for a number of reflexes which, again, are primitive responses to stimuli designed to protect the body against harm or even death. Such reflexes include the **gag reflex** (which prevents unwanted substances from entering the throat), the **corneal reflex** (which prevents injury to the front of the eye by shutting the lids if something touches the eye), and the **pupillary reflex** (which shuts down the pupil in bright light, preventing light-induced retinal injury).   *See page 30*

Some of these reflexes are used in neurological investigations to assess brain stem function.

Parts of the medulla, the pons, the midbrain and the upper cord contain discrete patches of small nuclei, referred to as the **reticular formation** (**RF**) (Figure 1.10) (Blows 2000d). These nuclei have connections with many parts of the brain. The reticular formation has the role of inhibiting those sensory stimuli entering the brain that can be considered as repetitive, weak or unnecessary, allowing only strong, significant or unusual impulses to pass. Other mechanisms such as vomiting, swallowing, coughing and sneezing are brain-stem RF-mediated functions, and are all linked to the function of respiration in some way. Part of the RF is the **reticular activating system** (**RAS**), i.e. those RF components that are responsible for the **sleep–wake cycle**. This cycle controls the timing of sleep in relation to light levels falling on the retina. The RAS has an **alerting centre**, part of the hypothalamus that sends out impulses to the conscious brain in order to maintain alertness when awake. The RAS also has a **sleep centre** lower down in the brain stem, which causes sleep through impulses sent to the conscious brain (cerebrum) via the thalamus. There is also a **postural inhibition zone** at the lowest point

See page 30

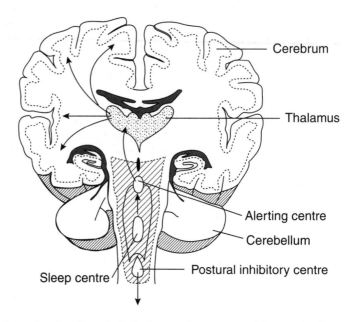

Figure 1.10 Coronal section through the brain stem showing area of the reticular formation (shaded) and the main centres of the sleep–wake cycle. Impulses from these centres are distributed either to the cortex via the thalamus or to the body via the spinal cord, as shown by the arrows.

of the brain stem where it meets the cord (Figure 1.10). This zone blocks muscle activity during sleep by sending inhibitory impulses down through the cord to the muscles in order to prevent individuals from acting out their dreams. Disturbance of the RAS is likely to cause abnormal changes in the sleep pattern associated with several mental health disorders.

The autonomic nervous system

The autonomic nervous system (ANS) is that part of the peripheral nervous system that functions automatically, i.e. without conscious control. The two parts of the ANS are the **sympathetic** and **parasympathetic** systems (Figure 1.11; see also Blows 2001b, p. 43). They act between them to stabilise many physiological parameters (for example, heart rate is stabilised at an average of 72 beats per minute), but the two parts allow the parameters to change when it becomes appropriate (for example, the heart rate can increase or decrease depending on the circumstances). The sympathetic component serves to increase those parameters, and this is useful for reactions to adverse stimuli, such as fear. Sympathetic responses to stimuli like fear result in, amongst other things, fast pulse rates, sweating and increased respiration, all of which are important in speeding up oxygen delivery to the tissues for a physical response to the cause of the fear. The parasympathetic component causes an opposite effect by reducing the physical parameters, e.g. slower heart and breathing rates, at times of rest. The range of functions for each system can be seen in Table 1.1.

See page 167

Table 1.1 illustrates the balance effect of the two systems working together to give *average* parameters, but averages that can shift in either direction as circumstances dictate. For example, heart rate averages at about 72 beats per minute but can rise to 120 or more in exercise or anxiety, or fall towards 60 during complete rest. Excessive sympathetic activity is seen in anxiety and phobic states when patients come into contact with their fears. Some parameters do not have an opposing parasympathetic activity.

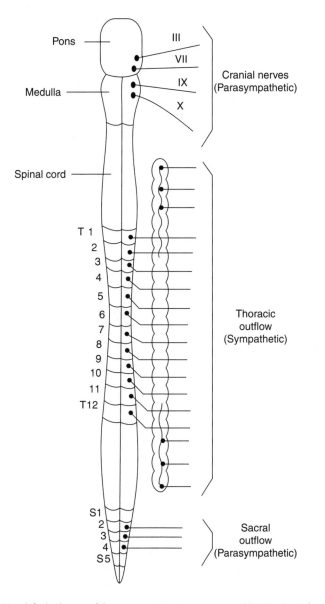

Figure 1.11 Simplified scheme of the autonomic nervous system (ANS). Cranial nerves (III, VII, IX and X) are shown in roman numerals. T = thoracic, S = sacral.

Table 1.1 Functions of the autonomic nervous system.

Target organ (or system)	Sympathetic function	Parasympathetic function
Mental alertness	Increases	No effect
Eye (pupil)	Dilates	Constricts
Heart muscle	Increased heart rate and force of contraction	Decreased heart rate
Coronary arteries	Dilated	Constricted
Blood pressure	Raised	Lowered
Bronchi	Dilated	Constricted
Digestive tract	Reduced peristalsis and increased sphincter tone	Increased peristalsis and decreased sphincter tone
Stomach	Reduces digestion	Increases hydrochloric acid
Liver/blood glucose	Glucose released from glycogen into blood	No effect
Kidney	Decreased urine produced	No effect
Bladder	Allowed to fill, internal sphincter closed	Emptied, sphincter opened
Adrenal medulla	Releases adrenaline	No effect
Metabolism	Increased	No effect
Skin	Increased sweating	No effect

Table 1.2 Brain pathways involved in mental health.

Pathway	Pathway		Importance to mental health
	From	To	
Mesolimbic pathway	Brain stem	Limbic system	Probably involved in psychotic symptoms, e.g. schizophrenia
Mesocortical pathway	Brain stem	Cerebral cortex	Probably involved in psychotic symptoms, e.g. schizophrenia
Nigrostriatal pathway	Substantia nigra	Corpus striatum	Site of extrapyramidal side-effects of drugs and of Parkinson's disease
Diffuse modulatory systems	Brain stem	Many parts of limbic area and cerebral cortex	Appears to be involved in depression and possibly eating disorders
Medial forebrain bundle	Brain stem	Frontal lobe of cerebrum	Involved in the brain reward pathways which are implicated in drug addiction
Dorsolateral prefrontal circuit	Frontal lobe (Brodmann 9 and 10)	Head of caudate nucleus (basal ganglia)	Involved in deficits of frontal lobe executive functions
Lateral orbitofrontal circuit	Prefrontal cortex (Brodmann 10)	Caudate nucleus	Involved in mood and personality changes
Anterior cingulate circuit	Anterior cingulate gyrus (Brodmann 24) of the frontal lobe	Several areas of brain stem and basal ganglia	Involved in speech and emotional loss, and apathy

See page 207

See page 207

See page 200

See page 219

See page 143

The pathways involved in mental health

Table 1.2 and Figure 1.12 show the major pathways of the brain that are chiefly involved in mental health disorders, **psychotropic** (affecting the mind) drug activity and drug side-effects. Further discussion of the pathways (or tracts) is given under the relevant neurotransmitter (Chapter 3), under the appropriate disorder and under the pharmacology involved.

The basic principles of brain pathologies affecting mental health

Pathology is the study of the nature and causation of disease. Disease is either **congenital** ('born with', i.e. the condition is present from birth, and therefore occurred before birth), or **acquired** (occurs at a later date after birth). Of the congenital causes, some may be **hereditary** (i.e. passed to the infant from the parent through gene errors, called **mutations**), or **teratogenic** (i.e. caused by a harmful chemical or viral agent passing through the placenta from mother to fetus, either a micro-organism, a drug or a toxin, causing harm or malformation of the fetus).

Of the acquired causes, there are a number of different categories which can involve the brain and therefore cause symptoms of mental health disorder, as follows:

- **Inflammatory**. Inflammation produces redness (rubor), swelling (tumor), pain (dolor) and heat (calor), with a corresponding loss of function. It may be due to an immune reaction to micro-organisms (**infection**) or other antigens, such as cancer cells (**sterile reaction**) (Blows 2005, Chapter 3). Inflammation involving the brain could be **meningitis** (inflammation of the meninges covering the brain) or **encephalitis** (inflammation of the brain itself).
- **Traumatic**. Physical injury, for example, damage to the brain from a blow to the head (Blows 2001a, Chapter 7). Long-term complications of brain injury include epilepsy and depression. *See page 285*

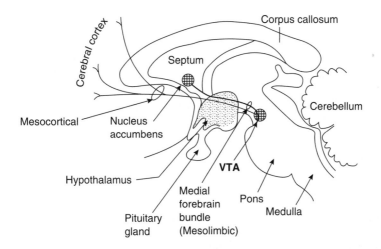

Figure 1.12 Sagittal section through the brain stem showing the ventral tegmental area (VTA) and the main dopaminergic pathways; the mesolimbic pathways (through the medial forebrain bundle) and the mesocortical pathways.

- **Neoplastic**. New growths of the brain, either **benign** or **malignant**, such as **meningioma**, a new growth of the meninges. Many malignant new growths in the brain are known as **secondaries** because they are formed from **metastases**, i.e. cells broken free from a **primary** growth elsewhere (Blows 2005, Chapter 9). New growths of the brain can cause confusion, personality changes and fits.

See page 37
- **Nutritional**. Deficiency or excess of a dietary nutrient, e.g. a vitamin or mineral, can cause, for example, a brain malformation or reduced level of neurotransmitter. An absence of adequate protein in the diet would reduce the amount of neurotransmitters in the brain that relied on a supply of amines, since amines are derived from protein.

- **Allergic**. The adverse reaction of the immune system to a foreign substance (called an **antigen**) (Blows 2005, Chapter 3). An antigen is any foreign substance, often a protein, that enters the body and provokes an immune reaction. Such reactions can affect the brain, causing fits, confusion or loss of consciousness.

- **Metabolic**. Abnormal changes in cellular **metabolism** which often produce toxic wastes, which can cause confusion, fits or reduced level of consciousness. An example of this is an excess production of urea which then enters the blood causing **uraemia**.

See page 261
- **Degenerative**. Deterioration and the ultimate death of cells due to age-related and other pathological changes. Degeneration of brain cells causes disorders such as **dementia** and **Parkinson's disease**.

- Age-related degeneration of the arterial walls supplying blood to the brain can cause **strokes** (also known as **cerebrovascular accidents**, or **CVA**), which can cause confusion, fits and loss of consciousness (Blows 2001a, Chapter 7).

- **Psychological**. Disorders caused by environmental **stress** and mental trauma, often over a long period, e.g. **anxiety states** and depression.

- **Iatrogenic**, health-related 'injuries' caused by the medical and nursing profession. Examples are: a drug side-effect, caused when a drug is prescribed by the doctor; a puncture wound caused by the nurse during the administration of an injection; or a pressure sore caused by a patient being immobilised in one position for too long. Some are inevitable, but others are preventable, and the medical and nursing staff should be working to minimise the harmful effects of their actions as much as possible.

- **Idiopathic**. This means 'of unknown cause'. Research has done much to reduce the number of disorders that fall into this category, and much progress has been achieved in finding the cause of many psychiatric disorders. However, there is still much more research to be done in order to remove some very important brain disorders from this category.

Key points

The meninges and cerebrospinal fluid

- The brain and the cord are covered by the meninges in three layers: the pia mater, the arachnoid mater and the dura mater.

- Between the arachnoid mater and pia mater is the subarachnoid space containing cerebrospinal fluid (CSF).
- Two lateral ventricles, the third ventricle and the fourth ventricle inside the brain are filled with CSF.
- Lumbar puncture is a method of collecting a sample of CSF from the subarachnoid space below the lumbar vertebra 2 (L2) level.

The cerebrum

- The cerebrum is the largest part of the brain, carrying out our cognitive and conscious processes.
- The frontal lobe is a major part of the brain involved in many mental health functions; in particular it is the site of consciousness of the 'self' and thinking.

The limbic system

- The limbic system below the cerebrum is involved in preservation of the individual and the species, and involves emotions and controlling behavioural patterns.
- The amygdala is the emotional centre of the brain.
- The function of the hippocampus are: short-term memory, learning and emotional behaviour and influencing thought.

The thalamus and hypothalamus

- The thalamus is the sensory relay station, passing sensations to the cerebrum.
- The hypothalamus has a wide range of functions, notably temperature control, regulation of eating, alerting the brain after sleep and controlling both the pituitary gland's hormones and the autonomic nervous system.

The basal ganglia and the cerebellum

- Below the limbic area are the basal ganglia and the cerebellum, areas involved in control of movement at a subconscious level (i.e. part of the extrapyramidal tract system).
- The function of the substantia nigra is the reduction of muscle tone.
- The functions of the cerebellum are fine control of balance, smoothing out muscle movement and synergy.

The brain stem

- The brain stem has the nuclei that control the cranial nerve functions and the vital centres, such as respiration, cardiac function and blood pressure.
- The brain stem houses the reticular formation and the reticular activating system that is involved in the sleep–wake cycle.

References

Blows W. T. (2000a) The nervous system, part 1. *Nursing Times*, **96** (35): 41–44.

Blows W. T. (2000b) The nervous system, part 2. *Nursing Times*, **96** (40): 45–48.

Blows W. T. (2000c) The nervous system, part 3. *Nursing Times*, **96** (44): 45–48.

Blows W. T. (2000d) The nervous system, part 4. *Nursing Times*, **96** (48): 47–50.

Blows W. T. (2001a) *The Biological Basis of Nursing: Clinical Observations*. Routledge, London.

Blows W. T. (2001b) The nervous system, part 7. *Nursing Times*, **97** (10): 41–44.

Blows W. T. (2002a) Lumbar puncture. *Nursing Times*, **98** (36): 25–26.

Blows W. T. (2002b) Electroencephalography. *Nursing Times*, **98** (38): 36–37.

Blows W. T. (2005) *The Biological Basis of Nursing: Cancer*. Routledge, London.

Carlson, N. R. (2010) *Physiology of Behavior* (10th edition). Allyn and Bacon, Boston.

Martini F. H. and Nath J. L. (2008) *Fundamentals of Anatomy and Physiology* (8th edition). Benjamin Cummings, San Francisco.

McPherson S. E. and Cummings J. L. (1999) The neuropsychology of the frontal lobes, in Ron M. A. and David A. S. (eds), *Disorders of Brain and Mind*. Cambridge University Press, Cambridge.

Raichle M. E. (2010) The brain's dark energy. *Scientific American*, **302** (3): 28–33.

2　Brain development

Introduction

The human brain is a remarkable structure, with functions that go beyond anything other organisms can achieve. However, although the human brain is fully in place at birth, with many of its functions working, it still has a lot more development to do, and will not be completely mature until about 22 years later. Being locked up inside a bony box (the **skull**) the brain relies entirely for much of that development on the sensory nervous system. It is through the senses that the brain keeps in contact with the outside world, and it is the outside world that has the biggest influence on the brain (Blows 2003). Therefore the brain can only make progress in development if the sensory systems are fully functioning. Fortunately, the sensory systems are always the most advanced at all stages of development.

The nervous system up to birth

The human nervous system starts as a groove forming along what will become the back of the early embryo. This groove deepens and closes over to form a tube, the **neural tube**. Forming this groove and the neural tube is a process called **neurulation** (Figure 2.1). The enclosed lumen within the tube is destined to become the **ventricular system** of the brain and cord, and will eventually contain a watery fluid called **cerebrospinal fluid** (**CSF**). The head (**rostral**) end of the tube and the tail (**caudal**) end initially remain open to the **amniotic fluid** that bathes the entire embryo. These tubal openings (called **neuropores**) will close between 26 and 28

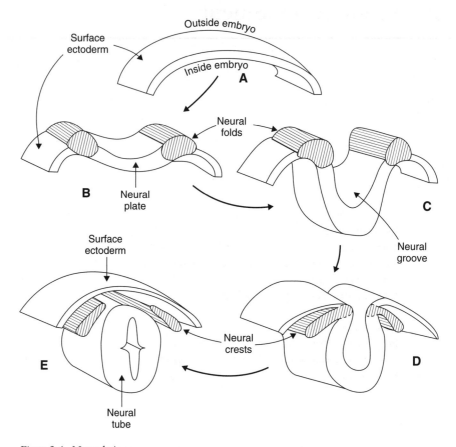

Figure 2.1 Neurulation.

days, the days counted from the start of pregnancy, i.e. conception (Figure 2.2). While the tube itself becomes the **central nervous system** (**CNS**, i.e. the brain and spinal cord), cells that originate from the tube form a crest (the **neural crest**) (Figure 2.1) between the tube and the embryonic surface, and these will develop into the **peripheral nervous system** (**PNS**, i.e. peripheral nerves).

Deep within the neural tube wall, in a cell layer next to the lumen called the **ventricular zone** (**VZ**), many millions of new cells are formed from **mitosis** (cell division), and these will eventually become mostly **neurons** (Figure 2.3). In the next zone out, the **subventricular zone** (**SZ**), more cells are dividing and these will become mostly **glia cells** (known as **neuroglia**), i.e. the support cells of the central nervous system.

See page 298   At first, these layers contain early **stem cells**, meaning these cells are not yet designated to become any particular cell type (i.e. they are **undifferentiated**). Cells of the VZ then pass through three stages of development to become neurons: 1. **neural epithelial cells**, 2. **radial progenitor cells** and 3. **intermediate neural precursors**. One key gene, called **GSK-3** (**glycogen synthase kinase 3**) has a major influence over radial progenitor cells, being responsible for these cells to move on

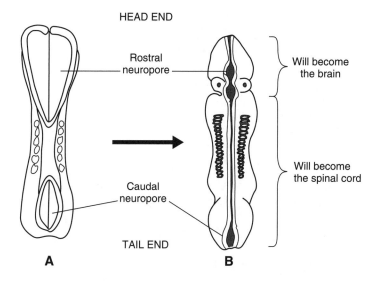

HEAD END

Rostral
neuropore

Will become
the brain

Will become
the spinal cord

Caudal
neuropore

TAIL END

A   B

Figure 2.2 The neuropores on days 26 and 28 gestation.

to neuronal status. Failure of this gene has been shown to prevent these cells from further development, and they simply continue to divide. The normal progress from intermediate neural precursors is to go on to become neuronal cell bodies. They are still in a very primitive state at this point; for example, these neurons are cell bodies only, and have no **axon**, **myelin** or **synaptic** connections.

Three waves of **neuronal migration** occur during the **second trimester** of *See page 199* pregnancy (i.e. third to sixth month of pregnancy). Migration involves the movement of millions of cells from the VZ inner layer of the tube to the surface. How they find their correct finishing point on the tube surface is not fully understood, but it involves a framework of glial projections extending from the lumen to the surface, and a critical protein coded by the gene called **srGAP2**. The protein produced from this gene has an active part called the **F-BAR domain**, which causes temporary finger-like extensions of the neuronal cell body, called **filopodia**, which then drag the cell to its new position on the tube surface. Once in their final destinations these primitive neuronal cell bodies form three cellular layers (Figure 2.3). The innermost layer is the product of the first wave, and the outermost layer is the product of the third wave. The position of these cells within these layers is both critical and irreversible, and, once placed, cells are ready to begin axon development and forming synapses. On completion, these neuronal migrations will never happen again. If cells are misplaced during migration, nothing can be done to correct this, and the brain will have some errors in synaptic connection. Mutations of srGAP2 and the incorrect positions and connections of misplaced neurons are now considered to be part of the problem in **schizophrenia** and **autism**. Correct axonal growth, guidance to its final destination and synaptic connections is due to the production of a large number of specific proteins; examples include the **Notch** cell signalling proteins and the **Netrin** and **Semaphorin** axonal guidance proteins.

The rostral end of the tube thickens and folds to form three primary brain vesicles, the **forebrain**, **midbrain** and **hindbrain** (Figure 2.4). The primitive brain

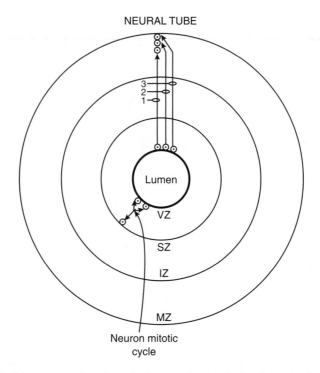

NEURAL TUBE

Neuron mitotic
cycle

Figure 2.3 Schematic section through the neural tube during the early development of
the nervous system. VZ is the ventricular zone near the tube lumen. The other
zones are SZ (subventricular zone), IZ (intermediate zone) and MZ (marginal
zone). Cell mitosis (division) takes place in the VZ, with the cell alternating
from close to the lumen (where it divides) to close to the SZ. At specific times,
three waves of cell migration out of the VZ into the MZ take place (labelled 1,
2 and 3). The first migration places cells short of the outer layer, but successive
migrations place cells closer to the surface.

also begins to fold; the start of the process of packing as much brain matter into the
skull as possible. These folds consist of two folds forward (the **midbrain** and **cervi-
cal flexures**) which are then separated by a fold backwards (the **pontine flexure**)
(Figure 2.4). The forebrain vesicle enlarges and expands in all directions to form the
cerebrum. This begins to engulf the parts behind (notably the **thalamus**, **hypothalamus** and **basal ganglia**), which will ultimately take up a position surrounded
by the rapidly developing cerebrum (Figure 2.4). The midbrain and hindbrain have
also grown, although not to the same extent, and between them these will form the
See page 16   **brain stem** and **cerebellum**.

The debate: when does consciousness start?

When do we first develop consciousness? This is a question that is often asked, and
is important when we have to consider what sensations a particular unborn fetus can
experience. The question is linked to the other problem in biology: How does the
brain create consciousness? This is known as *the hard problem* because it is just that,
virtually unsolvable (see Chapter 7 in Blows 2001).

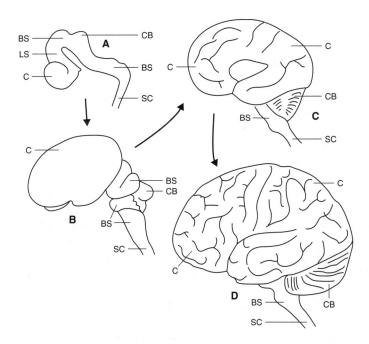

Figure 2.4 Left lateral views of the folding brain during development. A. At 5 weeks gestation, the upper (head, or rostral) end of the neural tube is folding forwards and backwards, and expanding, especially the cerebrum (C) B. At 13 weeks gestation the cerebrum is the largest component and is expanding backwards to encompass the limbic system (LS). C. At 26 weeks gestation the cerebrum is still expanding backwards and has encompassed the limbic system and part of the cerebellum (CB) and brain stem (BS) D. At birth the brain has completed its formation but has a lot of maturation to go. The remaining tube has developed into the spinal cord (SC).

Part of the answer may be determined by establishing at what point in gestation the pathways in the brain that are involved in consciousness are in place and functioning. The thalamus and cerebral cortex are the most important areas with regards to consciousness, and these are anatomically formed by between weeks 24 and 28 of gestation (Koch 2009). This is followed a few weeks later by evidence that both cerebral hemispheres are in communication with most parts of the brain. The groundwork for consciousness is therefore set up ready for the final trimester of pregnancy. However, it appears from multiple studies that the unborn fetus is alternating between two different sleep modes (called active and quiet sleep) throughout 95 per cent of this final trimester. The fetus is kept sedated and asleep by a mixture of chemicals secreted by the placenta. So, it would appear that the unborn child is not conscious enough to be aware of very much until the day of its birth, when it becomes detached from the placenta and is released into an environment rich in sensory stimuli.

The brain at birth

The major anatomical structures of the brain are all in place at birth, and a number of functions essential for keeping the baby alive are working. These functions are mainly those of the brain stem where the vital centres are located. The brain stem is the most developmentally advanced brain area at birth, and houses the **cardiac centre** (regulating heart function), the **respiratory centre** (controlling breathing) and the **vaso–motor centre** (stabilising blood pressure). The brain stem is also the centre for controlling **reflexes**, and again these are functioning from birth. There are two types of reflexes: the **avoidance** and **approach reflexes**. Avoidance reflexes are there to protect the baby against harm (e.g. the **blink reflex** protects against eye injury, the **pupillary reflex** protects against bright light) and they include the vomit, cough and sneeze reflexes. The approach reflexes help the child obtain food, e.g. the sucking and swallow reflexes (Figure 2.5). Other than these brain stem functions, the brain at birth is quite advanced in sensory perception.

The newborn can see, hear, feel pain and touch, as well as other senses, and these first started to happen before birth. However, the child at birth is lacking the motor skills we see in older children and adults. The motor system is well behind in terms of development at birth, and remains behind at all stages until near full maturity. The reason for this is threefold. First, the motor system is behind in physical development, i.e. it is slower in creating synaptic connections and forming myelin sheaths. Second, many of the motor skills involve **learning**, and this not only takes time but can only start to happen after birth. How much time learning takes depends on the skill in question, but is typically months or years. This is linked to the first reason because learning involves forming and strengthening synaptic connections. Third, motor development is heavily dependent on sensory **feedback**, and there is a distinct lack of sensory feedback before birth. Only after birth can sensory feedback

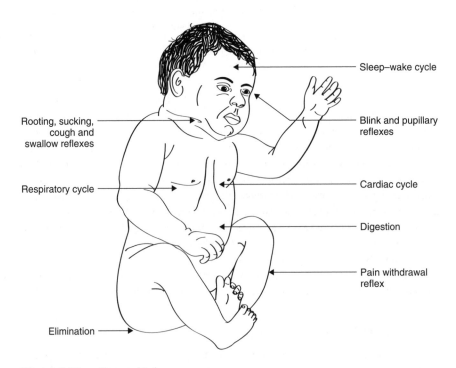

Figure 2.5 The reflexes at birth.

really begin to make a difference to the formation of motor skills. So the newborn can breathe, cry and move their limbs a little, but not much else. It's going to take years for the motor system to catch up with the rest of the brain.

The human brain at birth contains around 100,000,000,000 (100 billion) neurons, virtually the full complement of cells it is going to have, but it is just 25 per cent of the weight of the adult brain. However, it is already in the middle of a brain **growth spurt**. This started before birth and continues until about two years of age, i.e. the age when the brain weighs about 75 per cent of the adult brain weight.

Brain growth spurts do not generally involve the addition of new neurons. The child at birth will add very few new neurons after birth. A brain growth spurt involves the addition of new neuroglia cells, an increase in synaptic connections and myelination, and an increase in the protein content of the brain.

Infant and child brain development

Infancy has a number of definitions, but a good approach is to define infancy as the period from birth to the development of a language (i.e. the first few years of life, given there is considerable normal variation in the age of language development). During this time, three main processes are involved in brain growth: synaptogenesis, myelination and plasticity.

Synaptogenesis is the formation of new synapses; the connections between neurons. Each neuron is capable of having hundreds of synaptic connections with other cells, and these are forming daily from the time neuronal migration is complete (second trimester of pregnancy). Some of the unused synapses may be removed by a process called **synaptic pruning**, the purpose of which is to make the brain more efficient. Many unused synapses still remain, however, to allow for future new learning and adaptation to changed circumstances.

Myelination is the process of laying down a fat-based layer called myelin around the axons of neurons in order to provide some degree of insulation and to speed up transmission of nerve impulses. Some neurons are myelinated (called **'A' fibres**), and they have a speed of transmission up to 120 metres per second; while others are unmyelinated (called **'C' fibres**) and their speed is 2.3 metres per second.

Because myelination speeds everything up, this process improves brain efficiency, but is not fully complete until the early twenties.

Plasticity is defined as the brain's ability to adapt to new environments and new experiences. We are encountering new environments throughout our lives; new homes, new schools, even new countries, and with these new environments come new experiences. Childhood is no different, with new experiences each day. Plasticity is achieved by creating many more synapses than we actually use now, and not pruning them all away. This leaves us with considerable spare capacity which we can adopt for new environments, new events and new experiences. Plasticity is also linked to learning, and since everything new in our lives involves a degree of learning, plasticity allows for this. In this way the changing environment moulds the mind, making childhood a time when brains are set up for the future. At full brain maturity, plasticity is probably better than previously recognised. This is because neuronal differentiation (i.e. neurons becoming specialised in a particular function), axonal guidance (i.e. processes that ensure axons arrive where they should) and axonal branching continues on beyond full maturity. Certain proteins (notably **Notch**, **Mash**, **Netrin** and **Semaphorins**) control these neuronal developments, and these molecules are known to be produced well into the mature CNS.

Although behind in development, the motor system progresses rapidly through childhood, that progress being made possible by synaptogenesis, myelination and sensory feedback. The motor system is able to gradually adopt more functions, such as lifting the head, rolling over, crawling and eventually walking. These are all learned motor skills with the emphasis on sensory feedback through trial and error. You can witness this process when you see a child pull themselves up to stand for the first time. They will quickly fall, but eventually they learn to balance through many attempts, until they can stand properly. Once learnt, a motor skill will be stored as a motor memory in the brain for life, so that skill will never be lost unless that part of the brain is damaged.

Speech is partly a motor skill, since it involves muscular movements of the voice box (the **larynx**), the tongue, jaw and lips. It is also another good example of sensory feedback and learning, since in order to say words they must be heard first, then learnt (Hartshorne 2009). The first words usually appear between eight and eighteen months of age, but it should be noted that there is a considerable normal variation between individual children in the ages at which speech develops. After the first words, development is slow at first, e.g. only about ten words are mastered over the next three months or so. As soon as the child has a vocabulary of about fifty words, speech development increases. By about three years of age, the child should have a vocabulary of about one thousand words, and should be adding to this at the rate of about two new words per day. The first sentences appear at about two years of age and consist of two words (e.g. 'I do'). Prior to this children make themselves understood by **holophrasing**, i.e. by combining one word with a hand gesture (e.g. pointing at a biscuit and saying 'me'). **Telegraphic speech** is the first attempt to form true sentences, i.e. leaving out non-essential words. The ability of babies to learn speech eventually to adult levels of fluency appears not to be dependent entirely on brain maturity but is more to do with achieving a number of linguistic milestones, such as acquiring a certain number of words in the vocabulary. This is known as the **'stages of language hypothesis'** and is independent of brain maturity in all children (Hartshorne 2009). Two main areas of the brain involved in speech are **Broca's area** (the speech motor area, which controls the muscles of speech) and **Wernicke's** *See page 6* **area** (the language centre, or area of word processing).

Cerebral **lateralisation** is well underway by birth, and continues throughout life. This is the process by which new information, skills and experiences are assigned for storage in one side of the brain or the other. The cerebral hemispheres, left and right, are the sites of most long-term memory, and a learnt skill must be stored either on the left, or the right, or both. Males tend to lateralise more than females who usually assign skills to both sides. In practice, this makes no difference to carrying out the skill, but it helps to have stored the skill on both sides when trying to recover brain function after injury or disease to the brain. This helps us to explain why females tend to recover normal brain function better than males after disruption by disease or trauma.

Learning and memory

Childhood is all about learning, and memory is a major component of the learning process. Humans have the longest childhood, longer than any other species, and this length of time is as much about brain growth, learning and memory as it is about body development. Evidence is growing that higher intellectual abilities come with time, i.e. the longer the period before brain maturity the greater the intellect (see Table 2.1).

Children with different levels of intelligence, measured by **intelligence quotient** (**IQ**) tests, were shown to have variations in the thickness of the cerebral cortex, especially the prefrontal cortex. Table 2.1 suggests that the variations in the thickness and activity of the prefrontal cortex at different ages profoundly influence intelligence levels.

Learning and memory are products of strong synapses. Initially these synapses are formed from temporary proteins, but these are ultimately replaced by permanent proteins provided the synapse has been used enough. Usage of synapses therefore strengthens them, and they can then become permanent. This process will be improved by stimulating the brain, and by **rehearsal**, i.e. repeating the same learning multiple times, as actors do in learning their parts, and as students do before an examination. Synapses are also strengthened by excitement, a good reason why we tend to remember the exciting events in our lives. Strengthening synapses in this way is known as creating **long-term potentials** (**LTPs**); and therefore LTPs are the basis of the learning process. LTPs require activity through two types of **glutamate** receptors on the **post-synaptic membrane**, and these receptors are explained further in Chapter 4.

See page 68

Of the synapses not strengthened in this way, many (but not all by a long way) may be subject to synaptic pruning in order to improve brain efficiency.

There are a number of ways to classify memories (see Table 2.2), but the simplest is to consider two forms of memory: **long-term** and **short-term** memory. Short-term memory is one of the functions of the **hippocampus**.

See page 194

Within the hippocampus, a limited number of information bits can be held for a short period. To convert these to long-term memory requires rehearsal in order to establish LTPs. Long-term memory is held in many parts of the brain, the location depending on what is being memorised. For example, visual memory is stored in the

Table 2.1 Comparison of prefrontal cortex development, as determined by MRI studies, between children of different IQ test scores. Prolonged thickening of the cortex in Child A (from age 8 to 12) is possibly essential for development of higher intellectual cognitive circuits. Thinning of the cortex is happening in all teenage brains and is a mark of increased brain efficiency.

Child and IQ tests results	Brain at age 7 to 8 years	Brain at age 11 to 12 years
Child A High IQ test scores	This child has a thin prefrontal cortex which starts to thicken rapidly.	The cortex thickens rapidly to peak at 12 years old, then thins out slowly through teens.
Child B Average IQ test scores	This child has a thick prefrontal cortex peaking at 8 years old.	At 11 years old the cortex has already been thinning slowly from 8 years old and continues through teens.

Table 2.2 Types of memory.

		Type of memory		
Long-term	*Short-term*	*Explicit*	*Implicit*	*Declarative*
Permanently stored memory in various sites across the cerebrum, depending on the nature of the memory to be stored.	Limited number of facts stored temporarily in the hippocampus. Conversion to long-term memory requires rehearsal.	Memory involving conscious thought, e.g. remembering a relative's telephone number.	Sub-conscious memory, like knowing the route to the kitchen at home.	Memory for facts and events. Divided into **1. semantic** (memory for basic facts and figures; e.g. 9 is a number, fish have gills); and **2. episodic** (memory of the context in which these facts exist; e.g. 9 is the ninth number in a sequence of numbers starting with 1; gills are part of a system by which vertebrates extract oxygen from the environment).

See page 4

visual cortex of the occipital lobe, whilst **motor memory** is held in the **motor association cortex** of the **frontal lobe**, and so on.

The best years for acquiring and storing memory are between 13 and 25 years of age. Before this, memory is not fully mature, and after this period memory begins slowly to deteriorate. These years of best memory are known as the **reminiscence bump**, and are used for serious learning with good reason.

The teenage brain

The teenage years and the early twenties mark the final stages of brain development, with increasing skills far in advance of anything seen in the first decade of life. There is an improvement in attention span, due largely to increased myelination and synaptic changes of the frontal lobe. Information is processed faster by the teenager, using more logic and reasoning powers, and with a capability of abstract thought. The frontal lobe also shows changes in its organisation and function, eventually using less energy to do more work, i.e. it becomes energy efficient.

However, all these brain changes, in particular the frontal lobe changes, come at a cost. In the adult brain the frontal and temporal lobes have a major influence over the brain's emotional centres (the **limbic system**), but during teenage years the frontal lobe shows a marked reduction in this influence. Emotions then become controlled largely by the **amygdala**, the main limbic centre for emotions.

The loss of frontal and temporal lobe influence over emotions is far from the ideal situation. Starting at about 11 years of age, the frontal lobe loses some of its ability to read the social situation correctly. The teenager then finds it difficult to identify other people's emotions (about 20 per cent slower at doing this than during earlier years), and they become petulant, ill-tempered, sulky and have confused emotions.

Since one of the frontal lobe functions is to step in to control impulsive behaviour, this also is significantly reduced, and so impulsive behaviour increases, especially when influenced by alcohol or drugs. Two types of behavioural control are recognised: **exogenous control**, where the brain responds to external stimuli and uses reflexes to control behaviour, thus not allowing for much involvement of rational thought, and **endogenous control**, where control is based on a predetermined, thus logically thought through, voluntary plan. Endogenous behaviour can quite easily override exogenous control in the adult, but the adolescent finds this hard, and responds to situations more with exogenous control. Teenage behavioural patterns then seem more spontaneous and illogical, and the addition of stress, drugs and alcohol will make matters worse (Sabbagh 2006). When faced with a task to perform, part of the frontal lobe, called the **prefrontal cortex**, must work much harder in teenagers than the same brain area in adults in a similar situation. *See page 91*

It seems that the adolescent prefrontal cortex tries to solve the task single-handed, unlike adults where the prefrontal cortex calls upon other brain areas for help. The teenage prefrontal cortex can, in some extreme circumstances, become overloaded, an unlikely scenario in the adult brain, and this overload will impair the frontal lobes' abilities to carry out executive functions.

Frontal lobe changes, including synaptic pruning and myelination, will continue until the remodelling of the front lobe is complete, around 23 years of age. Synapses that are frequently used are strengthened whilst those that are never used may be lost by synaptic pruning (an example of synaptic pruning is the thinning of the prefrontal cortex identified in Table 2.1) while others are retained for plasticity. These changes show how important the environment is in providing the stimuli to strengthen synapses. It is true to say that, just as in early childhood, the environment moulds the teenage mind, and these changes offer a second opportunity for families and society to influence development of the brains of children. Providing positive stimuli (happiness, emotional support, education, freedom from want, music, and so on) will strengthen the brain in a positive manner, while negative stimuli (pain, fear, alcoholism, drug abuse, sexual abuse, crime, poverty) will strengthen the brain in a negative manner. The effects of strengthened brain pathways during early childhood, and during the teenage years, either in a positive or negative way, are generally for life, and negative pathways, once established, are very hard to change or eliminate. The life-long outcome of environmental influences on the brain is the responsibility of those who deliver that experience: the child carers. They provide the environment the child is exposed to. Every child should be provided with a positive, loving, caring, happy and stimulating environment from birth in order to guide brain development in the direction which will allow the resulting adult the best chances of a happy life, and success in meeting all the challenges life has in store. If the brains of children are moulded by exposure from an early age to crime, abuse, neglect and other physical and psychological hardships, these children find it very difficult, even impossible, to turn away from these negative effects later in life and lead a happy, fruitful life. Children with brains moulded in this negative manner may ultimately become parents who also provide a negative environment for their children, therefore perpetuating the problem (see drug abuse, Chapter 8). *See page 143*

Apart from the frontal lobe, changes also occur in the **corpus callosum** (which increases in size), **parietal lobe** (which decreases in volume), **occipital lobe** (which increases in volume) and **temporal lobe** (which reaches maximum volume at 16 to 17 years of age), although not to the same extent as the frontal lobe.

During late teenage years, a shift occurs away from the amygdala to the much improved frontal lobes for rational emotional influence. Ultimately, during the early twenties, the brain will complete its myelination and synaptic changes, reaching full maturity at about 23 years of age (Sabbagh 2006).

Hormone influences on brain development

The subject of hormonal and nutritional influences on the development of the brain has received much interest in the last decade since there is growing evidence that disorders such as **autism** and **schizophrenia** may be affected by such influences. During all the stages of brain development, from early embryo to full maturity, hormones are a key factor in the process, and abnormal hormonal production has a profound adverse influence on the brain. Hormones act on brain cells by first binding to receptors, therefore cells that are influenced by hormones must have these receptors present on the cell surface membrane.

See page 80

Testosterone, a hormone usually attributed to males, is produced in both sexes from an early stage of growth in relatively small quantities compared to puberty. The source of the hormones during fetal development is the **adrenal cortex**, the outer part of the **adrenal glands** which are found above the kidneys. These glands are formed and function long before the testes or ovaries. Both testosterone and oestrogen are produced from **cholesterol**. Boys produce surprisingly high levels of testosterone during fetal development, and for a short while after birth, but this level then drops until puberty, when is rises again. Girls produce much smaller quantities of testosterone before and after birth. The sex difference in testosterone levels causes different synaptic changes in the male brain to those of the female brain. Testosterone (and its derivatives) changes the synaptic connections to a form a male orientated brain.

See page 84

Oestrogen is produced from testosterone, and therefore is also originally from cholesterol. It also occurs in both sexes from the adrenal cortex. Oestrogen improves cell survival (this is known as a **neuroprotective** function) by altering gene expression that in turn changes the proteins in favour of cell survival. It also has some control over the formation and maintenance of neural networks by promoting synaptic connections.

Thyroid hormone is produced by the thyroid gland in the neck. The function of thyroid hormone is to stimulate and regulate cellular **metabolism**, the chemistry essential for cell function. Brain cells are busy metabolic factories, consuming glucose and oxygen to produce energy that will be used in many cellular functions, including the production of **action potentials** (nerve impulses). The principal hormonal activity appears to be by **triiodothyronine (T_3)** since most brain cells have T_3 receptors. Its counterpart **tetraiodothyronine (T_4)** appears to be less important. Thyroid hormone changes gene expression inside the nucleus, and that in turn changes the way cells grow and develop.

See page 82

Growth hormone, produced by the **pituitary gland**, works in conjunction with thyroid hormone in regulating growth in the brain's neural networks. A cascade of other hormones, including **insulin**, is involved in brain development, but their roles are not fully established. Most are likely to work through gene activation and regulation.

Nutritional influences on brain development

Nutriments have a part to play in brain development, so an adequate nutritious diet for the mother throughout pregnancy and for the child up to adulthood is essential. From birth to two years of age is a critical period for adequate nutrition, since the nervous system is particularly vulnerable to deficiencies during this time. Much has been said and written about the role of vitamins, minerals and fatty acids in childhood intelligence. Vitamins are summarised in Table 2.3, and minerals in Table 2.4.

Table 2.3 The vitamins involved in brain development and function (see also Ramakrishna 1999).

Vitamin	Notes
Vitamin A (Retinoids e.g. **Retinol)**	Essential for cell differentiation, proliferation and migration, gene expression and cell death. Excess and deficiency in the maternal diet during pregnancy can cause malformation of the fetal brain.
Vitamin B1 (Thiamine)	Thiamine is required for the activity of thiamine-dependent enzymes in the brain. These enzymes are involved in cerebral energy metabolism and myelin synthesis. Deficiency during critical stages in brain development results in permanent abnormal brain changes.
Vitamin B2 (Riboflavin)	Has a role in fatty acid metabolism, and a deficiency disrupts myelin synthesis.
Vitamin B3 (Niacin, Nicotinic acid)	Deficiency during fetal development causes irregularities in cell replication and differentiation, and cerebellar structure becomes particularly abnormal.
Vitamin B5 (Pantothenic acid)	A coenzyme required for energy production. Deficiency in humans is rare and evidence for involvement in brain development is hard to obtain. It is involved in neurotransmitter production, DNA replication and cell division, and therefore important in brain development.
Vitamin B6 (Pyridoxine)	Deficiency causes inadequate myelination, disruption of synaptogenesis and reduced brain cell organisation.
Vitamin B7 (Biotin)	Being widely distributed in food, and because the body can manufacture it, a deficiency of Biotin is rare. A lack of Biotin during pregnancy could be a possibility. Biotin is essential for carbohydrate and fat metabolism and a deficiency could disturb metabolism in the brain.
Vitamin B9 (Folic acid)	Prevents neural tube defects during very early fetal development.
Vitamin B12 (Cyanocobalamin)	Deficiency appears to affect basal ganglia function causing limb spasticity and involuntary movements. At least one brain enzyme, essential for brain development, is dependent on vitamin B12. Low B12 therefore causes infants to have poor brain development, and to be anorexic, irritable and to fail to thrive.
Vitamin C (Ascorbic acid)	Highly concentrated in brain cells throughout human development. Its role in brain development is not clear, but it may influence cell division.

	A deficiency during pregnancy may cause fetal brain cell losses, notably in the hippocampus.
Vitamin D (Cholecalciferol)	There is a wide distribution of vitamin D receptors in the brain. It influences proteins involved in learning, memory, motor control and possibly social behaviour. Metabolites of vitamin D are required for normal cerebellar development.
Vitamin E (Tocopherol)	Evidence of abnormal nervous system development has been shown in animal studies but it is not yet clear how this relates to humans.

Table 2.4 Some of the important minerals involved in brain development and function.

Mineral	Notes
Iodine (I) (a component to **thyroid** hormone)	Low levels associated with **hypothyroidism**, and causes infantile **cretinism**. This is associated with cerebral palsy, deafness and mutism. The critical stage of brain development affected by low iodine is after 14 weeks gestation. Both neuron and dendrite formation is affected, causing brain developmental failure.
Calcium (Ca)	Calcium ions play a central role in neuronal cell development, including cellular proliferation, differentiation, migration and maturation. Calcium is also essential for neurotransmission, and therefore critical for brain development.
Iron (Fe)	Maternal iron deficiency during pregnancy is not uncommon, and can seriously affect the fetal brain. Various regions of the fetal brain become dependent on iron at specific points in development, and deficiency at that time causes irreversible changes in myelination, neurotransmitters (especially dopamine) and neuronal networks.
Sodium (Na)	An essential component of nerve conduction, sodium is normally concentrated outside the neuronal cell body. Deficiency of sodium during pregnancy prevents normal neuronal function.
Potassium (K)	Potassium ions are an essential component of nerve conduction. Potassium is concentrated inside the neurons; all potassium outside the cell is controlled by **astrocytes**. Deficiency of potassium during pregnancy prevents normal neuronal function.
Zinc (Zn)	Zinc plays a role in neuronal replication and migration, brain growth, synaptogenesis and gene expression. Impaired memory and learning skills are evident in children born to mothers with low zinc.
Magnesium (Mg)	Magnesium is critical in activating over 300 enzymes, many of which are vital for brain function. It is also involved in the myelination of neurons, and so is vital to brain development.

Fatty acids

Omega-3 and **omega-6** are terms used to describe certain forms of fatty acid, one of the components of fat (Figure 2.6).

The 'essential' form of omega-3 is **alpha-linolenic acid (ALA)** ('essential' meaning the only source is the diet because the body cannot produce it), and the 'non-essential' forms are **docosahexaenoic acid (DHA)** and **eicosapentaenoic acid (EPA)** ('non-essential' meaning the body can manufacture these from other

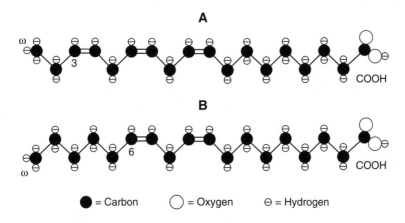

A

B

● = Carbon   ○ = Oxygen   ⊖ = Hydrogen

Figure 2.6 Omega 3 and 6 fatty acids.

forms). The 'essential' form of omega-6 is **linolenic acid** (**LA**), and the 'non-essential' forms are **gamma-linolenic acid** (**GLA**) and **arachidonic acid** (**AA**). As components of fats (or **lipids**), fatty acids in the brain are a part of fat-based structural elements, such as cell membranes and the myelin sheath around axons. DHA, for example, is widely found in these structures. Many claims are made for the improvement of mental health with the addition of essential fatty acids in the diet. For example, ALA in the diet improves the mood, promotes a sense of calm, increases learning ability and intellect and allows the brain to cope with stress better. There is substance to these claims, since many trials and clinical observations have strongly indicated links between the fatty acids and mental health. And DHA is a key player, since evidence now indicates that DHA is critical to optimum brain development at all stages of growth. Breast milk can have quite good levels of DHA (depending on the mother's diet), and long periods of breastfeeding, in some cases up to two years after birth, have resulted in children with fewer mental health problems. Infant milk formulas, until recently, have had very low levels of DHA, but this is now being corrected. Low DHA blood levels in children has been linked to **Attention Deficit Hyperactivity Disorder** (**ADHD**). *See page 305*

Trans-fats are chemical and physical distortions of unsaturated fatty acids. They can be caused by exposure to excessive heat, as in high-temperature cooking for long periods, but this actually produces only small quantities. The biggest quantities are produced artificially by manufacturers when normal fatty acids are changed under extreme high pressure. Producing trans-fat in this way converts liquid oils to solid fats at room temperature, and this is considered useful for long-term storage of fats and repeated use in cooking. However, consumption of trans-fats can result in disturbance of blood cholesterol causing an increase in heart disease. Recently, evidence is growing that trans-fats in the diet are getting incorporated into neuronal cell membranes, possibly during infant brain development. Cell membranes are critical in neuronal function because everything the cell needs must pass through the membrane by one means or another. Membranes incorporating the abnormally shaped trans-fats may not function properly, and distort what is passing into and out of the cell.

Key points

The nervous system up to birth

- The brain and cord is formed initially from a neural tube.
- Three waves of neuronal migration occur within the tube wall.
- Three primary brain vesicles, the forebrain, midbrain and hindbrain, form at the head end of the tube, and these become the complete brain.
- The sensory systems are always the most advanced at all stages of development.

The debate: when does consciousness start?

- The thalamus and cerebral cortex are the most important areas with regards to consciousness.
- These are anatomically formed by between weeks 24 and 28 of gestation.
- The unborn fetus is alternating between two different sleep modes, active and quiet sleep.
- It appears that, before birth, the child is not conscious enough to be aware of very much until the day of its birth.

The brain at birth

- The brain stem is the most advanced brain area at birth, and houses the vital centres and reflexes necessary for life.
- The newborn has all the senses functioning, but is lacking motor skills, mostly because the motor system is less well developed at birth.
- The brain is in a growth spurt at birth, which started before birth and continues until about two years of age, when the brain weighs about 75 per cent of the adult brain weight.

Infant and child brain development

- The environment has the biggest influence over brain development.
- Synaptogenesis is the formation of new synapses.
- Unwanted synapses may be removed by a process called synaptic pruning to improve brain efficiency.
- Myelination is the process of laying down myelin around the axons of neurons.
- Plasticity is the brain's ability to adapt to new environments.
- Cerebral lateralisation, the assignment of new skills to one side of the brain, is well underway by birth, and continues throughout life.

Learning and memory

- Learning is a product of strong synapses.
- Using synapses strengthens them and they can become permanent.
- Stronger synapses mean long-term potentials (LTPs) which are the basis of learning and memory.

- This process will be improved by rehearsal.
- Two main forms of memory are long-term and short-term memory.
- One of the functions of the **hippocampus** is short-term memory.

The teenage brain

- During the teenage years the frontal lobe shows a reduction in its influence over emotions which then become controlled largely by the amygdala.
- A partial shutdown of frontal lobe function is to improve myelination, synaptic pruning and energy efficiency.
- Between the years of 11 and 18 the teenager finds it harder to identify other people's emotions.
- During the late teenage years, a shift occurs away from the amygdala to the much-improved frontal lobes for rational emotional influence.

Hormone influences on brain development

- Hormones are a key factor in brain development, and abnormal hormonal production has a profound adverse influence on the brain.
- Hormones act by binding to cell surface receptors and influencing gene activity.

Nutritional influences on brain development

- From birth to two years of age is a critical period for adequate nutrition.
- The nervous system is particularly vulnerable to deficiencies during this time.
- There are strong indications that fatty acids in the diet are important in mental health.
- DHA is vital for optimum brain development at all stages of growth.
- Brain cell membranes incorporating the abnormally shaped trans-fats may not function properly.

References

Blows W. T. (2001) *The Biological Basis of Nursing: Clinical Observations*. Routledge, London.
Blows W. T. (2003) Child brain development. *Nursing Times*, **99** (17): 28–31.
Hartshorne J. (2009) Why don't babies talk like adults? *Scientific American Mind*, **20** (5): 58–61.
Koch C. (2009) Consciousness redux, when does consciousness arise? *Scientific American Mind*, **20** (5): 20–21.
Ramakrishna T. (1999) Vitamins and brain development. *Physiology Research*, **48**: 175–187.
Sabbagh L. (2006) The teen brain, hard at work. *Scientific American Mind*, **17** (4): 20–25.

3   Neural communication

The neuron

The functional unit of the nervous system is the neuron (Figure 3.1). All nerve impulses, or **action potentials**, originate in neurons. They travel along the neuron's extended cytoplasm, called the **axon**, to the point inside or outside the brain where an impulse is required. The impulse then initiates one of three possible actions, e.g. triggering another action potential within a second neuron, or a muscle contraction (in motor neurons), or possibly a glandular secretion (in neurons of the autonomic nervous system). Action potentials make things happen and therefore the cell generating the impulse has some control over that action. Strong or rapidly repeated impulses along a neuron result in powerful activities, such as muscle contraction.

We are born with 100 billion neurons, an amazing number by any standards, yet this vast mass of cells constitutes only about 10 per cent of the entire nervous system. The remaining 90 per cent is made up of 900 billion glial cells (also known as **neuroglia**), which have very different functions from neurons. There is a grand total of 1,000 billion cells in the nervous system, all derived from the same single fertilised ovum as the rest of the body. A very high rate of cell mitosis is required *before birth* to produce this vast number of neurons, i.e. about 250,000 new neurons *per minute* at the peak of cell mitosis! Although recent evidence indicates that some neuronal division can occur after birth in the hippocampus, the neuron cell mass in the brain is essentially complete at the time of birth. However, many *neuroglia* retain the power to replicate after birth and continue to do so throughout life.

See page 49   The neuronal connections, called **synapses**, are not complete at birth. They continue forming throughout childhood until the brain becomes fully mature in the late teens or early twenties. Synaptic development in childhood is promoted by stimulation of the senses and by education, and involves the creation of memory (see Chapter 2).

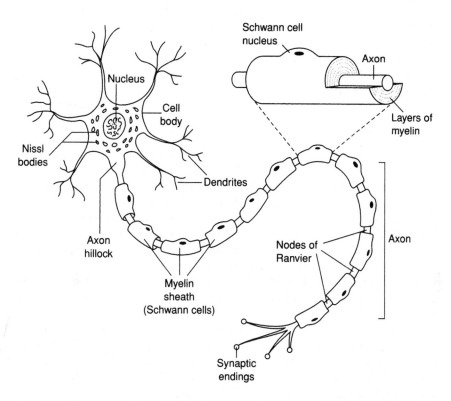

Figure 3.1 The neuron. The cell body shows a nucleus surrounded by Nissl bodies. The axon starts at the axon hillock and terminates at the synapse. Myelin covers the axon in segments with gaps between called the nodes of Ranvier. A myelin segment is shown enlarged. Each segment is laid down by a Schwann cell.

The neuron (Figure 3.1) has a relatively standard cell body, with a surrounding cell membrane, a cytoplasm with **organelles** such as **mitochondria** (for cellular energy) and **ribosomes** (for producing proteins), and a nucleus with its own nuclear membrane. It is distinguished from other cells by the presence of cell body extensions, called dendrites and axons, and by the presence of **Nissl granules** (or **Nissl bodies**) within the cytoplasm (see below).

Dendrites are mostly *afferent* pathways; that is, they convey impulses *towards* the cell body. There are usually many such dendrites, branching in a number of different directions, each branch covered by short processes called **spines**. The more dendrites or dendritic spines a neuron has, the greater is the surface area available for forming synaptic connections. Dendrites are the sites of many synapses, which are formed from the local connections they have with other neighbouring neurons. **Axons** are *efferent* pathways, carrying impulses *away from* the cell body. Most neurons have only one axon, but there are examples of neurons with more than one. They can be long and some are nearly the length of the body, and they have few branches, most of the branches occurring at the terminal end. The majority of neurons are myelinated and they make distant connections with other neurons, muscle cells or glandular cells (Blows 2000).

Nissl granules (or Nissl bodies) are patches of intracellular **rough endoplasmic reticulum** (**rough ER**) and are the site of protein synthesis carried out by **ribosomes** (protein factories) in the ER membrane. Nissl bodies are especially concentrated close to the nucleus, in the region of the cytoplasm known as the **endoplasm**. Proteins produced in Nissl bodies are used within the cell to create membranes or organelles.

Axoplasmic transportation

Proteins are also required at the synapse, the terminal end of the axon, but because ribosomes are not found in the axon the proteins must be transported there from their source within the cell body. This **axoplasmic transport** (Figure 3.2) of proteins is a function of part of the cell's **cytoskeleton**; the protein support framework of the cell. Three structures are involved in this framework: **microtubules** (20 nm in diameter), hollow tubules made from the protein **tubulin** (see also Alzheimer's disease); **microfilaments** (5 nm in diameter), cable-like structures made from two twisted proteins; and **neurofilaments** (10 nm in diameter), strong structures branching out in many directions. Like the bony skeleton inside the body, this protein framework of the cell provides shape, support and some movement to the neuron, as well as allowing the mechanism of axoplasmic transport.

Axoplasmic transport first involves the packaging of essential proteins into vesicles that are destined for the synapse. These vesicles are then attached to another protein called **kinesin**. Using cellular energy in the form of **adenosine triphosphate** (**ATP**), produced by another organelle, the **mitochondrion** (Blows 2001, Chapter 1), the kinesin moves down the axon. Kinesin acts like legs to 'walk' the vesicle along the microtubules, which extend in bundles along the full length of the axon. In the long journey to the synapse, two speeds of axonal transportation have been observed. **Slow transportation** moves the vesicles up to 8 mm per day,

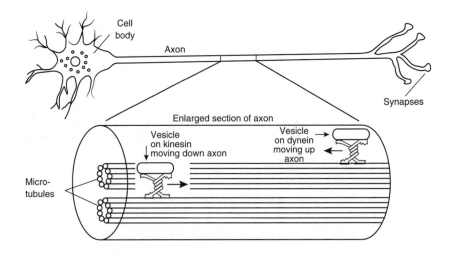

Figure 3.2 Axoplasmic transportation. The protein kinesin transports vesicles filled with other proteins along microtubules towards the synapse. Another protein called dynein does the same in the opposite direction.

while **fast transportation** moves them anything from 50 to 400mm per day. This is **anterograde** movement, i.e. from cell to synapse, involving the transportation of some neurotransmitters, but **retrograde** movement also occurs, from synapse to cell body, using the protein **dynein** in place of kinesin. Retrograde axoplasmic transport may be involved in feedback to the cell body related to the protein needs of the synapse (Figure 3.2). The whole axoplasmic transportation system is akin to the movement of goods by train along fixed tracks. It is important not to confuse axoplasmic transportation (protein movement along axons) with **neurotransmission** (the passage of an electrical impulse along axons). They are two very different concepts. Understanding neurotransmission is vital in grasping the main concepts of how the brain works and how drugs can modify its function.

Neurotransmission

Resting membrane potential

Neurotransmission is the passage of a nerve impulse (or **action potential**) along a neuronal axon. Before and after an action potential, the membrane is said to be in **resting membrane potential** (Figure 3.3). Resting membrane potential involves a very distinct concentration of **ions** on both sides of the membrane. Ions are charged particles, either positively charged (+) particles called **cations**, or negatively charged (−) particles called **anions**. The particles themselves are atoms of elements like sodium (forming a cation, Na^+), potassium (forming a cation, K^+), or chloride (forming an anion, Cl^-). The ionic concentrations on both sides of the axonal membrane are shown in Figure 3.3. There is a sodium concentration outside the membrane (i.e. in the extracellular fluid), and a potassium concentration inside the membrane (i.e. in the cell cytoplasm). In addition to ions, there are compounds that also carry an electrical charge, notably proteins and phosphates (PO_4), both

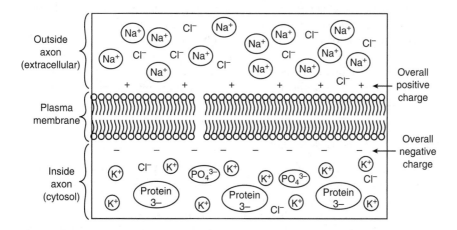

Figure 3.3 Resting potential in the neuronal membrane. Outside the membrane is a concentration of sodium, whilst inside is a concentration of potassium. The overall charge outside is caused mostly by the sodium, whilst the inside is negative because large negatively charged protein and phosphate (PO_4^{3-}) molecules cannot leave the axon.

of which have three negative charges each. Compounds are larger than ions, and because of this larger size these compounds cannot pass through the membrane, and are therefore confined to the cytoplasm inside the membrane. If all the charges on each side of the membrane are added together (with each negative cancelling a positive), the net charge which remains after such cancellation is negative on the inside and positive on the outside. The *difference* between this overall negative charge *inside* the membrane and the overall positive charge *outside* the membrane is minus seventy thousandths of a volt (**−70 mV**, or minus seventy millivolts). This is the electrical value for the resting membrane potential.

Diffusion

The membrane of the neuronal axon is semipermeable and as such it allows the occasional passage of ions one way or another. Sodium, for example, may tend to leak inwards, moving down its concentration gradient from a high concentration outside to a low concentration inside. Potassium on the other hand, moving down its concentration gradient, may leak a little in the opposite direction. This is a natural movement for particles, which pass from a high to a low concentration in an attempt to equalise the concentration on both sides of the membrane (the process of **diffusion**). Diffusion of particles is the driving force for the movement of many substances both into and out of cells in many parts of the body.

Threshold potential

While leakage causes small fluctuations to occur in the resting potential of −70 mV, an action potential delivered from elsewhere will cause a rapid change. In fact, as soon as the resting potential reaches −50 mV, a rapid opening of sodium channels in the membrane allows a massive influx of sodium into the axon, creating a new action potential. This figure of **−50 mV** is called the **threshold potential** (Figure 3.4), and marks the opening of many sodium channels in the membrane. Channels that open at specific voltages in the membrane, such as the sodium channels described here, are known as **voltage-gated channels**. The sodium floods into the axon because, as a positive ion, it is attracted to the overall negative charge on the inside of the membrane (an electrical effect). Also, it will move rapidly down its concentration gradient (a chemical effect). The sodium influx is therefore an **electrochemical** event.

Depolarisation and repolarisation

As a result of the sodium influx, the membrane potential moves further away from threshold potential to peak at **+30 mV**, and this is called **depolarisation** (Figure 3.4). As the membrane potential crosses **0 mV**, the membrane changes polarity – that is, the overall negative charge on the *inside* becomes positive, while the overall positive charge on the *outside* becomes negative (Figure 3.4). The inside of the membrane has gained many positive sodium ions and therefore becomes positive, while the outside has lost those same positive sodium ions and therefore becomes negative. At +30 mV (i.e. the peak of an action potential) potassium channels open and allow the rapid movement of potassium out of the axonal membrane. These

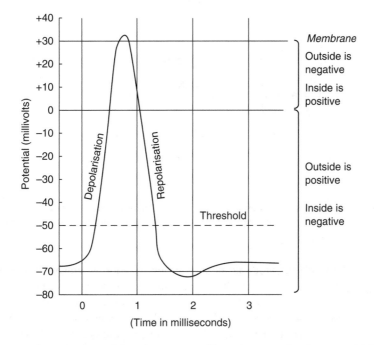

Figure 3.4 The action potential as seen on an oscilloscope screen. Resting potential is −70 mV. If sufficient depolarisation occurs for this value to reach −50 mV (threshold), an action potential will take place. Depolarisation is caused by sodium influx until +30 mV is reached. Repolarisation then occurs with a potassium efflux until resting potential is restored. As depolarisation and repolarisation cross 0 mV so the net charge on each side of the membrane reverses.

potassium channels are also voltage-gated, but they open at a different voltage to the sodium channels. Potassium moves out for the same electrochemical reasons that sodium moved in. The positively charged potassium is attracted to the negative charge outside the membrane and is also flowing down its own concentration gradient, from high inside to low outside. This mass movement of potassium returns the membrane to resting potential, i.e. from +30 mV down to −70 mV again, a process called **repolarisation** (Figure 3.4). As 0mV is crossed there is another reversal of membrane polarity, from the overall positive inside and negative outside of the action potential, to the overall negative inside and positive outside of the resting potential. However, this restoration of resting potential occurs with the main ions, sodium and potassium, in the reverse positions from when the process started. Before another action potential is possible, the sodium must be returned to the *outside* of the membrane and the potassium returned to the *inside* of the membrane. The membrane has sodium and potassium pumps (Figure 3.5) which pump these ions across the membrane, against their concentration gradients, and thus return the two cations to their former concentrations, sodium outside and potassium inside the axon. The period of time needed for this to take place, and for the sodium and potassium channels to close, is known as the **refractory phase** (Figures 3.4 and 3.5). During this period the axon cannot produce another action potential (Martini and Nath 2008).

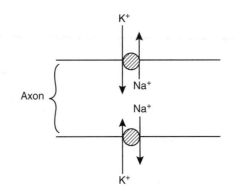

Figure 3.5 Sodium–potassium pumps are working during the refractory phase to restore the ions to the original positions; sodium is pumped out of the axon, potassium is pumped in.

Figure 3.4 shows the timescale, along the base axis, during which all these events take place. It is significant that the entire action potential occupies between two and three milliseconds (2–3 ms; i.e. two to three thousandths of a second), with a refractory phase lasting another millisecond. Thus, between one action potential and the next there is a time interval of about only four milliseconds, allowing a single neuron a capacity of up to 250 action potentials per second. The speed at which the nervous system works, in thousandths of a second, is faster than the blink of an eye, which to us appears to be instantaneous.

Myelinated and unmyelinated axons

The action potential described also has to pass along the axon from cell to synapse. In an unmyelinated axon, depolarisation at one part of the axonal membrane causes the membrane just ahead to reach threshold and begin the process of depolarisation there. Repeating this process continuously results in a wave of depolarisation that sweeps down the axon. This will be followed by a wave of repolarisation, immediately behind depolarisation, during which resting potential is restored (Figure 3.6).

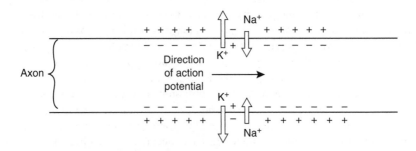

Figure 3.6 An unmyelinated axon. The impulse sweeps from left to right, caused by a sodium input, which reverses the membrane charge from resting to action potential, followed right behind by a potassium efflux, which restores the membrane resting potential charge.

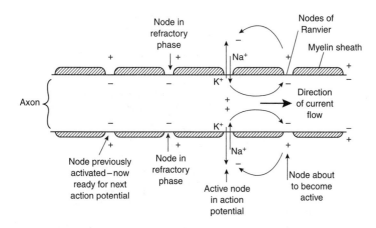

Figure 3.7 A section of myelinated axon showing saltatory action. The active node has a sodium influx followed immediately by a potassium efflux – i.e. an action potential. This positive input is attracted to the negative potential on the inside of the next node in the sequence, and this will rapidly reach threshold and action potential. The node behind the active node is in refractory phase.

In a myelinated axon a different process causes the spread of an action potential down the axon (Figure 3.7). Those segments of the membrane which are covered by myelin cannot allow the passage of ions, and so will not be involved in the movement of an action potential. However, the myelination has tiny gaps in it called the **nodes of Ranvier** where depolarisation and repolarisation take place. To describe what is happening, we will take a three-node sequence from a myelinated axon (see Figure 3.7). In Figure 3.7 the active node has reached threshold and will depolarise, i.e. reverse its polarity, while the other nodes are in resting potential. The positive sodium entering at the active node is attracted to the negative on the inside of the next node along, and will jump across the myelin internode to reach it. This movement of sodium causes the next node to reach threshold potential and depolarise. While sodium is entering this next node, the previous active node has reached repolarisation with the outflow of potassium. The process of sodium entering at a node and leaping over the internode to the next node is repeated along the length of the axon. This leaping over internodes is called **saltatory** ('jumping') action and speeds up the passage of an action potential down the axon. An action potential can pass along a fully myelinated axon at a speed of up to 120 meters per second compared to 2.3 meters per second along an unmyelinated axon. In either case the speed is fast, with action potentials passing through the full length of the body in a fraction of a second.

Synapses

Synapses (Figure 3.8) are the minute gaps (or **clefts**) occurring between the end of one neuronal axon and the membrane of the structure beyond. The **synaptic cleft**, which is between 20 nm and 50 nm across, separates the **presynaptic bulb** from the **post-synaptic membrane**. The presynaptic bulb is an expansion of the axon terminal. Within it there are many vesicles containing a chemical **neurotransmitter** destined to be released into the cleft. Neurotransmitters come in a variety of different forms

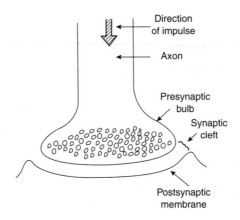

Figure 3.8 A synapse. The axon ends in a presynaptic bulb which is filled with vesicles
   housing a neurotransmitter.

(see Chapter 4), but they all have in common the ability to bind to protein receptors
attached to the postsynaptic membrane and thus cause a change within that membrane
and the cell beyond. This happens when the neurotransmitter is released from the
presynaptic bulb in response to the arrival of an action potential (Figure 3.9).

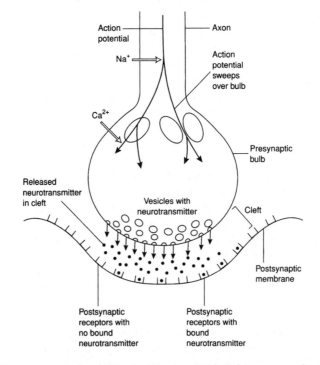

Figure 3.9 Events at a synapse during an action potential. Calcium enters the presynaptic
   bulb and the vesicles flood to the presynaptic membrane; the vesicles rupture and
   empty their contents into the synaptic cleft. Neurotransmitters can bind to receptors in the postsynaptic membrane and initiate a change in that membrane.

Action potentials sweeping down the axon involve the influx of sodium ions (Na⁺), but on arrival at the presynaptic bulb the ionic influx changes to a different ion, i.e. the calcium ion (Ca²⁺). This change to the double positive charge of calcium probably causes an even faster rise to +30 mV in the presynaptic bulb, triggering a sudden migration of the vesicles to the presynaptic membrane. Here they rupture and empty their neurotransmitter contents into the cleft. These chemicals then flood the cleft and bind to receptor sites on the postsynaptic membrane. The binding of a neurotransmitter, even for only one or two milliseconds, causes important changes in the postsynaptic cell. After binding, the neurotransmitters will be removed from the receptor. Some will be broken down and disposed of by excretion via the cerebrospinal fluid (CSF) and the blood to the kidneys. Others are also degraded but reabsorbed back into the presynaptic bulb and recycled. Some neurotransmitters are recycled in part via cells called astrocytes. *See page 53*

Excitation and inhibition

Some synapses are **excitatory** in function, while others are **inhibitory** (Figure 3.10). Excitatory synapses cause activity to occur beyond the postsynaptic membrane, often generating an action potential in the membrane of a second neuron. This is achieved by the binding of a neurotransmitter to receptors of the postsynaptic membrane which are linked to sodium channels in that membrane. The neurotransmitter causes the receptor to open the sodium channel; sodium then

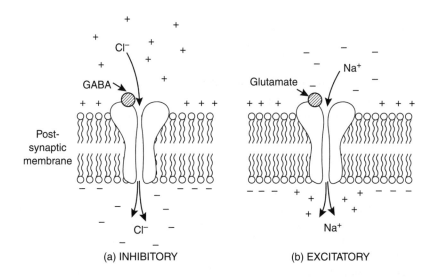

(a) INHIBITORY   (b) EXCITATORY

Figure 3.10 Two types of postsynaptic receptor. (a) An inhibitory receptor binding GABA (gamma-aminobutyric acid). This causes the opening of a chloride (Cl⁻) channel and chloride enters the postsynaptic membrane. The entry of this negative ion causes the resting potential to become even more negative, preventing any chance of an action potential in that membrane. (b) An excitatory receptor binding glutamate. This causes the opening of a sodium channel and sodium ions (Na⁺) to enter. The entry of a positive ion sets up an action potential in the postsynaptic membrane.

floods into the membrane from its high concentration outside the membrane, and starts a new action potential.

Inhibitory synapses do the opposite. The post-synaptic receptors are linked to chloride (Cl⁻) channels which open by the binding of neurotransmitter allowing chloride to enter the membrane. Chloride will move down its concentration gradient from the higher concentrations found outside the membrane (Figure 3.3). The resting potential of that membrane, i.e. negative on the inside, becomes even more negative, ensuring that any action potentials in that neuron are impossible (i.e. they are inhibited). At first sight this may seem surprising. After all, the nervous system is designed to generate action potentials, so the blocking (or inhibition) of action potentials appears to go against the very purpose of the system. However, think for a moment about a car. It is designed to move (a car that does not move is a waste of time), yet one of the fundamental components is a braking system, designed to prevent movement. Is that surprising? Of course not, since a car that cannot stop is deadly. And so it is with the brain. Uncontrolled, unchecked action potentials would be like a car going downhill with no brakes. Life for the person with no inhibitory synapses would be a living nightmare, and some mental health disorders are linked to low levels of inhibitory neurotransmitters (see Epilepsy). With no inhibition, every action potential would cause some form of activity; and this would cause a state of brain overactivity. Compare the inhibitory synapses with the 'off' switch on a computer, where activation of this switch causes a shutdown of the system. Every system, including the nervous system, needs a form of deactivation mechanism at some point.

Neuromodulators

Neurotransmitters and their receptor binding sites are critical, not only to the function of the entire nervous system but also to the mechanism of action of many psychotropic drugs, and therefore a more detailed discussion of these chemicals and their receptors is given in Chapter 4. However, in addition to neurotransmitters, chemicals called neuromodulators are also produced at the synapse. The term **neuromodulator** can be applied to various substances which are often released along with a neurotransmitter. These neuromodulators have a generally wider effect on neuronal function than neurotransmitters for the following reasons:

1   Neurotransmitters are released in small quantities and act locally within the synapse in which they are released. Neuromodulators are released in larger quantities and spread out beyond the synapse from which they are released. They therefore influence many other synaptic connections over a larger area of the brain.

2   Neuromodulators appear to modify the response of receptors to the neurotransmitter.

3   Some neuromodulators may act by binding to **autoreceptors**, which are receptors situated on the presynaptic membrane of the bulb, thus modifying the release of neurotransmitters (Breedlove et al. 2010).

Neuromodulators are mostly **neuropeptides**, i.e. small proteins of the nervous system. However, several substances usually classified as neurotransmitters may have a neuromodulatory role by acting beyond the synapse from where they were released, e.g. **enkephalin** and **cholecystokinin** (see Chapter 4). Several groups of **hormones** are also peptides. Hormones have an even wider influence over the activity of the brain (as well as the body) by being released into the blood circulation. Hormonal influence over brain activity is discussed in Chapter 5.

Neuroglia

Astrocytes

Neuroglia, or glial cells, are the support cells of the central nervous system. They outnumber the neurons by nine to one (there are an estimated 900 billion neuroglia compared with 100 billion neurons), but they do not create or transmit action potentials (impulses) as neurons do. Of this vast number, the commonest glial cells are the **astrocytes** (Figure 3.11), so called because of their star shape, created by many fine extensions pushing out in all directions. There are two forms of astrocyte: the **fibrous** form and the **protoplasmic** form. The fibrous form is largely found in the white matter of the brain. Fibrous astrocytes have fewer processes than their protoplasmic cousins, but their processes are long and straight, some with broad ends (like feet), which attach to blood capillaries or to the cells of the pia mater. The fibrous astrocytes respond to brain tissue injury by growing in large numbers (a process called **gliosis**). Unlike most neurons, both kinds of astrocyte retain the ability to go through mitosis (cell division) for the duration of the person's lifetime. The protoplasmic forms appear mostly in the grey matter of the brain. Their processes are shorter but more numerous than in the fibrous type, each process being more extensively branched.

Astrocytes generally have a very close association with neurons, surrounding the cell bodies and synapses, as well as blood capillaries, with their processes. They appear to have a role to play during the moment when neurons are transmitting an action potential. Neuronal action potentials cause the adjacent astrocytes to increase their metabolism and at the same time to partly depolarise, although they do not themselves achieve an action potential. Potassium ions (K^+) flood out from the axonal membrane of the neuron as the action potential sweeps down towards the synapse, and the astrocyte takes up this extracellular potassium in order to stabilise

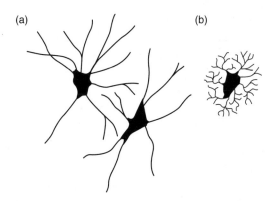

Figure 3.11 Astrocytes: (a) fibrous; (b) protoplasmic.

the ionic environment around the neuron. Excess *extracellular* potassium is dangerous to the brain and, if it got into circulation, it would be dangerous to the heart.
Potassium is normally kept concentrated *inside* the cells.

Astrocytes are also involved in the biochemistry of neurotransmitters. They are
often found surrounding the synapse, where they prevent neurotransmitter leakage and assist in the removal and, in some cases, the recycling of neurotransmitters
after these chemicals have fulfilled their task. One such form of neurotransmitter
recycling that involves the astrocyte is the production of glutamate from gamma-
aminobutyric acid (GABA) within the cytoplasm of an astrocyte close to the GABA
synapse. The glutamate thus created is passed back from the astrocyte to the neuron
for the further synthesis of GABA (Figure 3.12). This is a good example of the
supportive role of these cells.

Some astrocytes have been found to bind neurotransmitters to receptor sites
attached to the astrocyte membrane, although the purpose of binding of neurotransmitters to astrocytes is not fully known. In one example of this, glutamate,
an important neurotransmitter of several brain areas such as the cerebrum, was
able to bind to astrocyte receptors. Binding to these receptors caused the astrocyte to oscillate between high and low calcium levels within its cytoplasm. These
calcium waves within the cell have been seen to pass on to other cells through
membrane-to-membrane contacts between adjacent astrocytes. In one experiment,
a calcium wave induced in one astrocyte by adding glutamate was witnessed to
pass through 59 other attached astrocytes before it stopped. Such calcium surges
must indicate a form of cell signalling about which much is still to be learnt. Other
functions of astrocytes have been proposed from varying amounts of evidence. For
example, the broad feet resting on blood capillaries suggest a possible nutritional
role for these cells. It would not be possible for every one of 100 billion neurons to
receive its own blood supply. Many neurons rely on nutrients being collected from
the circulation by astrocytes and passed on to the neurons, with wastes possibly going in the opposite direction. Astrocytes also store glucose and pass this on to the
neurons for energy purposes.

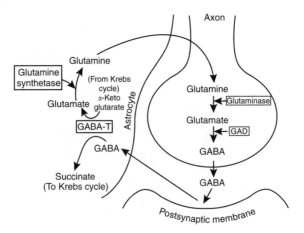

Figure 3.12 Astrocytes near a GABA synapse are partly involved in the GABA–glutamate
      synthesis cycle. The enzymes are in boxes: GABA-T = gamma-aminobutyric
      acid transaminase; GAD = glutamic acid decarboxylase.

The importance of studying astrocytes is highlighted by this large number of diverse functions. Gliosis (excessive growth of glial cells) is somehow involved in brain repair, and this mechanism may have implications for mental health, such as in dementia. Also, the role of astrocytes in neurotransmitter recycling could be of importance in depression or anxiety, and the fact that they have neurotransmitter receptors now makes them possible targets for psychotropic drugs. Such future drugs may be used to modify mental activity by affecting astrocytes, with or without neuronal involvement, and it is possible that some current drugs may already be influencing mental activity through astrocyte involvement.

Other glial cells

The glial cells that form myelin sheaths around axons fall into two types, the **oligodendrocytes** within the central nervous system only, and the **Schwann cells** within the peripheral nervous system only. Myelination, as identified earlier, is essential for the saltatory passage of action potentials. Some neurons remain unmyelinated but they are less numerous. Oligodendrocytes are small cells within the brain and cord, and during embryonic development each cell contributes myelination to several axons at once. Each Schwann cell, however, contributes myelination to only one segment of a single peripheral axon (Figure 3.1). Both types of cell leave gaps (the nodes of Ranvier) between the myelination patches where short sections of axon are exposed (Figure 3.1).

Glial cells include the following other types:

- The **microglia**, small phagocytic cells of the central nervous system (CNS, i.e. the brain and spinal cord), which engulf and remove not only invading organisms but also remnants and debris of dead cells.
- The **ependymal cells**, flat cells lining the brain's ventricular system and ducts, which provide a smooth surface for the cerebrospinal fluid (CSF) to flow over. They have cilia (minute hair-like processes) on the cell surface which produce a sweeping action that aids the circulation of CSF.
- The **satellite cells**, the smallest cells of the brain, associated with neuronal cell bodies and Schwann cells. They maintain the optimum chemical environment around neurons, and they appear to respond to inflammation and injury.

Ependymal cells fall into three main groups. The **ependymocytes** line the ventricles and central canal of the spinal cord. The **tanycytes** line the floor of the third ventricle and have processes touching blood capillaries; they may be involved in the movement of hormones from the blood to the adjacent hypothalamus. The **choroidal cells** cover the choroid plexus and promote the production of CSF.

During embryonic development of the nervous system, ependymal cells take on another role related to the migration of neurons within the neural tube (the embryonic stage of development of the central nervous system). They form a temporary framework along which the migrating neuron will move from its site of cellular mitosis. This framework is rather like a trellis along which a plant will grow. The process of neuronal migration is important for the correct location of neurons in the brain and the establishment of their subsequent synaptic connections (see Chapter 2).

See page 27

If the wrong route is taken by neurons along the ependymal framework, inappropriate synaptic connections will be formed. This malformation is implicated in several mental health disorders, notably schizophrenia, and is discussed further in Chapter 10.

Key points

The neuron

- Neurons are the functional unit of the nervous system. They have a cell body bearing dendrites and an axon.
- Axons are efferent pathways conveying action potentials to the synapse. They are mostly myelinated to speed up the passage of action potentials.

Neurotransmission

- The membrane begins in resting potential, with sodium concentrated outside the axon and potassium concentrated inside the axon.
- Action potentials are generated by a sodium influx into the axon, followed by a potassium output from the axon, which restores resting potential.

Synapses

- Synapses store neurotransmitters, which are released into the cleft on arrival of the action potential. Neurotransmitters then bind to the postsynaptic membrane and cause changes beyond that membrane.
- Synapses are either excitatory (causing changes such as action potentials in the postsynaptic membrane) or inhibitory (blocking such changes).

Neuroglia

- Neuroglia are the support cells of the nervous system. Astrocytes are the most numerous of the neuroglia, providing nutritional, ionic and neurotransmitter support to neurons.
- Oligodendrocytes (within the brain and cord) and Schwann cells (within the peripheral nerves) provide myelination to axons.

References

Blows W. T. (2000) Systems and diseases: The nervous system 1. *Nursing Times,* **96** (35): 41–44.

Blows W. T. (2001) *The Biological Basis of Nursing: Clinical Observations.* Routledge, London.

Breedlove S. M., Watson N. V. and Rosenzweig M. R (2010) *Biological Psychology: An Introduction to Behavioral, Cognitive and Clinical Neuroscience* (6th edition). Sinauer Associates, Massachusetts.

Martini F. H. and Nath J. L. (2008) *Fundamentals of Anatomy and Physiology* (8th edition). Benjamin Cummings, San Francisco.

4 Neurotransmitters and receptors

Introduction to neurotransmitters

Neurotransmitters are the chemical agents released from the presynaptic bulb into the synaptic cleft. They are sometimes referred to as the *primary messenger*, since they occur as free chemicals that move across a space (in this case, the cleft) and cause a change in another part (in this case, the postsynaptic membrane). Another term used for neurotransmitters is **ligand**, meaning a naturally produced agent that binds to a receptor and in so doing changes that receptor. The main change that occurs in receptors on binding of a ligand is an **allosteric** effect, i.e. a change of receptor *shape*. This change then has a further effect, the nature of which depends on which receptor is involved; it may be either within the membrane or beyond it in the cytoplasm of the cell.

Most neurotransmitters fall into three main groups: the **amines**, the **amino acids** and the **peptides**. Amines are compounds containing the **amino group** (NH_2) and have the general structure RCH_2NH_2 where R is a variable portion (known as a **radical**) (Figure 4.1a). Variations in the radical give rise to different amines. Amino acids, the building blocks of proteins, are amines in which a **carboxyl group** ($COOH$) replaces one of the hydrogens on a carbon atom (Figure 4.1b). A peptide is a small protein, i.e. a small number of amino acids bonded together in a linear chain. Acetylcholine is a neurotransmitter of different origin and is discussed separately. **Catecholamines** are amines combined with a **catechol group** (Figure 4.1c), which consists of a carbon ring with two OH branches. A discussion related to each of the better-known neurotransmitters follows, as this information is relevant to an understanding of the neuropathology of the various mental health disorders and to neuropharmacology. *See page 75*

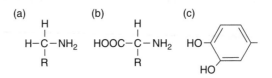

Figure 4.1 The structure of three compounds: (a) an amine; (b) an amino acid; (c) the catechol group. NH_2 is the amino group; COOH is the carboxyl group; R is the radical (variable portion).

Receptors

Specific activity at the synapse is not due to the function of any particular neurotransmitter but to the function of the receptor to which it binds. By binding to different receptors, the *same* neurotransmitter is often seen to produce *different* effects. Receptors for any given neurotransmitter fall into several types (or groups) according to structure and function, and each receptor type usually has distinct subtypes. A good example is acetylcholine, which binds to two main types of receptors, either nicotinic or muscarinic, and these have subtypes (e.g. muscarinic subtypes are M_1, M_2, M_3, M_4, M_5). Subtle variations in the way these subtypes respond to acetylcholine binding results in a wide range of activity for the neurotransmitter.

It is also important to recognise two other ways of classifying receptor sites:

1   According to their *location*. **Postsynaptic receptors** are part of the *postsynaptic* membrane of the cell that occurs beyond the cleft. Their purpose, when activated by neurotransmitter, is to effect some kind of change within that postsynaptic cell, such as the generation of a new action potential. Alternatively, **autoreceptors** are found on some *presynaptic* membranes or other parts of the neuron and therefore allow neurotransmitters to bind to the same neuron that releases it. Such autoreceptors are thought to provide feedback information to the neuron and the presynaptic bulb, in particular, to regulate (or control) any further neurotransmitter release.

2   According to their *function*. Some receptors are **ionotropic**. They control the opening or closing of a particular ion channel and can do this remarkably quickly, usually within milliseconds. When a neurotransmitter binds to a receptor, the receptor changes shape (the allosteric effect) and this opens a channel in the membrane, e.g. a sodium channel, allowing ions to pass through the membrane. The passage of sodium ions (positively charged cations) into a second neuron will initiate a new action potential and therefore occurs at **excitatory** synapses (Figure 3.10). The passage of chloride (a negatively charged anion) into a second neuron will prevent an action potential and therefore occurs at **inhibitory** synapses (Figure 3.10). Other receptors are **metabotropic** (Figure 4.2). They do not *directly* influence ionic channels but do cause changes in the metabolism of the postsynaptic cell.

The binding of a neurotransmitter to metabotropic receptors causes activation of a membrane-bound protein on the inside of the cell. This is the **G-protein**, abbreviated from *guanosine triphosphate (GTP) binding protein*, which may have an inhibitory (G_i) or a stimulatory (G_s) effect on cellular enzymes. In this way, metabotropic

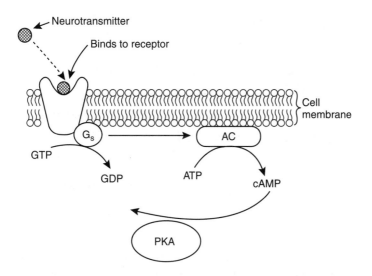

Figure 4.2 An excitatory metabotropic receptor. The neurotransmitter (first messenger) binds to the receptor outside the membrane. This activates a stimulatory G-protein (G$_s$), which binds guanosine triphosphate (GTP) and forms guanosine diphosphate (GDP). The activated G$_s$ protein moves along the inner membrane, and collides with and activates adenylyl cyclase (AC). This in turn binds adenosine triphosphate (ATP) to form cyclic adenosine monophosphate (cAMP). cAMP is free to move into the cell (it is a second messenger) and activate protein kinase A (PKA), which can have a multitude of different effects on the cell. Compare with Figure 4.3.

receptors, like ionotropic receptors, can also be excitatory or inhibitory. However, because they operate through a different mechanism, they are slower than ionotropic receptors and their effects remain over a longer period of time. When the G$_s$ protein is activated, it moves along the inside of the membrane until it contacts a membrane-bound enzyme called **adenylyl cyclase** (**AC**). Allosteric activation of AC then occurs and this enzyme binds and splits intracellular ATP to form **cAMP** (**cyclic adenosine monophosphate**). cAMP is known as a **secondary messenger** because it is free to move through the cell (unlike the G$_s$ protein and AC which are bound to the inside of the postsynaptic membrane). The primary messenger was the neurotransmitter, which was free to move around the synaptic cleft. The secondary messenger is free to move around the inside of the cell (within the **cytosol**). Secondary messengers like cAMP, and others such as **inositol triphosphate** (**IP3**) and **diacylglycerol** (**DAG**) produced by some metabotropic receptors, then go on to influence other cellular functions. IP$_3$ opens calcium channels, whilst cAMP and DAG activate an enzyme known as **protein kinase** (**PK**). When activated, PK regulates changes in the cell's metabolism. This may involve the opening of ion channels, causing changes in the ionic environment of the cell, the moderation of protein synthesis, or even the activation of specific genes leading to protein synthesis (**gene expression**) (Figure 4.2). Metabotropic receptors that activate G$_i$ proteins are inhibitory because they block any activity of AC (Figure 4.3).

Receptors are actually proteins set into the cell membrane and they have a specific role which is activated by the binding of neurotransmitter (Martini and Nath

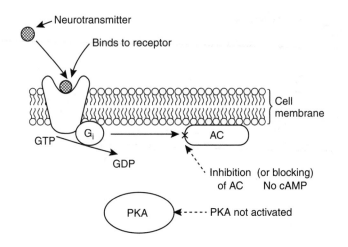

Figure 4.3 An inhibitory metabotropic receptor. The activated inhibitory G_i protein collides with adenylyl cyclase (AC), which is then deactivated and unable to form cyclic adenosine monophosphate (cAMP). As a result, protein kinase A (PKA) is not activated. Compare with Figure 4.2.

2008). Some receptors are attached to the outer surface of the membrane, while others are transmembranous (i.e. they pass right through the membrane, appearing on both sides). Cells can of course produce proteins, so they can also produce receptors when necessary. This means that cells can **upregulate** their receptors by producing more of them, increasing the receptor density of their membrane and therefore binding more of the neurotransmitter. This is likely to be the consequence of reduced quantities of available neurotransmitter.

Alternatively, cells can **downregulate** their membrane receptor density by slowing receptor production, especially if the neurotransmitter is in abundance. Measurements of receptor density on postsynaptic membranes give useful information about the levels of neurotransmitter present in the synaptic cleft. This is important because variations in the level of neurotransmitter can affect mental health, causing, for example, depression.

The amine neurotransmitters

Dopamine

Dopamine, noradrenaline and adrenaline are three **catecholamine** neurotransmitters that share a common pathway of production (Figure 4.4). The starting point for the production of dopamine is the dietary amino acid **tyrosine**, which is converted by the neurons to **dihydroxyphenylalanine** (known as **dopa**) by the enzyme **tyrosine hydroxylase**. Further conversion to dopamine is by another enzyme called **dopa decarboxylase**. After use, dopamine is broken down in two sites, within the cleft and in the presynaptic bulb, by several enzymes including one *See page 234* called **monoamine oxidase** (**MAO**) which is situated at the junction of the axon *See page 201* with the bulb. The final metabolite, **homovanillic acid**, is excreted via the CSF.

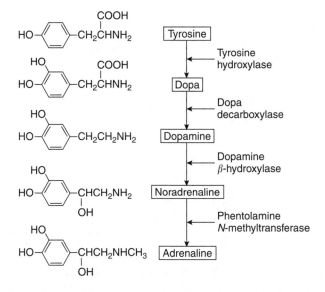

Figure 4.4 The formation of dopamine, noradrenaline and adrenaline from the amino acid tyrosine. The products are boxed, while the enzymes (unboxed) label the arrows. The chemical structure of each product is shown on the left.

Dopamine activates several important pathways of the brain (Figure 4.5). From the brain stem nucleus known as the **ventral tegmental area** (**VTA**), closely associated with the substantia nigra, two major dopaminergic (i.e. responding to dopamine) tracts pass out to specific brain areas. Tracts passing to the **cerebral cortex** form the **mesocortical pathways**, and others to the **nucleus accumbens** of the **limbic system** form the **mesolimbic pathways** (Martini and Nath 2008). Additional major dopaminergic pathways are the tracts from the **substantia nigra** in the midbrain to other main areas of the **basal ganglia**, forming the **nigrostriatal pathways**. Some authors join the nigrostriatal and mesolimbic pathways together under the term **mesostriatal system**.

In some sites of the brain, dopamine acts as an inhibitory neurotransmitter, although, as discussed, the function of neurotransmitters more often relates to the receptor that it binds to than to the ligand itself. In this capacity, dopamine is involved in inhibiting muscle tone, a function of the substantia nigra (see Parkinson's disease). It also inhibits breast milk production by blocking the release of the hormone **prolactin** from the anterior **pituitary gland** when the woman is not breastfeeding. Dopamine also plays a vital role in the function of the limbic system and here it is associated with brain arousal. It is implicated in psychotic disturbances such as hallucinations in schizophrenia and manic-depressive psychosis, as well as being involved in the reward pathways associated with drug addiction (Blows 2000).

See page 263

See page 143

Dopamine receptors

Dopamine receptors are all metabotropic, i.e. working through a G-protein system. At least five subclasses of dopamine receptor are identified (D_1, D_2, D_3, D_4

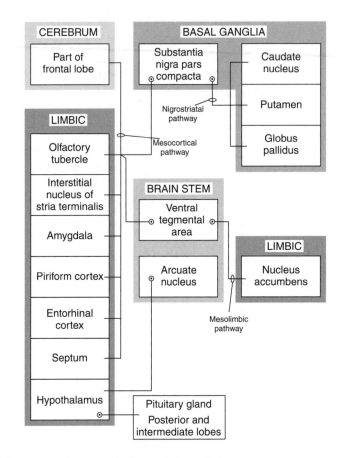

Figure 4.5 The main dopamine pathways of the central nervous system.

and D_5). They are often grouped as the D_1-like subgroup (D_1 and D_5), because they are both excitatory, and the D_2-like subgroup (D_2, D_3 and D_4), because they are all inhibitory. D_1 and D_5 are both excitatory because they increase the level of cAMP in the cell. D_1 is the most abundant dopamine receptor in the brain, especially the basal ganglia. D_2-like receptors are inhibitory because they reduce the level of cAMP in the neuron. D_2 is found in the basal ganglia, nucleus accumbens and the Ventral Tegmental Area of the brain stem. The D_3 receptor is inhibitory and is found in the limbic system and in particular the hypothalamus. D_4 is inhibitory and is mostly found in the cortex, hippocampus, amygdala and nucleus accumbens. D_5 is excitatory and is found in the thalamus. There may be a D_6 and D_7, although these are not yet fully established.

Noradrenaline

Noradrenaline (**norepinephrine**) is a catecholamine produced from dopamine by the action of the enzyme **dopamine β–hydroxylase** (**DBH**) (Figure 4.4). Noradrenaline is produced both as a hormone from the **adrenal medulla** and as a neurotransmitter in parts of the brain and at the **sympathetic** nerve terminals. The *See page 18* adrenergic brain pathways (i.e. those responding to noradrenaline) centre primarily on the **locus coeruleus** in the brain stem (Martini and Nath 2008). Tracts from this nucleus pass out to the cerebrum and limbic system (Figure 4.6) as part of the **diffuse** *See page 219* **modulatory systems** similar to serotonin pathways (see serotonin) (Blows 2000).

Adrenaline

Adrenaline (epinephrine) is the final stage in the production of catecholamine transmitters. Noradrenaline is acted on by the enzyme **phentolamine N-methyltransferase** (**PNMT**) to produce adrenaline (Figure 4.4). Adrenaline is well known as a *hormone* of the **adrenal medulla**, but as a *neurotransmitter* it is far less well understood. This is because it is found in low concentrations across many widespread sites in the brain. It does not usually occur in specific nuclei, and this pattern of diffuse distribution makes it difficult to study, resulting in a poor understanding of its role in the brain.

Adrenergic receptors

Adrenergic receptors, i.e. those that bind and respond to noradrenaline and adrenaline, are either alpha (α) or beta (β), with subtypes of each (α_1, α_2, β_1, β_2, β_3). They are all metabotropic, activating cellular changes through secondary messengers. The α_1 type is excitatory, and the activation of this receptor causes depolarisation by releasing calcium stored inside the cell. This receptor is found in the brain as a postsynaptic receptor and also in the vascular and intestinal smooth muscle and the heart. The α_2 type is inhibitory (i.e. it uses a G_i protein) and deactivates calcium channels, thus having the opposite effect to α_1 receptors. α_2 receptors are found in the brain as autoreceptors as well as postsynaptic receptors. They are also located in the same smooth muscles as α_1 and on the surface of platelets and nerve terminals.

Beta receptors, on activation by noradrenaline, increase the postsynaptic membrane response to other excitatory stimuli by indirectly affecting ion channels via a

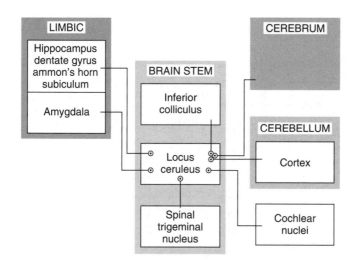

Figure 4.6 The main noradrenaline pathways of the central nervous system.

series of intermediate proteins which increase cAMP. Both β_1 and β_2 are found in the brain, whilst the β_3 type is located in adipose tissue.

Serotonin

See page 219

Serotonin, an important neurotransmitter, is part of the brain's **diffuse modulatory systems**. Nine nuclei (the **raphe nuclei**) in the brain stem send out serotonergic pathways (i.e. those responding to serotonin) to many parts of the cerebrum and limbic system (Figure 4.7). The serotonergic system has influence over a wide range of brain functions including regulation of mood, movement, appetite, sexual activity, sleeping and some glandular secretions (Blows 2000). It therefore plays a vital role in the maintenance of mental health and will be discussed again when considering a number of conditions, such as depression and eating disorders.

Serotonin is also known as **5-hydroxytryptamine (5-HT)** and is originally derived from the dietary amino acid **tryptophan**. This crosses the **blood–brain barrier** into the brain, transported by a molecule called the **large neutral amino acid transporter (LNAA)**. The blood–brain barrier is a layer of cells between the circulating blood and the brain tissue which acts like a filter, allowing some molecules to pass into the brain but not others. Since LNAA transports several amino acids into the brain across this barrier, particularly tyrosine, valine and leucine, the amount of tryptophan entering the brain is dependent on its concentration in the blood compared with the concentration of the other amino acids involved.

Neurons that use serotonin have the enzyme **tryptophan hydroxylase (TRPH)** in order to convert tryptophan to **5-hydroxytryptophan**, and this is further converted to serotonin by a second enzyme known as **aromatic amino acid decarboxylase (AAAD)**. **Vitamin B6 (pyridoxine)** is vital in the function of AAAD, and thus is important overall in the production of serotonin (Figure 4.8). After its release into the synaptic cleft and after it has bound to postsynaptic receptors, serotonin

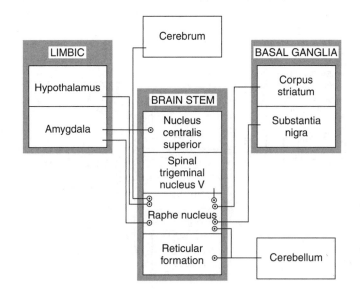

Figure 4.7 The main serotonin pathways of the central nervous system.

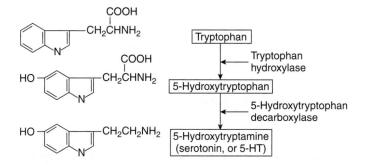

Figure 4.8 The formation of serotonin (5-hydroxytryptamine, or 5-HT) from the amino acid tryptophan. The products are boxed while the enzymes (unboxed) label the arrows. The chemical structure of each product is shown on the left.

is taken back into the presynaptic bulb (a process called re-uptake) and metabolised. The enzymes that are responsible for this are monoamine oxidase (MAO) and **aldehyde oxidase**, resulting in a **metabolite** (or waste product) called **5-hydroxyindoleacetic acid (5-HIAA)**. This is excreted first via the cerebrospinal fluid, then to the blood that carries it to the kidneys.

Serotonin receptors

Serotonin receptors form many classes and subclasses, all of which are metabotropic. Table 4.1 shows the main classes and subclasses and their intracellular action on binding serotonin, where known. These intracellular actions may be involved in various mental activities and disorders as follows (Nolen-Heoksema 2007; Carlson 2010):

- Addiction involves 5–HT1A, 1B, 2A, 2C and 3
- Aggression involves 5–HT1A and 1B
- Anxiety involves 5–HT1A, 1B, 1D, 2A, 2B, 2C, 3, 4, 6 and 7
- Appetite involves 5–HT1A, 2A, 2B, 2C and 4
- Cognition involves 5–HT2A and 6
- Impulsivity involves 5–HT1A

Table 4.1 Classes of serotonin receptors and their intracellular actions. (Ex) = excitatory; (In) = inhibitory.

Serotonin receptor class	Receptor subclasses	Intracellular role
5–HT1	5–HT1A, 1B, 1D, 1E, 1F	Decreases cAMP (In) with different effects. Some reduce AC activity
5–HT2	5–HT2A, 2B, 2C	Activates DAG and IP_3 (Ex)
5–HT3		Opens Ca^{2+} channels (Ex)
5–HT4		Increases cAMP (Ex)
5–HT5	5–HT5A	Decreases cAMP (In)
5–HT6		Increases cAMP (Ex)
5–HT7		Increases cAMP (Ex)

- Learning involves 5–HT1B, 2A, 3, 4 and 6
- Memory involves 5–HT1A, 1B, 2A, 3, 4, 6 and 7
- Mood involves 5–HT1A, 1B, 2A, 2C, 4, 6 and 7
- Sexual behaviour involves 5–HT1A, 1B, 2A and 2C
- Sleep involves 5–HT1A, 2A, 2B, 2C, 5A and 7.

The amino acid neurotransmitters

Glutamate and GABA

Glutamate and **gamma-aminobutyric acid (GABA)** are important neuro-transmitters found throughout the cerebral cortex and they share a common synthesis pathway (Figure 4.9, and see also Figure 4.12). Glutamate (glutamic acid) is a potent excitatory transmitter involved in consciousness. It is produced mostly during the daytime as a result of cerebral activity. The synthesis of glutamate is linked with the **tricarboxylic acid** (or **Krebs**) **cycle**, the energy cycle of the neuron. α-**Ketoglutarate**, a component of this cycle, is converted to glutamate by the enzyme **GABA transaminase (GABA-T)**. After use, glutamate is acted on by a second enzyme called **glutamic acid decarboxylase (GAD)** to produce GABA (Figure 4.9).

GABA is a major inhibitory neurotransmitter. After use it is converted to **succinate** by GABA-T (the same enzyme that acted on α-ketoglutarate). Succinate

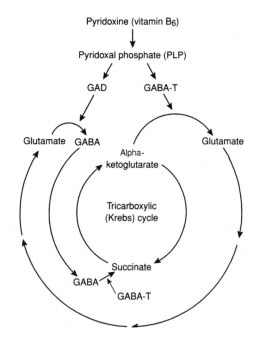

Figure 4.9 The synthesis of glutamate and gamma-aminobutyric acid (GABA). The two main enzymes involved are gamma-aminobutyric acid transaminase (GABA-T) and glutamic acid decarboxylase (GAD). Notice that vitamin B$_6$ is required to form pyridoxal phosphate (PLP), which is essential for both enzymes. Note also the involvement of the tricarboxylic (Krebs) cycle.

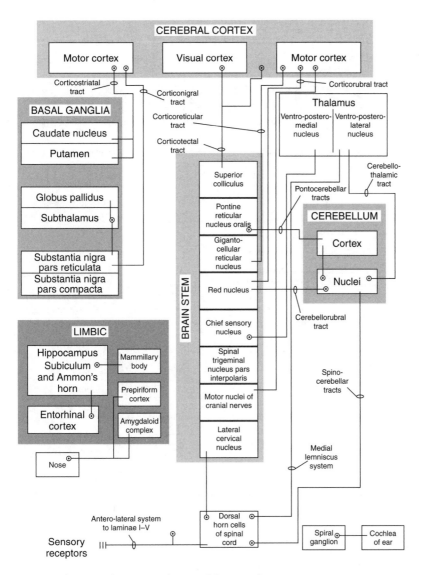

Figure 4.10 The main glutamate pathways of the central nervous system.

becomes another component of the tricarboxylic cycle. Both enzymes, GABA-T and GAD, rely on a co-factor called **pyridoxal phosphate** (**PLP**) in order to function. PLP itself relies on a supply of **pyroxidine** (**vitamin B₆**), and thus glutamate and GABA are both indirectly dependent on vitamin B₆ in the diet. GABA-T is most active in astrocytes located close to GABA synapses, while GAD is active in the pre-synaptic bulb of glutamate neurons (see Figure 3.12). The major glutamate pathways of the brain are shown in Figure 4.10 and the major GABA pathways in Figure 4.11. A low GABA level in some areas of the brain is implicated as part of the cause of epilepsy, and some drug treatments of epilepsy (anticonvulsants) target the enzymes that regulate GABA production, and therefore increase GABA levels at the synapse.

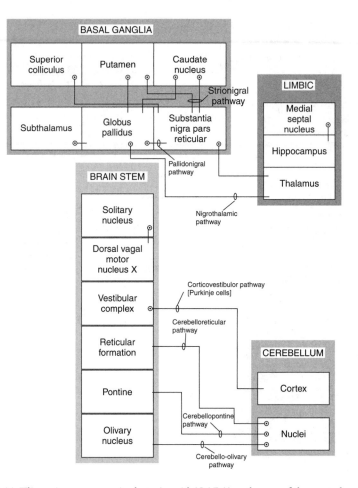

Figure 4.11 The main gamma-aminobutyric acid (GABA) pathways of the central nervous system.

Glutamate receptors

The term 'glutamate receptors' is used for those receptors that bind glutamate, but in reality other excitatory amino acids, such as aspartate, can also bind to and activate the same receptors. **Glutamate (*excitatory amino acid*) *receptors*** occur in seven known different classes (Carlson 2010), but only five classes are currently well understood. Each of these five is named after the artificial substance that is used as a ligand to bind to it in laboratory conditions. They are mostly ionotropic excitatory receptors linked to positive ion channels.

The **AMPA (α-amino-3-hydroxy-5-methyl-4-isoxazoleproprionate)** receptors are the most common type of receptor found in the brain. These ionotropic receptors are not specific to any particular positive ion, and will allow the passage of calcium, potassium and sodium.

The **K (kainic acid,** or **kainate)** receptor is a nonspecific ion channel receptor allowing the passage of sodium and potassium, and causing depolarisation in the cell when activated. Their distribution is more limited in the brain than AMPA and NMDA receptors, and they have both a pre- and post-synaptic activity.

The **NMDA** (**N-methyl-*d*-aspartate**) receptor (Figure 4.12) is the most potent and best-understood of the excitatory amino acid receptors. It is mostly in the cerebral cortex, especially in areas concerned with learning and memory, such as the hippocampus. When inactivated, the ion channel that forms part of the receptor is both closed and blocked by a magnesium (Mg^{2+}) plug on its inner surface. Activation of the receptor requires the binding of both glutamate and glycine, which together cause allosteric changes that open the channel. Removal of the Mg^{2+} plug is achieved by voltage changes across the membrane, occurring when AMPA or K channels are opened farther along on the same membrane. In this way, NMDA receptors function in harmony with other excitatory amino acid receptors. Calcium movement through the open channel causes the biggest depolarisation, with sodium and potassium movements also occurring (Figure 4.12).

The **metabotropic glutamate receptors** are classified into 8 subtypes (labelled $mGluR_{1-8}$) (Carlson 2010). These include the **ACPD** and the **L-AP4** receptors, named after specific drugs which bind to and activate some of these receptors. They exist mostly within the central nervous system on neuronal dendrites, as well as on astrocytes and oligodendrocytes.

GABA receptors

GABA receptors are of two subtypes, $GABA_A$ and $GABA_B$. The $GABA_A$ receptor (Figure 4.13) is ionotropic, where GABA opens a chloride channel in the postsynaptic membrane. When chloride (Cl^-) enters the cell, it hyperpolarises the membrane and therefore prevents action potentials (Figure 4.13). By blocking action potentials in this way, GABA is said to be inhibitory, and therefore reduces the overall activity of the brain. The $GABA_A$ receptor is the site of binding for several important drugs used in psychiatry, the benzodiazepines and the barbiturates, as well as binding alcohol.

See page 184
See page 154

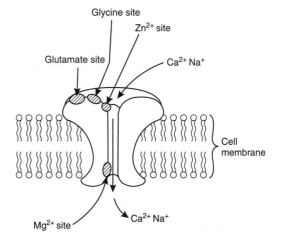

Figure 4.12 The NMDA glutamate receptor. Ca^{2+} is the calcium ion, Na^+ is the sodium ion, Mg^{2+} is the magnesium ion and Zn^{2+} is the zinc ion.

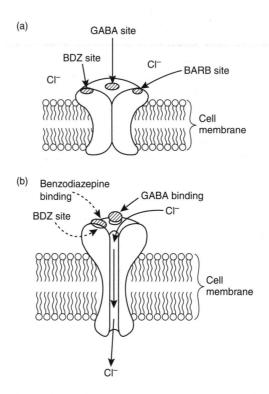

Figure 4.13 The gamma-aminobutyric acid (GABA) inhibitory receptor (GABA$_A$). (a) The closed receptor with no GABA binding. Notice the BDZ (benzodiazepine) and the BARB (barbiturate) binding sites. (b) The open receptor with GABA and benzodiazepine binding. The opening through the cell membrane is a chloride (Cl⁻) channel.

The GABA$_B$ receptor is metabotropic, causing reduced AC activity and reduced levels of intracellular calcium.

Aspartate and glycine

Aspartate (Figure 4.14) and **glycine** are two nonessential amino acid neurotransmitters and neurons can synthesise them as required (i.e. they are not directly obtained from the diet). Aspartate is, like glutamate, another excitatory neurotransmitter, acting through the NMDA receptor. Although aspartate is widely distributed throughout the brain, aspartate concentrations are generally weaker than those of glutamate, except in the ventral motor pathways of the cord. Glycine is, like GABA, another mostly inhibitory neurotransmitter. The distribution of glycine in the central nervous system is similar to that of aspartate, being less widely distributed than GABA and somewhat less well concentrated in spinal motor neurons than aspartate.

The peptide neurotransmitters

Generally, peptide neurotransmitters are produced from **precursors** – that is, protein gene products from which the final neuropeptide is obtained by enzymic

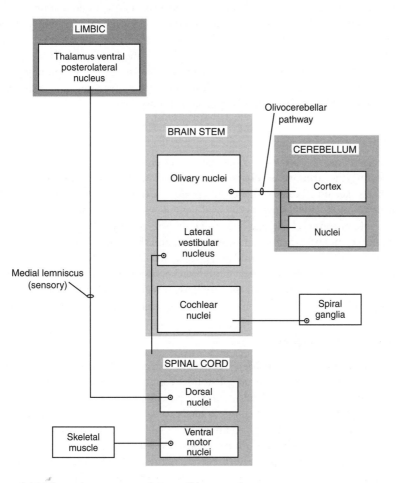

Figure 4.14 The main aspartate pathways of the central nervous system.

action. These peptides are often found in both the digestive tract and the brain. In the brain they appear to be concentrated mostly in the hypothalamus. The hypothalamus is known for many functions, one of which is the control of appetite.   *See page 12*

Cholecystokinin

Cholecystokinin (**CCK**) is a peptide found both in the digestive tract (where it regulates emptying of the gall bladder) and in the brain. It is derived from the precursor **procholecystokinin**, which is found in the cerebral cortex and the hypothalamus. A number of different cholecystokinins are produced from this precursor, the best ones studied in the brain being CCK4 and CCK8. Cholecystokinin in the hypothalamus is involved in regulating the inhibition of food intake once the stomach is full (a process called **satiation**, controlled by the **satiety centre** of the hypothalamus). The function of cholecystokinin in the cerebral cortex is less understood, but is linked to memory, cognition, the mother–infant relationship and pain threshold regulation. CCK8 is also concentrated in the hippocampus, amygdala and the spinal cord. It is often found associated with dopaminergic neurons, notably in the nigrostrial pathway and the nucleus accumbens, where it must have a function related to the role of dopamine. Two receptor types are known, CCK_A (mostly found in the digestive tract, less in the brain) and CCK_B (mostly found in the brain, less in the digestive tract). Cholecystokinin is generating greater interest now since there is evidence linking this neurotransmitter to several mental health disorders, notably anxiety, depression and psychosis.

Neuropeptide Y

Neuropeptide Y (NPY) is a neurotransmitter known to occur in pathways connecting the **arcuate nucleus** (part of the basal **hypothalamus**) to the lateral hypothalamus. Release of neuropeptide Y causes an increase in eating, the neurotransmitter itself being a powerful stimulator of food intake. There are two groups of neurons in the lateral hypothalamus activated by NPY: those that secrete **melanin-concentrating hormone (MCH)** and those that secrete **orexin**, both of which are peptides that stimulate appetite and lower body metabolism. Since NPY has some control over normal food intake, disturbance of NPY may be related to some eating disorders. Of the five known receptors for NPY, only four (Y_1, *See page 180* Y_2, Y_4 and Y_5) are found in humans. They are metabotropic inhibitory receptors.

Vasoactive intestinal peptide

Vasoactive intestinal peptide (VIP) is a digestive system peptide that is also located in some neurons that use acetylcholine (e.g. the parasympathetic nervous system stimulation of salivary glands), where it potentiates the action of acetylcholine. It would appear that VIP in the brain is likely to have a neuromodulatory role, not causing direct effects itself but modifying the effects of other neurotransmitters. It appears to be active within the **suprachiasmatic nucleus**, a small area of the brain which controls the **circadian rhythms** (the natural daily rhythms of the body), in particular those linked to external light levels, e.g. the sleep–wake cycle.

Substance P (neurokinin-1) and neurokinin A (neurokinin-2, previously substance K)

Substance P (neurokinin-1) and **neurokinin A (neurokinin-2)** are two peptides derived from the same precursor molecule, the protein **protachykinin**.

Substance P was the first neuropeptide discovered. It is the neurotransmitter of the grey matter at the back of the cord (called the **dorsal horn**). Here it functions on the main pain pathways from the periphery to the cord (i.e. the first sensory, or afferent, neuron). In the brain, substance P is mostly concentrated in the substantia nigra, where it activates dopaminergic neurons, and in the hypothalamus; it is also found in association with serotonin neurons originating in the raphe nucleus (see serotonin). Both substance P and neurokinin A bind to **NK receptors (NK = neurokinin)**. Three such receptors are known, NK_1, NK_2 and NK_3, all of which are metabotropic. Substance P may have some influence on mood and thus on depression. Using drugs to block specific substance P receptors, particularly NK_1, could therefore become a useful line of treatment in mood disorders (NK_1 is found in brain areas involved in stress and emotions). Neurokinin A (neurokinin-2),
See page 64

although isolated and chemically analysed and with at least one receptor found in the brain, is poorly understood in terms of brain activity.

Somatostatin

Somatostatin is a peptide found in various sites within the nervous system, such as the sympathetic nervous system (along with noradrenaline) and the thalamus (along with GABA). It is also present in the dorsal root ganglion of the first (peripheral) sensory neuron, the cerebral cortex, the limbic system, the hippocampus, the hypothalamus and parts of the brain stem (Figure 4.15). It is also a peptide of the digestive system, where it inhibits the release of several digestion-related hormones. In the brain, somatostatin has a sedatory effect and increases the action of sedatory drugs such as the barbiturates. It appears to reduce the rate of firing of neurons, suppresses motor activity and inhibits the release of growth hormone from the pituitary gland. Several forms of the molecule are known to have activity in humans, notably somatostatin-14, somatostatin-25 and somatostatin-28, where the number represents the amino acid content of the molecule.

Endogenous opioids

The chemistry of the brain involves the production of opiate-like substances called **endogenous opioids**, proteins produced under pain or stress conditions which

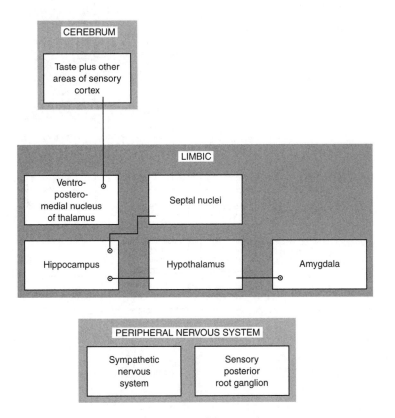

Figure 4.15 The main somatostatin pathways of the central nervous system.

block pain at either **spinous** (spinal cord) or **supraspinous** (brain stem) levels. Several classes of endogenous opioids are now known.

The **enkephalins** (Figure 4.16) are small peptides called **met-enkephalin** and **leu-enkephalin,** which are produced in response to minor pain, having an analgesic effect of about two minutes. **Beta-endorphin** (β-endorphin) is a larger peptide produced in response to more severe pain with an analgesic effect of around four hours or so.

The **dynorphins** (**dynorphin A**, **dynorphin B** and others) are intermediate sized peptides, and the **endomorphines** (**endomorphine-1** and **endomorphine-2**) are both small peptides. All of these naturally produced chemicals bind to opiate receptors in the upper cord and brain stem called **mu** (μ), **delta** (δ) and **kappa** (κ) receptors. Mu receptors may exist in two subtypes, μ_1 and μ_2, a distinction based on possible variations that may occur between the mu receptors of the brain stem and the mu receptors of the respiratory centre. Delta and kappa receptors

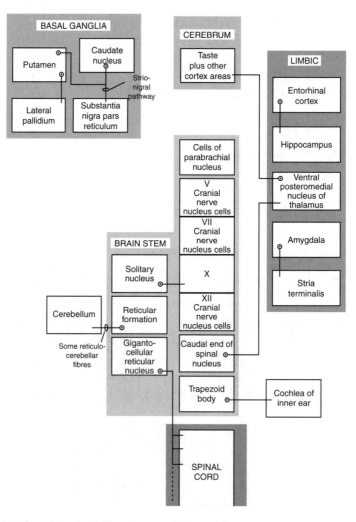

Figure 4.16 The main enkephalin pathways of the central nervous system.

are similarly subdivided, with δ_1, δ_2, δ_{cx} and δ_{ncx} proposed for delta, and κ_1, κ_2, κ_3 proposed for kappa. The delta receptor subtype δ_{cx} is said to form a complex with mu receptors, whilst the δ_{ncx} does not form a complex with any other receptors.

Kappa receptor subtypes, κ_1 and κ_2, have become a complex issue, with other further subdivisions of each subtype proposed. Research will continue in this area, mainly because of the devastating problems caused by heroin and other opiate addictions and the need to find a solution to this problem. The dynorphin receptors, for example, are somehow involved specifically in cocaine addiction. This work will eventually identify and classify many more subtypes of the opiate receptors with a view to finding antagonist drugs that will prevent the addictive opiate drugs from binding. The affinity of the endogenous opiates for the various opiate receptors, where this has been established, is shown in Table 4.2.

Other neurotransmitters

Acetylcholine

Acetylcholine (ACh) is one of the earliest known synaptic ligands. Its production requires the enzyme **choline acetyltransferase (ChAT)**, which uses **choline** derived immediately from the extracellular fluid around the neuron and transfers to it an **acetyl group** to form ACh (Figure 4.17). Choline from dietary sources must be delivered to the brain by the blood, and therefore the supply of choline determines the amount of ACh that can be produced. Only **cholinergic** neurons (i.e. those that respond to ACh) contain ChAT and are therefore capable of producing ACh. These include **lower motor neurons (LMNs)** that use ACh at the **neuromuscular junction** (i.e. synapses between LMNs and muscle cells). ACh is produced in the neuronal cell body and moved to the synapse by axoplasmic transportation.

Table 4.2 The affinity of endogenous opiates for opiate receptors.

Endogenous opiate	High affinity	Low affinity	Negligible affinity
Enkephalin	δ	μ	κ
β- Endorphins	μ, δ, κ_2	Other κ	
Dynorphins	κ	μ, δ	
Endomorphine	μ		

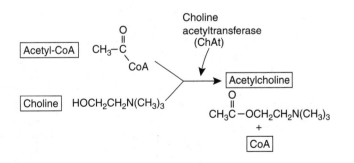

Figure 4.17 The synthesis of acetylcholine. The products are boxed with their chemical structure shown. The only enzyme (unboxed) labels the arrow.

After release into the synapse and binding to receptors, ACh is broken down while still within the cleft by another enzyme, **acetylcholinesterase (AChE)**. This releases the choline again from the molecule and much of this choline is returned to the presynaptic bulb and reused. The remaining **acetic acid** is excreted.

In the brain, acetylcholine is concentrated in the corpus striatum, with some found in the cerebrum, the nucleus accumbens, the limbic system including the hippocampus, and parts of the brain stem, especially some of the cranial nerve nuclei (Figure 4.18).

Cholinergic receptors

Cholinergic receptors, i.e. those which bind acetylcholine, occur in two forms, **nicotinic** and **muscarinic**. Muscarine and nicotine are plant alkaloids which bind to the respective receptor *under laboratory conditions*, and are therefore used to

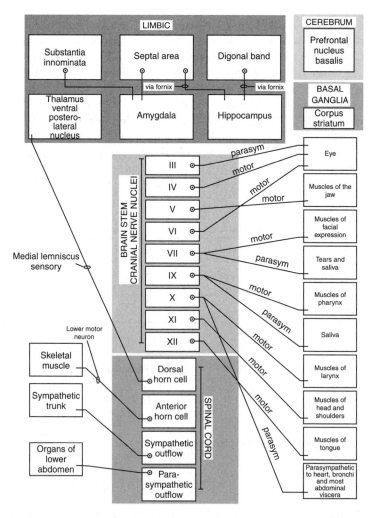

Figure 4.18 The main acetylcholine pathways of the central nervous system.

distinguish one receptor from the other. Obviously, *plant* alkaloids are not natural ligands of these receptors in the brain, they are just used to distinguish one receptor type from another. The nicotinic (N) receptor is ionotropic, causing the *direct* opening of membrane channels used by a range of cations, mostly sodium (Na^+) and calcium (Ca^{2+}). Nicotinic receptors are found mostly within the spinal cord, in the autonomic nervous system (ANS) and at the neuromuscular junction, but are less commonly found in the brain. Subtypes of nicotinic receptors are the N-m (muscle type), found at the neuromuscular junction, and the N-n (neuronal type), found at the ganglion synapse of the ANS.

The muscarinic (M) receptors are metabotropic; they regulate potassium ion channels *indirectly* by first affecting the secondary messenger **cAMP**, and this in turn affects the ion channels. The subtypes of muscarinic receptors are M_1, M_2, M_3, M_4 and M_5. The functions of these subtypes vary, but they generally cause excitation in the postsynaptic membrane. They are more common than nicotinic receptors in the brain, occurring both as postsynaptic and autoreceptors.

Histamine

Histamine is known as a chemical agent outside the brain that induces inflammation when released from storage in mast cells or platelets. It is synthesised from the dietary amino acid **histidine** using the enzyme **histidine decarboxylase**, which requires **vitamin B6 (pyroxidine)** to function. Histamine is also known as a neurotransmitter in the brain, but because it cannot cross the blood–brain barrier from the body to the brain, histamine must be synthesised within the brain. The hypothalamus has the greatest concentration of histidine decarboxylase found in the brain. Since the amino acid histidine can cross the blood–brain barrier, histamine can be produced in areas of the brain that have this enzyme, particularly the hypothalamus. Histamine is also found in a pathway extending from the brain stem to the cerebral cortex via the median forebrain bundle and in the hippocampus *See page 143* (Figure 4.19). Histamine is involved in the brain's control of alertness, in part of

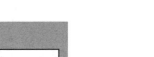
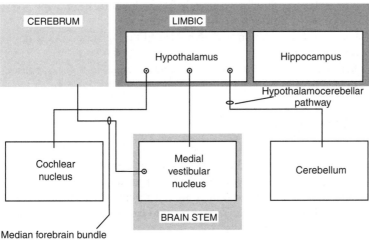
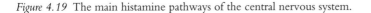

Figure 4.19 The main histamine pathways of the central nervous system.

the sleep–wake cycle, and in the mechanisms that regulate nausea and vomiting in the brain stem.

Histamine receptors

Histamine receptors are of four known classes, H_1, H_2, H_3 and H_4. They are all metabotropic and some are found in brain tissue. The H_1 receptor is found in both the brain stem and the cerebral cortex, the two areas linked by the histaminergic median forebrain bundle mentioned above. Because of histamine's role in the control of alertness of the cerebrum, antihistamines (or H_1 antagonists), which are able to cross the blood–brain barrier, can cause drowsiness as a side-effect. The H_1 receptor is also involved in regulation of circadian rhythms. H_2 receptors are found largely outside the brain on hydrochloric acid (HCl)-producing cells of the stomach wall, where the binding of histamine increases HCl production. In the brain, H_2 receptors are found in the same sites as H_1. H_3 receptors are found in the brain as a presynaptic autoreceptor on histaminergic neurons, allowing feedback to the presynaptic bulb to inhibit histamine release. H_4 is not involved in brain activity but controls histamine release from mast cells.

Key points

Neurotransmitters and receptors

- Neurotransmitters are the chemical agents released from the presynaptic bulb into the synaptic cleft.
- Most neurotransmitters fall into three main groups: amines, amino acids and peptides.
- The same neurotransmitter is often seen to produce different effects by binding to different receptors.
- Some receptors are postsynaptic, part of the *postsynaptic* membrane, others are autoreceptors on the *presynaptic* membranes or other parts of the neuron.
- Autoreceptors are thought to provide feedback information to the presynaptic bulb to regulate further neurotransmitter release.
- Some receptors are ionotropic; they control the opening or closing of a particular ion channel.
- Other receptors, called metabotropic, cause changes in the metabolism of the postsynaptic cell.

Amine neurotransmitters

- Dopaminergic neurons and receptors are found in the basal ganglia (the nigrostriatal pathway) and the limbic system (mesolimbic pathway), and are involved in mental health symptoms and drug treatments.
- Serotonergic and adrenergic neurons and receptors are found in the diffuse modulatory pathways of the brain stem, and are involved in the cause and drug treatment of mood disorders.

Amino acid neurotransmitters

- Gamma-aminobutyric acid (GABA) is an important inhibitory neurotransmitter, which is partly implicated in epilepsy.
- Enzymes that control GABA levels are targets for some anticonvulsant drugs.
- The $GABA_A$ receptor is a major site for the action of some drugs used in psychiatry.

References

Blows W. T. (2000) Neurotransmitters of the brain: serotonin, noradrenaline (norepinephrine) and dopamine. *Journal of Neuroscience Nursing*, **32** (4): 234–238.

Carlson N. (2010) *Physiology of Behavior* (10th edition). Allyn and Bacon, Boston.

Martini F. H. and Nath J. L. (2008) *Fundamentals of Anatomy and Physiology* (8th edition). Benjamin Cummings, San Francisco.

Nolen-Heoksema S. (2007) *Abnormal Psychology*. McGraw-Hill, Boston.

5 Hormones and behaviour

Introduction: hormones, form and function

Hormones are chemical messengers: they move from one part of the body to another in the blood and have an effect, often stimulatory, on a *target* organ or tissue. The brain is the target organ for a range of hormones that have influence over neuronal growth and development as well as function.

Hormones are the products of **endocrine glands**, which are glands that secrete their products directly into the blood. Hormones are of two basic types, the protein hormones (the **peptides**) and the lipid (or fat-based) hormones (the **steroids**). In order to work, a hormone must first bind to a receptor site that is associated with the target cell. Cells without receptors for a specific hormone are not targets for that hormone. Peptide hormones are too large to penetrate the cell membrane and must therefore bind to receptors on the cell surface. Steroid hormones can pass through the membrane and bind with receptors within the cell cytoplasm or the nucleus (Figure 5.1). Receptors for hormones, like those for neurotransmitters, are usually proteins, coded by and synthesised from gene sequences within the target cell **DNA** (**deoxyribonucleic acid**). DNA is the molecule housed inside the nucleus of most cells and forms the genes, the blueprints on which all cellular proteins and other characteristics are based. Cells therefore have the ability to increase (upregulate) or decrease (downregulate) their receptor numbers by activating or deactivating the appropriate genes. This affects the sensitivity of that cell to the effects of the hormone; since upregulation can bind more hormone, downregulation binds less hormone.

On binding to the receptor, the hormone–receptor complex effects changes within the cell, usually by binding to a **gene promoter** sequence on the DNA

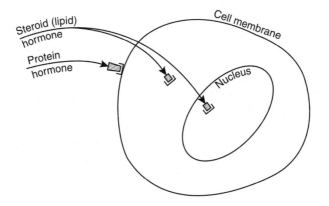

Figure 5.1 Hormones and receptors. Protein hormones are too large to enter the cell, so they bind to surface receptors. Steroid (lipid) hormones are smaller and so they can enter the cell and bind to receptors inside the cytoplasm or nucleus.

and initiating transcription of the gene (Figure 5.2). **Gene transcription** involves the assembly of an **RNA (ribonucleic acid)** molecule, the first step in protein synthesis. In this way hormones arriving at the cell trigger a wave of protein synthesis which will alter in some way the activity of that cell. In neurons this change in activity is likely to influence the response of the cell to action potentials or to neurotransmitters, or alter the cell's metabolism in some way.

As the functional component of the endocrine system, hormones are regulated by **feedback mechanisms** that influence their production and release from the gland. This feedback is mostly of the **negative** kind, i.e. a rise in the blood levels of the hormone causes the production and release of the hormone to fall. The opposite is also true, where low blood hormone levels allow greater production and release of the hormone. In this way, a stable blood level should be achieved. Such feedback mechanisms are a part of general **homeostasis** by which the body maintains a stable internal environment that promotes optimum function of its organs.

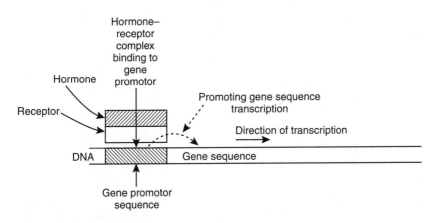

Figure 5.2 The complex of hormone and receptor affects gene transcription by interacting with the gene promoter sequence of the deoxyribonucleic acid (DNA).

Homeostasis is critical in many areas such as temperature control, electrolyte, fluid and acid–base balance. Many nursing observations are carried out in order to monitor the function and effectiveness of specific homeostatic mechanisms; observations such as recording of the pulse rate, blood pressure and temperature (Blows 2001). Homeostasis operates through the two major communication systems of the body, the endocrine and nervous systems. Close collaboration between these two systems is responsible for regulating most of the functions of the cells and tissues through a wide variety of situations, a collaboration known as the **neuroendocrine response**. Disturbance of homeostasis causes biochemical and other imbalances which seriously upset the normal functioning of various organs, not least the brain. Some disorders of homeostasis involving hormones can cause mental symptoms for which the hormonal levels of the blood require investigation.

The pituitary hormones

See page 12 The pituitary hormones were listed in Chapter 1 because they are subject to hypothalamic control.

As will be seen in the following pages, some disorders of the pituitary gland can disrupt the function of other endocrine glands and the resulting change in hormonal levels can cause mental symptoms. Important examples of this are changes in **thyroid-stimulating hormone** (**TSH**), which controls levels of thyroid hormone in the blood, and in **adrenocorticotropic hormone** (**ACTH**), which influences adrenal cortex function by stimulating cortisol production (Figure 5.3).

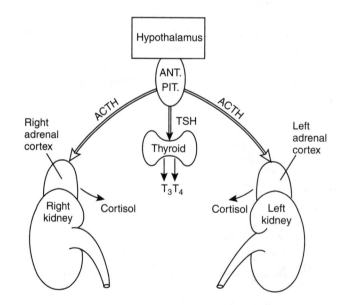

Figure 5.3 The hypothalamo–pituitary–adrenal (HPA) axis, where adrenocorticotropic hormone (ACTH) from the anterior pituitary stimulates cortisol production. The hypothalamo–pituitary–thyroid (HPT) axis, where thyroid-stimulating hormone (TSH) stimulates the release of the thyroid hormones T_3 and T_4.

The thyroid hormones

The thyroid hormones are produced by the thyroid gland, which is situated in the neck, on top of the trachea and below the larynx. Hormones from this gland occur in two forms, **triiodothyronine (T3)** and **tetraiodothyronine (T4)** (Figure 5.3). **Iodine** is a major component of these hormones and the two forms have respectively three and four atoms of iodine per molecule. Production of T3 and T4 is dependent on the levels of **thyroid-stimulating hormone (TSH)** produced by the pituitary gland. Thyroid hormones (T3 and T4) are essential for the growth, development and metabolic function of many tissues, not least the brain.

In normal tissues, these hormones maintain a normal metabolic rate, but changes in mental function appear if the levels of thyroid hormone are too low or too high. Disorders of thyroid level may be *primary* (i.e. affecting the gland itself), or *secondary* (i.e. caused by abnormal changes in TSH level from the anterior pituitary gland). Blood tests for T3\T4 plus TSH will indicate which is the problem.

Hypothyroidism, in which the blood level of thyroid hormone is too low, is sometimes called **myxoedema**. It is most common in females over the age of 40 years. Failure to produce enough of this hormone can result in a number of symptoms which could be misinterpreted as a true mental disorder. Patients with myxoedema suffer lethargy, depression, personality changes and psychotic episodes known as *myxoedema madness*. This is manifested as paranoia, hallucinations and delirium.

Hypothyroid disorders are occasionally associated with depressive mood disorders and about 10 per cent of depressed patients with lethargy are also hypothyroid. Thyroid hormone treatment is sometimes used in addition to antidepressant drugs to improve the patient's response to the antidepressant therapy. Such a combination is sometimes used in those patients who quickly rotate between the depressed and manic phases of bipolar depression. The antimanic drug *lithium* can predispose to hypothyroid states, especially if used for long-term therapy, and therefore monitoring of thyroid function during lithium treatment is important to avoid complications. Neonatal hypothyroidism puts the newly born infant at risk of developmental brain function failure, known as **cretinism**, a serious problem that can be corrected if recognised from birth and treated with thyroid hormone. *See page 214*
See page 237

Hyperthyroidism is the production of excess thyroid hormone by the thyroid gland. **Thyrotoxicosis** is an umbrella term incorporating a number of disorders involving high thyroid levels. It refers to the release of excess hormone into the blood at very high toxic levels. These disorders, such as **Grave's disease**, are either **primary**, i.e. caused by a problem with the thyroid itself, or **secondary**, i.e. resulting from a response by a normal thyroid to too much TSH from the pituitary gland. In either case the patient shows anxiety, agitation and delirium, with nervous excitability, irritability, insomnia and other psychotic manifestations, largely due to excessive overactivity of the sympathetic nervous system. If the hormone excess is severe, memory loss and disorientation can occur, with manic excitability, delusions and hallucinations. Stress seems to be a causative factor, theoretically owing to excessive use of the endocrine system during childhood trauma (e.g. loss of parents, economic hardship, rivalry with siblings) (Sadock et al. 2010). It becomes important, therefore, for all patients suffering from 'anxiety' to have their blood thyroid hormone and TSH levels measured to exclude a thyroid problem. *See page 167*

Hormones from the adrenal cortex

The adrenal glands, situated on top of the kidneys, have an *outer* **cortex** and an *inner* **medulla**. The cortex produces several steroidal hormones based on cholesterol derived from the blood (Figure 5.4). There are several hormonal groups produced by the cortex, including the **mineralocorticoids** (those hormones active on minerals); the **glucocorticoids** (those hormones influencing blood glucose levels); and the sex hormones for males (**androgens**) and females (**oestrogens**) (Figure 5.4).

Cortisol is a glucocorticoid, the production of which is stimulated by ACTH from the anterior pituitary gland. Cortisol has several functions, notably raising the blood glucose level by its anti-insulin effects, and it helps to protect cells against the adverse effects of stress.

Excess cortisol occurs in the disorder **Cushing's syndrome** or as a result of prolonged corticosteroid drug treatment. Treatment by drugs is of course a medical activity, and when the action of doctors or nurses causes disease it is known as **iatrogenic**, i.e. disease caused by medical intervention. Iatrogenic disorders should be avoided as much as possible, but some iatrogenic problems are unavoidable. In the case of disorders caused by drugs this can be avoided or reduced by adjusting the dose level.

Cushing's syndrome occurs more often in women than in men and causes a similar state to that of bipolar depression (Breedlove et al. 2010), with insomnia, loss of emotions and energy, and attempted suicide in about 10 per cent of untreated patients. Alternatively, the patient's mood may swing into euphoria, agitation, mania or delirium, with psychotic symptoms such as hallucinations. Depression may also follow withdrawal from long-term steroid therapy, this being one of several reasons for a keeping steroid treatment as short as possible and reducing the dose gradually rather than suddenly. Some women with Cushing's syndrome may show a degree

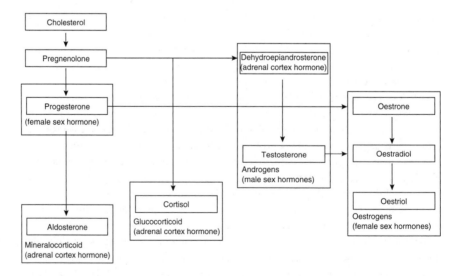

Figure 5.4 Flow diagram of the production of various steroidal (lipid-based) hormones from cholesterol in the adrenal cortex, including cortisol, aldosterone, the female oestrogens and the male androgens.

of **masculinisation**, growing unwanted hair and losing their menstrual periods (**amenorrhoea**), and this can add to their depression. Men with this condition can become impotent and lose their hair.

Addison's disease is an insufficiency in cortisol production from the adrenal cortex. Lack of cortisol results in the patient becoming tired, lethargic and depressed and sometimes showing psychotic symptoms. This person may also develop delirium and confusion. Generally the mental symptoms are milder that those seen with Cushing's syndrome. The problem may not reside in the adrenal gland itself *See page 12* but could be a failure of adrenocorticotropic hormone (ACTH) from the pituitary gland. Treatment with corticosteroid supplements is essential for life.

Production of cortisol is also severely reduced in a condition called **adreno-genital syndrome** (Figure 5.5). The poor secretion of cortisol can be caused by low activity of either of the enzymes **21-hydroxylase** or **11β-hydroxylase**, both of which are essential for the metabolic pathway that leads to cortisol (Figure 5.4). The loss of these enzymes is a **congenital** defect; that is, the person is born with the enzyme error, the consequences of which are a corresponding increase in the synthesis of androgens. In the female fetus this causes Addison's disease, the excess androgens having a masculinising effect at the same time. The 'girl', while being genetically female, develops male-like external genitalia, making gender difficult to determine (**pseudohermaphroditism**). The excess testosterone produced may *See page 87* also have a masculinising effect on the girl's brain, causing a mental conflict of identity or 'self'. In a male fetus with this condition, Addison's disease is accompanied by advanced sexual development, i.e. puberty, at an early age.

A similar condition, **adrenogenitalism** (Figure 5.6), occurs in the fetus when the pituitary gland produces too much ACTH. The excessive stimulation of the adrenal cortex results in higher than normal production of testosterone, the main male androgen. Cortisol production in this situation remains normal since all the enzymes involved in the steroid hormone pathways are functioning. The stimulation of the cortex causes **hyperplasia** (excessive cellular growth) within the cortex of the gland. This is an **autosomal recessive** disorder, again causing masculinisation of the female fetus (pseudohermaphroditism) with male-like external genitalia. The male fetus with this condition has excessive sexual development, except for smaller-than-average testes, which remain underdeveloped owing to the negative feedback from the high adrenal testosterone. Testosterone stimulates growth, so androgenital children of both sexes are generally taller than their peers, but as bone

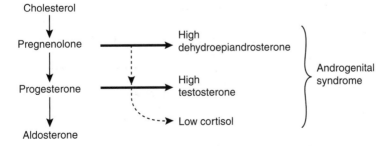

Figure 5.5 Adrenogenital syndrome, caused by excessive androgens (testosterone and dehydroepiandrosterone) in conjunction with low cortisol.

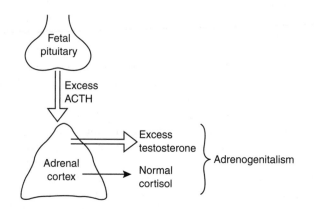

Figure 5.6 Adrenogenitalism, caused by excessive ACTH driving testosterone production to excess, while cortisol remains normal.

growth is stopped prematurely they are therefore shorter than average as adults. The mental effect is again one of conflict concerning sexual identity and this may need to be addressed by both physical and psychological treatment.

Hormones from the adrenal medulla

See page 57

See page 18

The hormones produced by the adrenal medulla are the **catecholamines**, adrenaline and noradrenaline. Adrenaline has sympathomimetic activity, that is, it increases the functions of the sympathetic nervous system (Figure 5.7). The physical

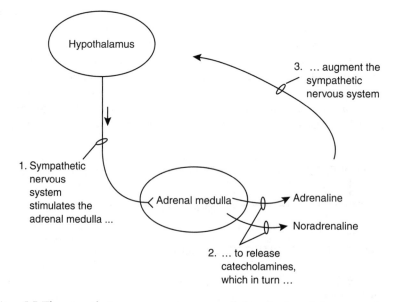

Figure 5.7 The sympathetic nervous system, controlled by the hypothalamus, can increase the production of catecholamines (adrenaline and noradrenaline) from the adrenal medulla. These, in turn, augment the sympathetic nervous system.

symptoms of excessive stimulation of the sympathetic nervous system include an increase in the heart rate, sweating, tremor and insomnia. The mental symptoms include apprehension or even fear leading to panic, all of which give a clinical picture of anxiety attacks. Differentiation between excessive catecholamine production and true anxiety may be achieved by measuring the blood adrenaline levels, although anxiety itself may cause increased release of this hormone. A rare cause of high levels of adrenaline in the blood is an adrenaline-producing tumour of the medulla called a **phaeochromocytoma**.

See page 174

Sex hormones and the differences between male and female brains

The **oestrogens** and **androgens** are the sex hormone groups for females and males respectively. There are three oestrogen hormones and several androgen hormones. The female oestrogens are **oestradiol**, **oestrone** and **oestriol**. The male androgens are mainly **testosterone** and **dehydroepiandrosterone** (DHEA). However, besides testosterone, other androgens include **androstenedione**, **androstenediol** and **androsterone** (Figure 5.4). Oestradiol is the most potent of the oestrogens, while testosterone is the most potent of the androgens. They are all synthesised from **cholesterol** via a pathway which includes the production of the other steroidal hormones, **cortisol**, **progesterone** and **aldosterone** (Figure 5.4). Following puberty, the female ovary produces most of the oestrogen, while the male testes produce most of the testosterone. However, in addition, trace quantities of both the oestrogens and the androgens are produced and released from the **adrenal cortex** in both sexes. Females produce small quantities of androgens and males produce small quantities of oestrogens. This is a vestige of the past life of the growing fetus, when the adrenal cortex was the only producer of these substances. Both these hormonal groups have a multitude of target tissues and organs around the body, including the brain, where they have a profound influence on functional and sexual organisation. A lack of testosterone, supported by oestrogen, influences a 'feminine' brain, while testosterone forms a 'masculine' brain. It is important to note that these hormonal organisational effects happen at very precise and critical moments in fetal brain development. After this critical point the hormonal influence over the brain is of a different nature; that of influencing behavioural patterns, in particular sexual behaviour, and mood. High levels of testosterone are known to influence aggression in males, while oestrogen reduces aggression. Low levels of testosterone appear to result from stress and are linked to nervousness, bad temper and depressed moods in men (the **irritable male syndrome**) (Nowak 2002). Postmenopausal loss of oestrogen in women can lead to anxiety, loss of confidence, forgetfulness and even depression.

See page 124

See page 89

Hormones, mostly the androgens and oestrogens but others also, influence from before birth the sexual differences that are noted between male and female brains. The environment also has a massive impact on the way that gender variations in the brain are moulded throughout childhood (see also Chapter 2) (Eliot 2010). The physical differences in the brain are generally small but significant. Males have larger brains than their female peers throughout all the stages of life, and female brains reach full development earlier than male brains. The hypothalamus is involved in sexual behaviour and perinatal exposure to androgens in the male causes a larger

preoptic region of the hypothalamus than in females. In fact, the anterior hypothalamus shows significant **sexual dimorphism** (dimorphism = *two shapes*, i.e. two
different shapes between the sexes) in the *pattern of synaptic connections* found there.
This part of the brain has been called the **sexually dimorphic nucleus**. Structural
variation is achieved through exposure to sex hormones before, during and after
birth. It is also important to note that at such an early stage of development the
source of the oestrogen or testosterone cannot be the ovaries or testes, as they only
begin production much later in life. Early production of the sex hormones relies on
the adrenal cortex, which begins releasing significant levels in early life but reduces
production later.

The differences between the brains of men and women are demonstrable in
various tests that male and female subjects are asked to perform. However, it is not
possible to say exactly how each hormone effects changes in neural tissues. The
results of the tests show a trend in the types of skills each sex is better equipped to
do (Table 5.1). While male brains are physically larger than female brains, women
have a greater concentration of grey-matter cells (or neurons) in the areas concerned with communication. These areas are the dorsolateral prefrontal cortex (involved in memory and initiative: 23 per cent more cells) and the superior temporal
gyrus (involved in listening: 13 per cent more cells).

Male brains show a greater degree of lateralisation than those of females, des-
ignating one hemisphere for a task rather than both. On a day-to-day basis this
makes no difference, but it could be a handicap in circumstances where the designated hemisphere becomes damaged. In this situation in males the task is often lost
altogether, while females can switch to the other hemisphere. A typical example is
damage to the speech centre in the left hemisphere, where **aphasia** (loss of speech)
occurs four times more often in males (who cannot switch to the right side) than in
females (who can often make the switch). Lateralisation does not necessarily make
the performance of a skill any better or worse. In female brains there is increased
overlap between the hemisphere functions for the verbal skills and women do better in these skills than men. There are also other physical differences in the brain
between the sexes, the significance of which is not entirely understood:

- Females have longer temporal lobes than males.
- The female posterior corpus callosum (connecting the left hemisphere with
  the right hemisphere) is bulbous and wide compared to that in the male, which
  is cylindrical and uniform in width throughout its length.
- The female brain is more tightly packed with grey matter.

Table 5.1 Sex differences in the brain in terms of task performance.

MALE orientated brain (skills at which males are better than females)	FEMALE orientated brain (skills at which females are better than males)
• Spatial tasks, especially rotational skills	• Perceptual speed, i.e. rapid identification of matching items
• Mathematical reasoning	• Arithmetical calculations
• Navigational skills (e.g. map reading)	• Precision manual skills (e.g. embroidery)
• Target-directed skills, such as guiding or intercepting projectiles (e.g. dart throwing)	• Verbal fluency
	• Recall of landmarks along a route

Behaviour

Many aspects of life have some control or influence over behaviour, and the role of biology is now recognised as a major factor in the way we behave. Behaviourists are scientists who identify a particular behaviour that is of interest, or of social significance (e.g. drug abuse) and try to find causes. Physiologists and geneticists investigate the biology of specific behaviours.

The brain is the governing organ that determines our behaviour, and this is influenced strongly by developmental aspects (especially environmental stimuli), hormones (some aspects of hormonal influence on behaviour have been looked at above) and genes.

Genes do not directly determine behaviour. Their role is to code for many varied proteins which are components of much of the body's structure and metabolism. Genes in the brain code for a large number of different protein receptors which bind hormones and neurotransmitters, and changing these receptors has significant influence on brain function, especially behaviour. A good example is a variation of a gene that codes for a dopamine D2 receptor called the **A1 allele**, associated with one specific behavioural pattern, alcoholism. The behaviour patterns of alcoholism and drug abuse are examined in more detail in Chapter 8.

Developmental aspects have been discussed in Chapter 2, where the influence of **environmental factors** moulds the mind. For example, consider a child and its mother playing on the floor when a spider runs out from under a chair. The child's mother is scared of spiders and climbs on the chair, screaming. The older child may infer from this that the correct response to a spider is to climb on a chair and scream. This is called **learned behaviour**, where children learn how to behave in various situations by copying from example. Children and adults both learn aspects of behaviour from good or bad experiences. A child knocked over in a park by a large dog may, as a result, fear dogs for life, and adjust their behaviour to avoid them. The opposite is also true, as in drug addiction, where initial exposure to drugs may lead to further drug-seeking behaviour. As seen in Chapter 2, both good and bad experiences, especially in early life, have profound good or bad influences on both brain development and future behaviour. When considering both ends of the behavioural spectrum, i.e. good and bad, both charitable and criminal activities can be seen to be influenced by learned behaviours.

Aggression and testosterone

As seen in this chapter, exposure of the fetus to androgens such as testosterone causes masculinisation of the brain (**prenatal androgenisation**). However, the highest testosterone levels in males occur between the ages of 16 and 30 years, peaking around 25 years of age. Testosterone has been described as the fuel that drives a number of behaviour patterns, especially aggression. **Innate drives** are those built in from birth, i.e. those from within, and testosterone fulfils that in relation to aggression. Evidence has linked violent crime with high testosterone levels. At puberty, exposure to high levels of testosterone causes males to increase their aggressive tendencies, including sexual aggression. Apart from this innate drive, other theories of aggression include 1. the frustration model, where a frustrated need leads to aggression to satisfy that need, and 2. aggression as a learned behaviour.

There is probably some a combination of all these factors in any act of aggression. The three types of aggression are:

1. **Offence**, where aggression is used against another person, often without provocation;
2. **Defence**, where aggression is used as protection against offence;
3. **Predation**, where aggression is used to gain something. In the animal world aggression is used to gain food (e.g. the lion attacks a gazelle), but in the human world predation is used mostly to gain money or goods (e.g. theft and mugging) or to satisfy other needs (e.g. rape).

Aggression is also strongly linked to the levels of serotonin in the brain. All the evidence indicates that serotonin has a calming (inhibitory) effect on an individual, reducing impulsive behaviour in particular, and therefore aggression is linked to low levels of serotonin. Reduced levels of serotonin correlate particularly well with aggression to oneself (i.e. suicide) and with impulsive aggression towards others. Corresponding changes in serotonin receptors, consistent with serotonin receptor structural abnormalities, have been found in the frontal lobes of those committing violent suicide. Such receptor changes reduce the effectiveness of the serotonin present. The poor function of the serotonin system may be due to an error in the gene that codes for **tryptophan hydroxylase**, a key enzyme in the synthesis of serotonin.

The areas of the brain involved are also becoming apparent (Figure 5.8). The effect of androgens on aggression between males appears to be mediated through a part of the hypothalamus called the **pre-optic area**. Androgens early in life (prenatal testosterone in males) appear to organise and sensitise this and other areas

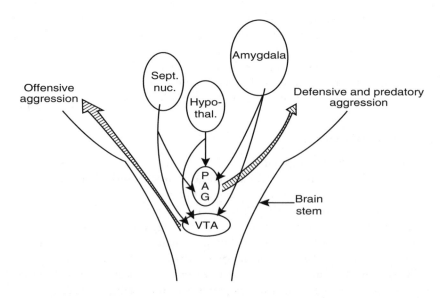

Figure 5.8 Aggression. Inputs from the septal nucleus (Sept. nuc.) and amygdala to the periaquaductal grey (PAG) cause defensive and predatory aggression; inputs to the ventral tegmental area (VTA) cause offensive aggression.

of the brain involved in aggression later in life. Testosterone later in life (pubertal testosterone, again in males) appears to activate these same areas. Offensive aggression appears to be mediated through the **ventral tegmental area** (**VTA**) in the brain stem, while different parts of the **periaquaductal grey** (**PAG**) are associated with defensive and predatory aggression. These areas are themselves moderated by inputs from the hypothalamus, the septum and the amygdala (Figure 5.8). Examples of this are defensive and predatory aggression. Defensive aggression can be activated by stimulation of the medial hypothalamus, while predatory aggression can be activated by stimulation of the lateral hypothalamus. The frontal lobe inhibits impulsive behaviour including aggression to some extent, but this is reduced during puberty (Chapter 2).

Antisocial behaviour appears to involve problems with the **dorsal and ventral prefrontal cortex**, the **amygdala**, and the **angular gyrus** (brain areas required for making moral decisions).

While testosterone is significantly lower in females than in males, some women receive exposure to higher levels than others, and the women thus exposed, either as a fetus or later in life, show increased aggressive tendencies towards others. Excessive alcohol often induces higher levels of testosterone in women who then misbehave in public, often aggressively, as a result.

Pregnant women with higher testosterone levels than average are more likely to have daughters described as **tomboys**, i.e. interested in male-orientated, rather than female-orientated lifestyles. The opposite also appears to be true, with higher-oestrogen mothers having daughters with very feminine ways. Clearly the child is being influenced by the **teratogenic** effect of the mother's hormone, and in the case of testosterone this organises and sensitises pathways involved in aggression.

Oestradiol, the main female oestrogen, causes a reduction in aggression and a general calming effect on the brain. It is possible that hormonal shifts which result in a lowering of oestradiol just prior to menstruation may have some bearing on the **premenstrual syndrome**, a state of irritability and increased aggression that occurs a few days before a menstrual period.

A neurotransmitter called **arginine–vasopressin** (AVP) which is active in the amygdala helps to regulate maternal aggression, a behavioural pattern aimed at making sure the child survives. Stress is also directly related to aggression, since violence is a very stressful social experience for both the aggressor and the victim. Brain neurotransmitters and immune cytokines change alarmingly during stress, and this increases vulnerability to depression and immune-related disorders. Women react to stress as much as men, and this applies particularly to couples in a relationship, where women can display **relational aggression** towards their partners. This involves less belligerent aggressive attacks, such as social manipulation, spreading rumours and gossip, refusing to speak to their partners, damaging their property and other such activities (Lilienfeld and Arkowitz 2010).

Murder, especially *serial murder*, is a form of offensive aggression that has also sparked a great deal of interest. Neuroscientists want to be able to answer the question: *What goes on inside a serial killer's mind?* Now some answers are coming to light. Murderers appear to lack the level of **prefrontal lobe** activity seen in law-abiding subjects. In the absence of adequate prefrontal lobe activity, the emotions are unmodified in any way by conscious reasoning. Some work carried out on male murderers has shown an actual loss of prefrontal neurons, particularly those neurons responsible for learned remorse, conscience and social sensitivity. These men have been categorised as suffering from **aggressive impulse personality disorder**, or **antisocial personality disorder** (**APD**) (Carlson 2010; Nolen-Hoeksema 2007).

APD is characterised by:

*   impaired relationships with other people;
*   deceitfulness, lying;
*   lack of emotion, fear and danger;
*   life-long antisocial behaviour and irresponsibility;
*   violent crime;
*   little, if any, remorse for harm caused to others, and indifference to their suffering;
*   low tolerance for frustration; becoming bored easily and inability to endure boredom.

About 3 per cent of the population are thought to suffer APD, most of them being men. There is a strong genetic influence, with **monozygotic** (identical) twin studies indicating 50 per cent concordance, and **dizygotic** (non-identical) twin studies showing 20 per cent concordance.

Deficits in the frontal and temporal lobes in APD (causing poor concentration and an inability to form concepts and goals, and to perform sound reasoning) coupled with low serotonin (where low levels are linked to impulsiveness and aggression) appear to be the main pathological problems. Because of this, these people tend also to be of a lower educational status.

Psychopath is the term often used to describe those persons who are generally more disturbed than those with APD. They show no emotions, being cold and callous towards other people. They can gain pleasure from inflicting suffering on others; they are often violent, cruel and malicious. They are also dogmatic in their opinions, and engage freely in unacceptable and criminal activity. About 0.5 per cent of the UK population are thought to be psychopathic (but between 15 and 20 per cent of the UK prison population). Psychopaths have been found to have a malfunctioning amygdala (the brain's emotional centre) so they are not processing emotions correctly. There are also anomalies in the frontal and temporal lobes, especially the prefrontal cortex which normally restrains impulsive and aggressive behaviour. It appears that this restraint is lost in psychopaths. The result of this is a malfunctioning circuit involving the amygdala and the frontal areas of the brain. Normally this circuit allows the amygdala and frontal lobes to work together controlling emotions and behaviour, but this fails to happen in psychopaths. Dopamine levels are also significantly raised in psychopaths. The brain appears to be structured towards obtaining constant reward at any cost, through the dopaminergic pathways, and this is often achieved by antisocial behaviour which involves taking risks.

Murderers also show altered levels of chemicals in the brain. Testosterone also appears to be the fuel that drives predetermined behaviour in men as well as aggression. That predetermined behaviour pattern is probably controlled by other factors such as genetics. If the behaviour pattern involves aggression, high levels of testosterone can drive the aggression to the point of murder. Alarmingly high levels of testosterone in some men have been associated with violence involving the rape and murder of women, sometimes multiple women, a problem called **sexual sadism**. The neurotransmitter serotonin normally has an inhibitory effect on such violent behaviour. Killers often have low levels of serotonin, and the combination of high testosterone with low serotonin becomes an explosive mixture that can result in particularly nasty impulsive violent murders that may be repeated multiple times. Low serotonin in an adult appears to be associated with disruption of the family during that person's childhood. Separation of the child from the mother is the key disrupting factor. As indicated in Chapter 2, environmental factors, in particular bonding of the child with its mother, appear to *mould the mind*, providing stimuli for synaptic connections within the serotonergic pathways of the brain. Without this maternal love and support, the brain becomes devoid of vital serotonergic pathways and the effects of serotonin remain low.

Some murderers also have high levels of a substance called **cryptopyrol**, a chemical normally found in the liver and obtained from the breakdown of **erythrocytes** (red blood cells). Increased levels of cryptopyrol have a similar effect in the brain to that seen with the use of the drug **lysergic acid diethylamide** (**LSD**). LSD has the effect of a hallucinogen, i.e. distorting the sensory systems, causing the subject to see the world as a jumble of abnormal sensory inputs. *See page 158*

The fact that there are brain changes related to aggression raises issues such as: *Can murderers be held responsible for their crimes if they have errors in their brain?* and, *If there is no cure from their brain disorder, should murderers ever be released from custody?* This is an ethical debate beyond the scope of this book, but these issues will be of greater importance as more pathological discoveries are made. This is just the kind of debate that nurses are in an excellent position to be able to contribute to.

Cannibalistic behaviour, which is rare, may be simply a response to the need for food in a situation where there is a risk of starvation. Cannibalistic tendencies have been associated with some modern murders and evidence of cannibalistic practices has recently been found in some ancient archaeological sites (McKie 1998). Cannibalism may be caused by physical damage to the frontal lobes, possible from a head injury. It does not seem likely at present that any of this neuroscientific 'evidence' creates the grounds for excusing the perpetrators of their crime by claiming they are 'sick' (Ahuja 2002).

Nurses need to be able to manage aggression effectively for their own safety and the safety of others, particularly children, who are unable to protect themselves. Aggression in the public arena and in the workplace is now an escalating problem, and nurses are in the front line for physical and verbal abuse (Liu 2004). The **CASE de-escalation model** for coping with a potentially violent situation is an initiative of Sheffield University, and involves an education programme for health-care workers. Walker et al. (2002) describes the CASE (Calming, Assessing, Self, Enabling) de-escalation model and gives instructions on the prevention and safe management of aggressive situations. Much aggression and violence is associated with excessive consumption of alcohol and drugs, and this complicates the situation. The emphasis must be placed on personal safety and getting help at the earliest opportunity.

Key points

Hormones

- Hormones are chemical messengers; they have an effect on a *target* organ or tissue.
- The brain is the target organ for many hormones, influencing neuronal growth, development and function.
- Hormones come from endocrine glands, and are of two basic types: proteins and lipids (called steroids).
- A hormone must bind to a receptor site on the target cell.
- The hormone–receptor complex changes the cell by binding to DNA, and causing transcription of a gene.

Thyroid hormones

- Thyroid hormone occurs in two forms: triiodothyronine (T_3) and tetraiodothyronine (T_4). Iodine is a major component of this hormone.
- Hypothyroidism (or myxoedema) is too low a blood level of thyroid hormone, which causes depression, lethargy, personality changes and psychotic episodes (myxoedema madness).
- Lithium can cause hypothyroidism, and patients should be monitored for thyroid function.
- Neonatal hypothyroidism, leading to brain developmental failure, is known as cretinism. It is corrected by treatment with thyroid hormone.
- Hyperthyroidism (thyrotoxicosis) is excess thyroid hormone in the blood causing memory loss, disorientation, manic excitability, delusions and hallucinations.

Adrenal cortex hormones

- Cortisol is a glucocorticoid from the adrenal cortex. Production is stimulated by adrenocorticotropic hormone (ACTH) from the anterior pituitary gland.
- Excess cortisol causes Cushing's syndrome with depression-like symptoms, insomnia, energy loss and emotional flattening. Sufferers may have mood swings with euphoria, and delirium with hallucinations.
- Addison's disease is a lack of cortisol, causing tiredness, lethargy and depression, and sometimes delirium and confusion.
- Oestradiol is the most potent of the female oestrogens, whilst testosterone is the most potent of the male androgens.
- An absence of testosterone, coupled with oestrogen, creates a 'feminine' brain, whilst the presence of testosterone forms a 'masculine' brain.

Adrenal medulla hormones

- The hormones produced by the adrenal medulla are the catecholamines, adrenaline and noradrenaline.
- Adrenaline has sympathomimetic activity, that is, it increases the functions of the sympathetic nervous system.

Differences between male and female brains

- The brain differences are created by both hormonal and environmental exposure.
- The sexually dimorphic nucleus is part of the hypothalamus which shows differences between the sexes.

Behaviour

- Behaviour is determined by multiple factors, notably developmental aspects, environmental stimuli, hormones, neurotransmitters and genes.
- The three forms of aggression are offence, defence and predation.
- Aggression is influenced by hormones such as testosterone and oestrogen, and neurotransmitters, especially serotonin.
- Nurses need to be able to manage aggression effectively for their own safety and the safety of others, particularly children.
- Frontal and temporal lobe problems plus low serotonin appear to be the main pathological problems in antisocial personality disorder.
- A malfunctioning circuit involving the amygdala and the frontal areas of the brain is the main problem in psychopaths.
- Testosterone appears to be the fuel that drives aggression.

References

Ahuja A. (2002) Bad brain or bad person? *The Times* (T2 Science) 22 April: 10.

Blows W. T. (2001) *The Biological Basis of Nursing: Clinical Observations.* Routledge, London.

Breedlove S. M., Watson N. V. and Rosenzweig M. R (2010) *Biological Psychology: An Introduction to Behavioral, Cognitive and Clinical Neuroscience* (6th edition). Sinauer Associates, Massachusetts.

Carlson N. R. (2010) *Physiology of Behavior* (10th edition). Allyn and Bacon, Boston.

Eliot L. (2010) The truth about boys and girls. *Scientific American Mind,* **21** (2): 22–29.

Lilienfeld S. O. and Arkowitz H. (2010) Are men the more belligerent sex? *Scientific American Mind,* **21** (2): 64–65.

Liu, J. (2004) Concept analysis: aggression. *Issues in Mental Health Nursing,* **25** (7): 693–714.

McKie R. (1998) The people eaters. *New Scientist,* **157** (2125): 43–46.

Nolen-Hoeksema S. (2007) *Abnormal Psychology* (4th edition). McGraw Hill International Edition, New York and Boston.

Nowak R. (2002) Men behaving sadly. *New Scientist,* 173 (2332) (2 March): 4.

Sadock B. J., Sadock V. A. and Ruiz P. (2009) *Kaplin and Sadock's Comprehensive Textbook of Psychiatry* (9th edition). Lippincott, Williams and Wilkins, Baltimore.

Walker J., Wren J. and Skalycz A. (2002) Safety first. *Nursing Times,* **98** (9; 28th Feb): 20–21.

6 Genetic disorders affecting mental health

- **Introduction**
- **Chromosomes and genes**
- **Disorders of inheritance**
- **Autosomal disorders**
- **Sex chromosome abnormalities**
- **Genetic disorders**
- **Key points**

Introduction

A better understanding of the genetic component of many diseases is crucial to unravelling the pathology of the disease and improving its management. This is particularly true in the case of mental health disorders. As key persons in the management of these disorders, nurses will need a good working knowledge of the subject if they are to participate in counselling, drug therapy and research intended to improve treatment and care. This chapter therefore provides a brief introduction to human genetics and an overview of the genetic aspects of disorders that nurses will encounter.

Chromosomes and genes

The human **karyotype**, or chromosome 'set', is made up of the 46 chromosomes normally found in the cell's nucleus, but arranged as shown in Figure 6.1. Forty-four of these chromosomes (1–22) pair up to make 22 pairs of **autosomes**, which regulate many different body activities. The chromosomes making up the final pair are the **sex chromosomes** – X and Y in males, X and X in females. All the chromosomes carry our **genes**, some of the largest carrying more than 4500 genes!

Of each pair of chromosomes, one is inherited from the mother, the other from the father, i.e. 23 chromosomes from each parent. Each pair of autosomes therefore consists of two chromosomes that are structurally the same, carrying an identical arrangement of corresponding genes. For this reason they are known as **homologous autosomes** (homologous = similar, corresponding to). The genes that occur on one chromosome of a pair also occur in the same positions on the other

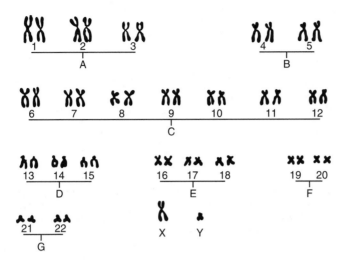

Figure 6.1 The normal human karyotype (this is a male, as denoted by the Y chromosome). A normal karyotype has 46 chromosomes, 22 pairs of autosomes (1 to 22) and one pair of sex chromosomes.

chromosome of the same pair. Within any homologous pair of chromosomes, the gene pairs are alternate versions of the same gene on each chromosome. The word **allele** is used to represent alternative versions of the same gene, one on each chromosome pair. They are the same gene, but because they come from different parents they are likely to carry different **traits**. The difference between *genes* and *traits* is highlighted by the following example: the gene for eye colour carries different traits according to which parent it comes from. One gene, from the mother, could carry the trait for blue eyes, whilst the other gene, from the father, carries the trait for green eyes. So, eye colour is the gene, while blue or green are the traits. The green eye gene is the allele (alternative version) of the blue eye gene, and vice versa. If two different eye colour traits are present in the same karyotype, which one will become the true colour of the eye in that individual? In other words, which gene will be expressed into the **phenotype** (phenotype means the features of the physical body)? The answer to the question depends on which gene is **dominant** and which is **recessive**. Dominant genes are always expressed into the phenotype when present at either one or both alleles (i.e. from one or both parents) (Figure 6.2). The gene traits of dominant genes therefore become a physical feature of the person. When the same genes (and the same traits) are present at both alleles they are described as **homozygous**. When different genes (and therefore different traits) are present at the alleles they are known as **heterozygous**. Recessive genes are only expressed into the phenotype when they are present at both alleles, i.e. when no dominant gene is present (Figure 6.3). A recessive gene at only one allele will not be expressed and the alternative dominant gene will determine the physical trait. However, the recessive gene will be passed on to the next generation. Two different dominant traits, one at each allele, may both be expressed into the phenotype as **codominant** genes, resulting in some kind of mixture of both traits in the phenotype of the individual.

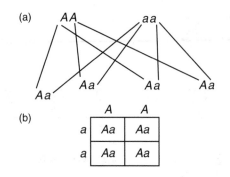

Figure 6.2 Dominant gene inheritance. Capital letter equals dominant gene, small letter equals recessive gene. Homozygous parents (*AA*, i.e. both dominant genes; or *aa*, both recessive genes) will have offspring that are all mixed (*Aa*, i.e. mixed dominant and recessive). Shown as a crossover and as a Punnett square.

Genes demonstrate varying degrees of **penetrance** – that is, the extent to which each individual gene contributes to the completed body (the phenotype). Genes showing complete penetrance achieve maximum influence over the phenotype. Incomplete penetrance occurs where the gene's activity is reduced, resulting in a weaker influence on the phenotype. Dominant genes will often show a high degree of penetrance whenever they are present, but recessive genes will have little or no penetrance unless they exist at both alleles (i.e. no dominant gene is present). The amount of penetrance that a *mutated* (or abnormal) gene demonstrates is an indication of its influence on the severity and course of several important mental health disorders. However, those genes of low-level penetrance may still be passed on to future generations of the same family where the gene's penetrance may be altered and increased.

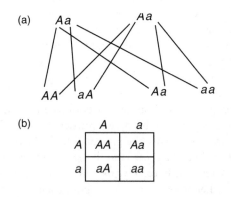

Figure 6.3 Recessive gene inheritance. Capital letter equals dominant gene, small letter equals recessive gene. Heterozygous parents (*Aa*, i.e. mixed dominant and recessive genes) have a 25 per cent chance of having an *AA* offspring (i.e. pure dominant genes), a 50 per cent chance of having an *Aa* offspring (i.e. mixed genes), and a 25 per cent chance of having an *aa* offspring (purely recessive). This last child shows recessive traits (or a recessive genetic disorder) that has missed one or more generations. Shown as a crossover and as a Punnett square.

Genes are stretches of **deoxyribonucleic acid** (**DNA**) found within the **chromatin** that makes up the chromosomes, and this DNA provides a code for producing specific proteins. Through the DNA, genes determine three important things about proteins:

- the type of proteins that will be produced;
- the amino acids that will be present in the final protein;
- the sequence of those amino acids in the protein.

DNA comprises four chemical **bases**: **adenine** (**A**), **thymine** (**T**), **guanine** (**G**) and **cytosine** (**C**), usually represented by their first letter as shown in brackets here. These bases form groups of three along the DNA called **codons**, and each codon codes for one specific amino acid in the final protein; for example, the codon GCA (guanine, cytosine and adenine) codes for the amino acid **alanine** (Figure 6.4). The types, numbers and sequence of the codons determine the type, numbers and sequence of the amino acids in the completed protein.

Genes have a particular site where they are found on the chromosome, called the gene **locus** (or **gene slot**). This locus is specified by giving the chromosome number first, followed by the arm of the chromosome (p = short arm; q = long arm), and then the banding number which is the site along that arm where the gene is located (see Figure 6.5). The arms of chromosomes show light and dark bands, and the banding number is the number of the band, counting away from the centromere, where the gene is located. The **centromere** is the point where the two chromatin strands join. This gives us the final number of the locus. As an example, take the gene locus 15q21.3, which means it is on the 15th chromosome, in the long arm (q) at the site found at band numbered 21.3 counted away from the chromosome's centromere. The higher the number, the further from the centromere the gene is sited (see Figure 6.5).

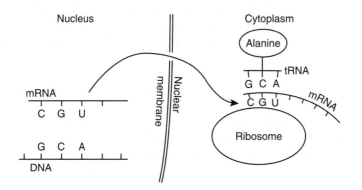

Figure 6.4 The genetic code for alanine. GCA (guanine–cytosine–adenine) on the DNA codes for the amino acid alanine by first forming the opposite code on messenger RNA (mRNA). The opposite of G is C, but the opposite of A is U (uracil) in RNA. U replaces the T (thymine) used in DNA. The mRNA leaves the nucleus and binds with a ribosome. Transfer RNAs (tRNAs) bear the same codes of bases as the original DNA codons (triplets of bases) in the DNA in the nucleus; of the case shown here it is GCA, coding for alanine. Repeating this along the DNA molecule, with different codes for different amino acids, forms a string of amino acids at the ribosome called a protein.

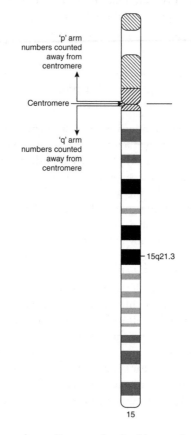

Figure 6.5 The gene locus. Genes are localised by a code using first the chromosome number (here it is chromosome 15), then the arm, represented by 'p' for the short
arm, 'q' for the long arm, and then the number counted away from the centromere. So 15q21.3 identifies the long arm of the 15th chromosome at point 21.3
from the centromere.

The proteins derived from the genetic code are of various types. They could be,
for example:
* structural proteins involved in building the cells of the body;
* enzymes involved in the metabolism of cells;
* hormones involved in the regulation of body functions;
* antibodies involved in the defence systems of the body.

This list is incomplete, but it shows the vital importance of genes in the construction, function and defence of the body and why gene errors can be so devastating to
the individual. Most gene errors are **mutations**, where changes occur in the bases
of the DNA resulting in a false code and therefore an error in the protein produced
from that code. This faulty protein will no longer function properly. Mutations
occur as a result of damage to DNA, caused either by chemicals or by radiation,
that is beyond the capabilities of the DNA repair enzymes. These excellent enzyme
systems (which we share in common with the elephant!) can repair most of the

mutations that occur, but sometimes the damage involves DNA that is missing or is beyond repair. Mutations that are inherited from generation to generation are rarely repaired and may often go on to cause diseases. Mutations include the following DNA errors (Figure 6.6):

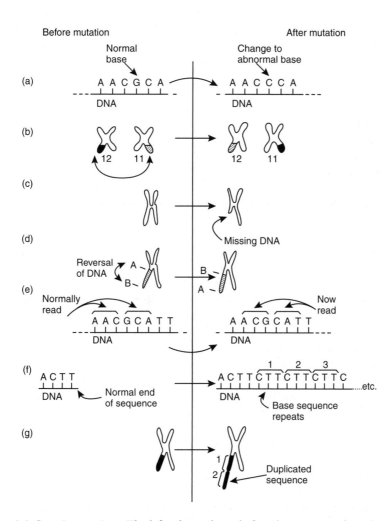

Figure 6.6 Genetic mutations. The left column shows before the mutation, the right column is after the mutation. (a) In a point mutation one base on the DNA is changed to a different one, creating a different code which introduces a different amino acid into the protein. (b) Translocation, in which a DNA sequence is swapped over between two chromosomes (shown here as an 11:12 translocation). (c) Deletion, in which a DNA sequence is lost entirely. (d) Inversion, in which a DNA sequence is reversed on the same chromosome (and thus will be read backwards). (e) Frame shift, where the normal DNA reading is moved one or more bases along (shown here as a single base shift normally read AAC, but now read ACG). This changes the amino acids in the protein. (f) Repeated base sequence, where the same base code is repeated many times (here it is CTT), resulting in a long tail of one kind of amino acid on the protein. (g) Duplication, where a DNA sequence is copied and attached to the end of a chromosome.

1　**Point mutations**, where a single base is swapped for another, incorrect, base. These have the effect of coding for the wrong amino acid in the protein, which therefore suffers a loss of function to varying degrees (Figure 6.6a).

2　**Translocations**, where some DNA of one chromosome has switched position with another stretch of DNA from a second chromosome. As an example, a 9:21 translocation means that chromosomes 9 and 21 have switched parts of their DNA with each other. The DNA is now in the wrong place and activation of these codes is likely to cause either a faulty protein or no protein product at all (Figure 6.6b).

3　**Deletions**, where some DNA is lost and chromosomes are therefore incomplete. The loss of some, perhaps many, genes will be detrimental to the function of the body, since some vital proteins cannot be produced (Figure 6.6c).

4　**Inversion**, where DNA is turned upside down in the chromosome and may be coded backwards, causing disruption of both the code and the protein that results (Figure 6.6d).

5.　**Frame shifts**, where the codon is read incorrectly one base to the left or right of the correct reading frame. As an example, if the DNA sequence was . . . AACGCATT . . . , the normal codon reading might be AAC, then GCA, and so on. However, a frame shift might read ACG, CAT, and so on, i.e. it would be read one base along to the right. It could also be read one base along to the left, i.e. CGC, ATT, and so on. The result of either shift is the incorrect reading of the codes, leading to the wrong amino acids being selected and the protein being wrongly constructed (Figure 6.6e).

6　**Base sequence repeats** (the so-called **stuttering gene**), where one codon is repeated many times – often hundreds of times – resulting in a long chain of one type of amino acid on the end of the protein. This is seen in several mental health and neurological conditions, notably Huntington's disease and possibly schizophrenia. The mechanism by which this error causes neurological and mental health problems is not fully determined. Not only do base sequence repeats occur as **familial disorders** (passed on through multiple generations of the same family), they also show the phenomenon of **anticipation**, an addition of further repeats to the DNA with each successive generation. This causes the disorder to start earlier with each new generation of that family, who also show increasingly severe symptoms as the repeat sequence gets longer (see Huntington's disease) (Figure 6.6f).

See page 272

7.　**Duplication**, where a sequence of DNA is copied (as part of a chromosome) and added onto the previously existing arm of a chromosome (Figure 6.6g).

8.　**Unstable sequence**, where a very large repeated base sequence, similar to but much longer than that found in (7) above, causes a complete loss of gene function. Fragile X syndrome is such a condition, resulting in some degree of mental retardation.

See page 113

Disorders of inheritance

Autosomal gene mutations are responsible for a number of genetically **inherited** disorders (i.e. those resulting from genes present at birth) and genetically **acquired** disorders (i.e. those where an individual develops a gene error during their life due to the damage and mutation of a previously normal gene). However,

Table 6.1 Proportions of genes in common between relatives of different degrees.

Relationship to affected person	Approximate percentage of shared genes
Monozygotic (MZ or identical) twin	98
Dizygotic (DZ or non-identical) twin	50
First-degree relative (sibling, parent, son, daughter)	50
Second-degree relative (grandparent, aunt, uncle)	25
Third-degree relative (e.g. cousin)	12.5

environmental factors are also likely to play an important role in some mental health disorders and these disorders are therefore usually classified as **polygenic**, where several genes are seen as interacting with one or several environmental factors to cause the disorder. In this sense, genes play a role that *increases the susceptibility* of an individual to develop a particular disorder, rather than causing the disorder directly. Whether the person develops the disorder or not may depend on the environmental factors they encounter.

Inherited genetic disorders are said to be **familial**; that is, they are found in successive generations of the same family. In the case of *inherited* disorders, the gene error is passed on from parents to offspring through the sperm or ovum. In studies involving families affected by an inherited gene disorder the researcher will look at percentage risks between **first-degree relatives** (parents, brothers, sisters, sons or daughters) of an affected person. Studies of **second-degree relatives** (grandparents, aunts or uncles), or even **third-degree relatives** (e.g. cousins) of an affected person may also be of value in understanding the nature of the gene and its inheritance pattern. Studies of twins are particularly important when studying genetic inheritance, especially of **monozygotic (identical) twins** who have about 98 per cent of their genes in common. Table 6.1 shows the approximate proportions of genes shared between an affected person and their various relatives. From this it can be seen that **dizygotic (non-identical) twins** share the same amount of genes as ordinary brothers or sisters.

For a discussion on the genes related to a specific mental disorder, see the chapter on that disorder; for example, the genes involved in depression are discussed in Chapter 11, those for schizophrenia in Chapter 10, and those for dementia in Chapter 14. Genes involved in Huntington's and Parkinson's diseases are discussed in Chapter 13.

The most important difference between a genetic disorder and a chromosomal disorder is the number of genes involved (i.e it becomes a problem of magnitude, or numbers of genes involved). In genetic disorders there may be one or just a few genes at the root cause of a particular disease, whilst chromosomal disorders involve abnormalities of a whole or part of a chromosome, adding up to perhaps several thousand genes.

Autosomal disorders

Two major chromosomal errors can result in mental health disorders: those that involve whole chromosomes and thus affect the number of chromosomes in the karyotype (e.g. trisomies and monosomies), and those that affect part of individual chromosomes without influencing the karyotype number (e.g. deletions).

Several chromosomal abnormalities can occur that result in an abnormal karyotype chromosome count (the normal value being 46 chromosomes). A **trisomy** is the occurrence of one extra chromosome attached to a pair, giving a karyotype of 47 chromosomes (Figure 6.7). A **monosomy** is the occurrence of only one chromosome instead of a pair: one chromosome is missing, giving a karyotype of 45 chromosomes (Figure 6.7). People with some trisomies or with most monosomies do not survive; those bearing these chromosomal abnormalities are subject to spontaneous abortion during pregnancy, i.e. a miscarriage caused by nature. This is because either too much genetic material is present (trisomies) or not enough is present (monosomies) to be compatible with life. It is possible that individual cells within one person can differ in the presence or absence of a trisomy. Those sufferers with all their cells containing a trisomy are called '**full trisomies**', and those with a mix of trisomy and non-trisomy (normal) cells are called '**mosaic trisomies**'.

The trisomies that can *survive* to birth are those of autosomes **8**[1], **9**, **13**, **16**[2], **18**, **20**[2], **21** and **22**[1] (1= survival is rare; 2= survives as a mosaic only). Autosomal monosomies are almost entirely fatal as a fetus. The only exception may be monosomy 21. Only a handful of full monosomy 21 cases have been reported, and only one lived beyond their first birthday. Mosaic monosomy 21 cases have survived more often.

Most of the phenotype abnormalities associated with surviving trisomies include some degree of mental retardation, and therefore may be seen by the psychiatric nurse at some time.

Trisomy 8 or **Warkany syndrome 2** (three number 8 chromosomes) results in an individual who is abnormally shorter or taller than average (due to variations in growth patterns), no facial expressions, multiple physical abnormalities, especially of the muscular-skeletal system (e.g. a large skull) and some mental retardation. Most sufferers are mosaic for trisomy 8, with full trisomy 8 causing early death.

Trisomy 9 (three number 9 chromosomes) can be in full or mosaic form. The symptoms vary widely but include abnormal skull shapes, disorder of the nervous

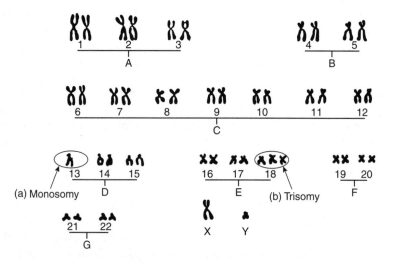

Figure 6.7 The human karyotype showing monosomy (here seen at chromosome 13) and trisomy (here seen at chromosome 18).

system and a degree of mental retardation. The heart, kidneys and musculo-skeletal system may be involved.

Trisomy 13 (three number 13 chromosomes) is called **Patau syndrome**. This occurs about once in every 5,000 live births and (like Edwards and Down syndromes) the risk of Patau syndrome is increased with advancing maternal age at the time of pregnancy. It causes a wide range of severe physical abnormalities with profound mental retardation. Half of those born with this syndrome die within one month of their birth.

Trisomy 16 (three number 16 chromosomes) occurs in full or mosaic form. Full trisomy 16 is incompatible with life and causes most of the miscarriages from chromosomal errors occurring during pregnancy. Trisomy 16 live births are mosaics only. The features of mosaic trisomy 16 are premature birth, defects in growth, lung and heart abnormalities, a short neck, high forehead and scoliosis (a specific curvature of the spine).

Trisomy 18 (three number 18 chromosomes) is called **Edwards syndrome**. This is more common than Patau syndrome, and second only to Down syndrome in prevalence, being present in one in 3,000 live births. The incidence increases with increased maternal age at the time of pregnancy. It causes various physical abnormalities (heart, kidney and other organs), failure of growth (developmental delay) and mental retardation. **Microcephaly** (a small head) with other cranial abnormalities are characteristic. Survival rate is poor, most dying before birth (due to cardiac malformations) with about 30 per cent of those surviving up to birth dying before their first birthday.

Trisomy 20 (three number 20 chromosomes) occurs in full or mosaic form, with full trisomy 20 causing early fetal death and miscarriage. Mosaic trisomy 20 is often detected prenatally, but the resulting child usually appears normal at birth. However, a consistent set of abnormalities have now been established. These are spinal abnormalities, sloping shoulders, poor muscle tone, recurrent constipation, and significant learning disabilities despite normal intelligence.

Trisomy 21 (three number 21 chromosomes) is known as **Down syndrome** (Figure 6.8). This is more common than other trisomies, occurring on average in about one in 600 live births. The incidence of a Down syndrome child being born increases with maternal age: the older the mother is at the time of pregnancy the greater is the risk of Down syndrome. A typical risk pattern is seen in Table 6.2.

The extra chromosome is caused mostly by a **non-dysjunction**, where ovarian cell division results in abnormal separation of the chromosomes and one ovum retains both of the chromosomes 21. The older the woman, the greater the risk of non-dysjunction. The single ovum then has two chromosomes 21, and the addition of a third chromosome 21 from the sperm on fertilisation completes the trisomy. Incidentally, should the normal sperm fertilise the other half of that ovum division – the half with no chromosome 21 – it would generate a monosomy 21 (having only the paternal chromosome 21).

Down syndrome results in a wide range of physical abnormalities and varying degrees of mental retardation. The physical abnormalities include a round skull on a short, broad neck, a flattened face and a prominent epicanthus of the eye (the upper lid fold close to the nose is anchored lower down giving an oriental or 'Mongolian' appearance, a feature responsible for the term *mongolism* which is sometimes inappropriately used). Other features are a large, furrowed tongue in a small mouth,

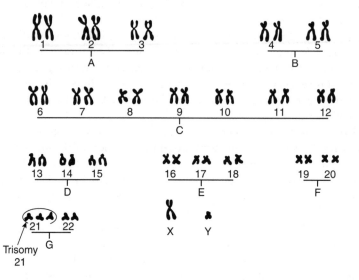

Figure 6.8 Down syndrome karyotype, showing trisomy at chromosome 21.

a single crease in the palm of the hand (known as a **simian crease**) and a long **plantar crease** down the sole of the foot extending from an enlarged gap between the first two toes. There may also be increased extensibility of the limbs due to poor muscle tone. Varying degrees of congenital heart defects can occur, and cataracts (opacity of the lens of the eye causing blindness), squints and nystagmus (rapid uncontrollable lateral eye movements) are more common in trisomy 21 than in the average person.

The mental retardation can be anything from very mild to quite severe (Sadock et al. 2009). At the mild end of the spectrum, Down syndrome children communicate and learn quite well and become relatively independent adults. They can perform quite intricate tasks and cope with jobs that are not too demanding. They are often happy and enjoy participating in activities such as learning a musical instrument, singing and dancing. Before the advent of modern social conditions and life-saving treatments such as antibiotics, Down syndrome children often died from neglect, undernutrition and infections. Now, many are living into adulthood, when they begin to face another problem. The middle-aged Down syndrome adult (i.e. 30 to 40 years of age) often shows evidence of dementia of the type related to Alzheimer's disease. Chapter 14 explores Alzheimer's disease in some detail, and *See page 286* the connection with chromosome 21, relating this to Down syndrome.

Table 6.2 Changes in the incidence of Down syndrome with maternal age (Nussbaum et al. 2001).

Maternal age at conception of child	Approximate incidence of Down syndrome
15 to 29 years old	1 in 1,250 to 1 in 1,100 live births
30 to 34 years old	1 in 900 to 1 in 500 live births
35 to 39 years old	1 in 385 to 1 in 140 live births
40 to 44 years old	1 in 100 to 1 in 40 live births
45 years old and over	1 in 25 live births

Trisomy 22 (three number 22 chromosomes) occurs in full or mosaic forms. Full trisomy 22 is the second commonest cause of spontaneous miscarriage during pregnancy after full trisomy 16. Mosaic trisomy 22 causes a long list of physical abnormalities including microcephaly, intrauterine growth retardation, craniofacial malformation (abnormal development of the head and face), limb deformities, heart and vascular disorders and arrested mental development.

Mosaic monosomy 21 cases (with only one number 21 in some cells) rarely survive as live births, with only a few cases reported. They have a collection of medical problems including microcephaly, skull, brain and facial deformities, abnormalities of the digits, poor muscle tone and retardation of both intellectual and physical development.

A constant physical abnormality in many of these disorders is **craniofacial malformation**, such as **cleft lip and palate** (incomplete closure of the upper lip and roof of the mouth), or more rarely **cyclopia** (a single eye in the forehead often associated with an absent forebrain). Cleft lip and palate is a birth defect that is encountered regularly, and the majority of these occur in otherwise normal babies (i.e. they are not suffering from a chromosomal syndrome, and therefore they are 'non-syndromic'). In chromosomal 'syndromic' cleft lip and palate, the upper jaw defect forms part of the multiple features that make up the syndrome.

The formation of the head and face is a complex biological phenomenon which is controlled by multiple genes, most of which are only now being discovered. Since the brain, head and face develop together as a unit, any defect in the development of one will impact on the development of the others. Whilst the brain forms from the head end of the neural tube, the bones, cartilages and connective tissue of the skull, and the peripheral nervous system of the head, are all derived from cranial **neural crest** cells. The face grows forward from both sides and fuses down the midline. It is the failure of this midline fusing process which causes cleft lip and palate.

New work is revealing the genes and their protein products that link the development of the brain with embryonic skull and facial construction (Cohen 2000). It is beyond the scope of this chapter to discuss them all, but one important gene involved in this process has several vital roles. This is the **SHH** (**sonic hedgehog homolog**) gene, which is one of three so-called *hedgehog* proteins. SHH acts as a **morphogen**, i.e. a cell signalling molecule that governs the nature of tissues, e.g. controlling cell differentiation, during embryonic development. SHH is involved in the development of many embryonic systems, in particular the midface (e.g. controlling the width of the face) and frontal areas of the brain. Mutations of SHH cause a collection of disorders called **holoprosencephaly**, i.e. failure of development of the face and frontal brain lobes, which includes cleft lip and palate.

Sex chromosome abnormalities

The genetic determination of an individual's sex relies on the inheritance of a combination of the **sex chromosomes**, **X** and **Y**. The **XX** combination produces a female and the **XY** combination produces a male. 'Maleness' therefore requires the presence of the Y chromosome, while 'femaleness' requires the absence of the Y chromosome.

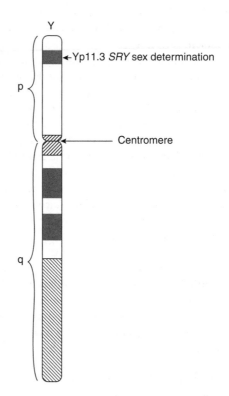

Figure 6.9 The male Y chromosome, showing the *SRY* (sex determination) gene locus at Yp11.3.

Several genes are involved in creating the male condition, one of which is very close to the **centromere** on the Y chromosome (Figure 6.9). This is the **SRY gene** (i.e. the **sex-determining region Y**), a gene that codes for a **transcription factor**. Transcription factors are proteins that bind to DNA and begin to trigger the process of RNA assembly, the process called **transcription**, leading to protein synthesis.

The *SRY*-encoded transcription factor switches on testicular development in the primitive gonad, which up to that point has been undifferentiated, being neither testes nor ovary. In addition, there are indications that *SRY* genes are also expressed in parts of the male brain, notably the hypothalamus and the midbrain, suggesting that this may trigger sex-determination within these brain structures (Lahr et al. 1995). H-Y antigen is another factor that predisposes towards the male condition, by promoting testicular development in the primitive, undifferentiated gonads. The gene that codes for the structure of H-Y antigen is on an autosome (chromosome 6), but its expression is suppressed (or inhibited) by factors coded on the X chromosome. Other Y chromosome factors block the X chromosome factors, a case of inhibiting the inhibitor, and this allows the expression of the H-Y antigen (Figure 6.10). There is about 1000 times more male H-Y antigen than female H-Y antigen due to the Y inhibition of the X factor in males.

XXY males are described as having **Klinefelter syndrome** (Figure 6.11). The additional X chromosome changes the normal karyotype of 46 chromosomes into

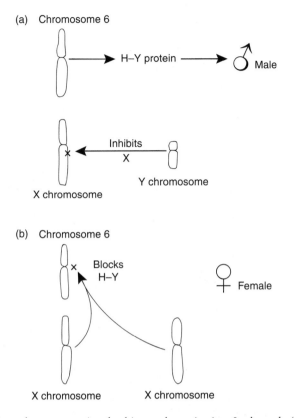

Figure 6.10 Three chromosomes involved in sex determination. In the male (a), chromosome 6 has the gene for the H–Y protein that causes masculinisation. The
presence of a Y chromosome produces an inhibiting factor that blocks the X
chromosome. In the female (b), the absence of a Y chromosome allows both X
chromosomes to block the H–Y protein from chromosome 6, and the female
condition will develop.

the abnormal number of 47. Klinefelter syndrome is the result of fertilisation involving either **diploid sperm** or **diploid ova**. Diploid in this context means
that the sperm or ovum carries *both* the sex chromosomes instead of just one; thus
one ovum would carry XX, or one sperm would carry XY. On fertilisation with
a normal Y sperm, the XX ovum would become XXY. Fertilisation between an
XY sperm and a normal X ovum would also result in XXY (see Figure 6.12).
Klinefelter syndrome occurs in 1 in 600 live births and, because the Y is present,
the child is always male. Males with this condition are usually tall, often thin, with
poor sexual development and are mildly mentally retarded. It would appear that if
more extra X chromosomes are present, e.g. XXXY or XXXXY, the degree of
mental retardation is greater (McCance et al. 2010).

Figure 6.11 also shows an XXX combination, which is the inappropriately
named **superwoman syndrome**. This is another 47-chromosome karyotype,
caused by a **trisomy X**. As for the male in Klinefelter syndrome, the XXX female
sometimes has poor sexual development and a mild mental retardation, but people

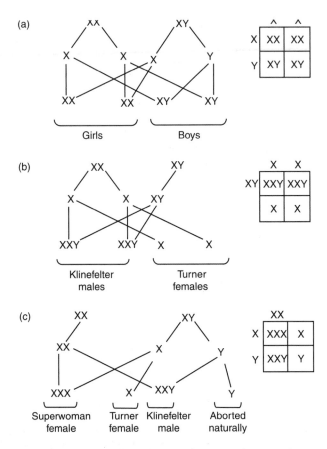

Figure 6.11 Inheritance patterns of sex determination. (a) The normal cross-over of the female XX and male XY to produce a 50 per cent chance of either sex. (b) Abnormal male clustering together of the XY chromosomes, giving sons with Klinefelter syndrome, or daughters with Turner's syndrome. (c) Abnormal female clustering together of the XX chromosomes, giving sons that either are Klinefelter syndrome or are incompatible with life and will spontaneously abort, or giving daughters who may be superwoman syndrome or Turner's syndrome. All three are shown as crossovers or **Punnett squares**.

with this syndrome are able to live relatively normal lives in society. Superwoman syndrome is rarer than Klinefelter syndrome, occurring in 1 in 1,600 live births. Again, as with Klinefelter's syndrome, any additional X present causes a greater degree of mental retardation. Very rare cases of XXXX and XXXXX syndromes have been reported, where more X chromosomes cause much greater degrees of mental retardation (Visootsak et al. 2007).

As shown in Figure 6.11, the single X (**monosomy X**) female also occurs, giving a 45-chromosome karyotype. Monosomy X is **Turner's syndrome**, characterised by a short female with poor sexual development and some minor physical abnormalities, including a depressed sternum and a webbed neck. However, with one X present these females have normal mental development. Turner's syndrome happens in about 1 in 3,000 live births.

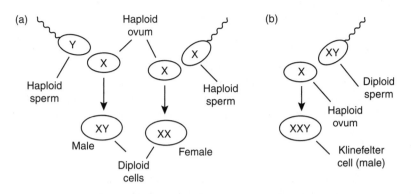

Figure 6.12 Sperm meets ovum. (a) Normally the sperm carries one sex chromosome (either X or Y) and this meets the ovum that carries one X chromosome to produce a fertilised ovum with XX or XY. (b) Sometimes an abnormal sperm carries both XY and meets a normal ovum to give a fertilised ovum with XXY. Normal sperm fertilising abnormal XX ovum to give either XXX or XXY also occurs occasionally (not shown).

XYY males do occur as well, since nearly 1 per cent of all sperm carry the YY chromosome combination which may fertilise a normal single X ovum to cause XYY. It perhaps happens in 1 in 1,000 live births. These males have attracted a great deal of research because this particular genetic combination was associated with aggression and criminal behaviour. The XYY combination was first reported in 1961 and its association with violent criminal behaviour was made in 1965. Today, much of this original work on XYY is seen to be inappropriate and flawed because of sample bias, since most of the work focused on male prison populations. We now know that less than 1 per cent of all XYY men become prisoners and that less than 2 per cent of male prisoners are XYY. Leaving prison populations aside, XYY may cause some small increase in antisocial behaviour when compared to the normal XY or even XXY combinations. Other characteristics of the XYY male include above-average height – XYY are around 1.82 metres compared to the XY average of 1.67 metres. Even as a child of six years, the XYY male is taller than 90 per cent of his peers of the same age. Sexual development is normal, but there will be poor coordination, delayed language skills and some learning difficulties. These males generally perform less well in intelligence quotient (IQ) tests than their XY counterparts, approximately on a par with XXY males.

Very rarely, XYYY and even XYYYY males have been reported, but unlike the additional X chromosomes, the additional Ys have little or no effect on mental development.

The X chromosome is much larger than the Y chromosome and this means that it carries many more genes. It is the source of significantly large numbers of rare but important mental retardation syndromes (Figure 6.13). The mental health nurse, who is in the best position to encounter them, should be aware of these syndromes. Table 6.3 lists the better-known X-linked syndromes that result in some degree of mental retardation and also illustrates the large number of mental retardation syndromes associated with the X chromosome. Notice in Figure 6.13 that there are a number of mental retardation syndromes positioned in clusters on the chromosome, the **loci** of the major ones being Xp22.3–p22.2; Xp11.3–p11.21 (close to the centromere); Xq21.3–q24 and Xq28.

An important point concerning the X chromosome is the fact that females have two X chromosomes whilst males have only one. This means that any particular gene error on one X chromosome is likely to be matched by a normal gene on the other X chromosome in females (the mutation occurring at only one allele), whilst in males the X chromosome gene error has no such normal counterpart. This results in X-linked gene disorders being generally much more severe in males than in females. Males suffer the full disease which may prove fatal in some cases. On the other hand, females may have only mild symptoms or even remain **asymptomatic** (having no symptoms at all). However, females will still be able to pass on the faulty gene to their offspring, and if this is a son he is likely to suffer the severe form of the illness. It is very rare (and very unlucky) for a female to have the faulty gene on both X chromosomes (i.e. at both alleles). This only happens if both parents have the disorder, i.e. they both carry the same faulty gene. In this case, the disorder in this female would be severe.

The term **phenotype** refers to the physical features caused by the **genotype**, or genes present in the cell. Another way of stating this is to say that the genotype

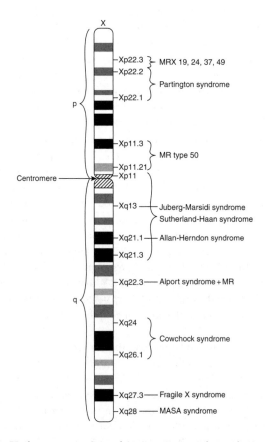

Figure 6.13 The X chromosome. Several important mental retardation (MR) syndromes are located on both the p (short) and q (long) arms.

Table 6.3 X-linked syndromes involving mental retardation.

Gene locus	Syndrome name or code (if any)	Phenotype
Xp22.3–22.2	MRX19, 24, 37	
Xp22.3–22.2	MRX49	Mild to moderate MR
Xp22.3–21.3		MR in males only
Xp22.2–p22.1	Partington syndrome	Male only, mild to moderate MR, dystonic hand movements, dysarthria
Xp21–q13		Varying degree of MR
Xp11–q21.3	Sutherland–Haan X-linked MR syndrome	Short stature, small testes, microcephaly, brachycephaly, MR
Xp11.3–p11.21	MR type 50	Moderate MR
Xq13	Juberg–Marsidi syndrome	Probably males only. Growth delay, facial anomalies, deafness, MR and microgenitalism
Xq21.1	Allan–Herndon syndrome	Severe MR, muscle and movement anomalies, head abnormalities
Xq22		Female epilepsy, MR
Xq22.3		Alport syndrome (multiple physical deformities and disorders, worse in males) with MR, elliptocytosis, midface hypoplasia
Xq24–26.1	Cowchock syndrome	Neuropathy, deafness and MR. Worse in males
Xq26–27		Male moderate MR, facial abnormalities and large testes
Xq27.3	Fragile X syndrome	See text
Xq28	MASA syndrome	MR, aphasia, shuffling gait, adducted thumbs
X	Chudley MR syndrome	Moderate to severe MR, short stature, mild obesity, hypogonadism, facial abnormalities

MR = mental retardation. X = X chromosome (MRX with a number refers to a specific mental retardation syndrome). p = short arm, q = long arm. See text for other definitions of terms.

consists of the genes locked up in the cell nucleus, while the phenotype is the bodily features (tall, short, etc.), created by expression of the genes. Other terms included in Table 6.3 are **adducted thumbs**, where the thumbs lie bent inwards across the palm of the hand; **aphasia**, the inability to speak; **brachycephaly**, a congenital skull malformation in which the head is short but wide; **dysarthria**, a difficulty with speech due to poor speech muscle control; **dystonic (dystonia)**, an abnormal posture of a limb or the trunk with slow and twisting movements; **elliptocytosis**, an increase in the number of **elliptocytes** (oval instead of round **erythrocytes**, red blood cells) in the blood; **gait**, the method of walking; **hypogonadism**, underdevelopment of either testes or ovum; **hypoplasia**, reduced numbers of cells causing underdevelopment of an organ; **microcephaly**, a small head with a small brain; and **neuropathy**, a disorder of the nerves.

Fragile X syndrome (Figure 6.14) is a mental retardation syndrome caused by a **trinucleotide repeat**, where the same three genetic bases are repeated many times. The repeated bases in this case are **CGG** (i.e. **cytosine–guanine–guanine**), where CGG codes for the amino acid **arginine**. Up to 54 such repeats occur normally, but any number of repeats from 52 to more than 200 are found in this syndrome. When expressed, the normal gene would code for a protein, known

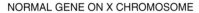

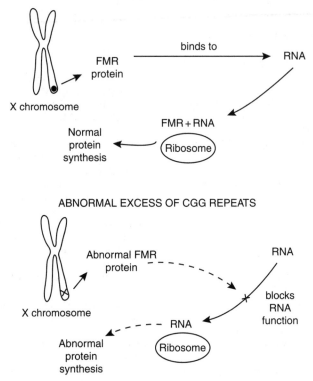

Figure 6.14 Fragile X syndrome. A gene on chromosome X codes for the FMR protein, which appears to be important for RNA binding at the ribosome (top). In fragile X syndrome faulty DNA at the FMR gene causes failure of normal FMR protein which in turns reduces RNA's ability to bind at the ribosome (below). Failure of RNA binding reduces the cell's protein production ability, and the neuron will suffer from the loss.

as the **FMR protein**, which binds with **RNA** (**ribonucleic acid**). RNA locks onto a **ribosome**, where **translation** of the RNA code into a protein (**protein synthesis**) takes place. FMR is required for the successful binding of RNA to a ribosome. In fragile X syndrome, however, the excessive CGG repeats block gene expression, with the consequent loss of the normal FMR protein and a subsequent loss of RNA binding ability. This leads to failure of the cell's protein synthesis functions, and in neurons this causes varying degrees of mental retardation (Figure 6.14). Males appear to be more affected than females (only 30 to 40 per cent of affected females have some degree of mental retardation). Less commonly, other symptoms occur, notably enlarged testes at puberty, large ears, a prominent jaw, some enlargement of the head in a few affected males, finger joints that extend further than expected owing to loose connective tissues, and aortic and heart valve disorders. Speech may be delayed and high pitched. Trinucleotide repeats, which are also sometimes called **stuttering genes**, are of growing importance in mental health, and are implicated in other disorders such as **Huntington's disease** and **schizophrenia**.

See page 270
See page 118

Genetic disorders

Apart from whole chromosomes or parts of chromosomes, a single gene or a few genes, on autosomes or the X chromosome, may be responsible for specific disorders involving mental health disturbance. The types of abnormal genes (mutations) are listed on page 000. **Deletions** involve the loss of a genetic sequence, i.e. a number of DNA bases, often due to breakages during cell division.

Cri-du-chat (cry of cat) syndrome involves the deletion of part of the short arm of chromosome 5 (5p15.2) (Faraone et al. 1999). This gene codes for **catenin delta-2**, a protein that is specific to neurons and is involved significantly in neural motility during the very early stages of nervous system development. Children born with this condition show mental retardation and severe physical abnormalities such as microcephaly (small head and brain), low-set ears and oblique palpebral fissures (openings of the eye). The disorder gets its name from a cat-like crying sound they make, but this gradually disappears as they get older.

Williams syndrome is caused by the loss of a small fragment of genetic material from one of the 7th chromosomes, a loss of about 15 or so genes at 7q11.23. The other 7th chromosome is present and complete. The incidence of this condition is about one in every 20,000 births worldwide. It causes a minor degree of mental retardation, resulting in lower than average intelligence test scores. The surprise, however, is the remarkable musical talent that many with the disorder display. Williams syndrome people can often perform, remember and even compose music to a very high degree of competency (Lenhoff et al. 1997). Several genes that are missing from the deleted segment are involved in brain development, but their mechanism of action is not fully known. The musical ability can be partly explained by studies of the brains from Williams syndrome people that show an extensive expansion of part of the temporal cortex called the **planum temporale**. This expansion is also found in gifted musicians without this syndrome (see music, Chapter 9). However, other areas of the brain in Williams syndrome are reduced to below normal size.

Prader–Willi and **Angelman syndromes** are both caused by deletion of part of chromosome 15, i.e. the gene locus 15q11. The deletion in Prader–Willi syndrome appears to be limited to 15q11, while in Angelman syndrome the deletion is wider, to include 15q11 and 15q12, and sometimes part of 15q13. It appears that the difference depends on which parent the deletion was obtained from. If the deletion is inherited from the mother (the maternal line of inheritance), the resulting syndrome in the offspring is Angelman; if from the father (the paternal line of inheritance) it is Prader–Willi. This is possible because of a molecular process called **imprinting**. Imprinting is the process of switching a gene on (activation) or off (deactivation) by control from a genetic **imprinting centre** (**IC**) which is found a short distance along the genetic base sequence from the gene being controlled (Figure 6.15). At 15q11–q12 there is a gene called *SNRPN* (small nuclear ribonucleoprotein N), controlled by a nearby IC. *SNRPN* codes for a protein called **SmN** (a small nuclear ribonucleoprotein sub-unit), which is involved in the processing of messenger ribonucleic acid (mRNA), the molecule required to carry the DNA code to the ribosome for protein synthesis. SmN is particularly expressed in the brain. Disturbance in the activation of this gene could be a cause of inappropriate protein synthesis in specific neurons, leading to abnormal development

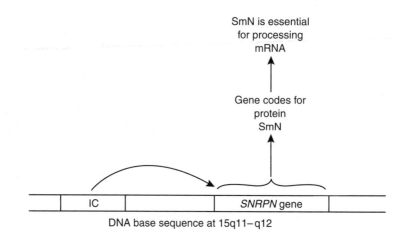

Figure 6.15 Angelman and Prader–Willi syndromes. The gene (*SRPN*) located at 15q11–
q12 is controlled by an imprinting centre (IC) further along the DNA sequence. The gene codes for the SmN protein, which is important in processing
mRNA. Mutations in the IC affect protein production, and this error is passed
on to the offspring, through successive generations, from either the maternal
line (Angelman) or paternal line (Prader–Willi).

of the brain or malfunction of those neurons. Mutations in the form of deletions in
the IC of this gene appear to result in the fixing of the gene activation on a single
parental line only. The deletions are probably due to the fact that this particular
DNA sequence has two points that are susceptible to breakage.

Angelman syndrome is characterised by severe motor impairment, e.g. **ataxia**
(poor coordination of movement and loss of balance), **hypotonia** (loose, floppy
muscles), and mental retardation, including failure of speech and epilepsy. Other
abnormal characteristics include a large mandible, which may protrude forward
(**prognathism**), a large open mouth (**macrostomia**) with protruding tongue,
excessive laughter (appearing happy), puppet-like movements and hyperactivity.

Prader–Willi syndrome also shows symptoms of hypotonia and mental retardation. In this syndrome the sufferer develops what appears to be a **hyperphagia**, i.e.
an excessive appetite, which could lead to overeating and obesity. In fact, they appear to eat anything, even to the point of eating clothing, curtains, paper and other
non-edible substances. However, the current opinion is that these patients are not
actually eating these inedible substances, they are using the mouth as another sense
organ, i.e. taste is as important to recognition of objects as is sight and touch.
People with this condition have small hands, small feet and a short stature, coupled
with reduced levels of gonad function (**hypogonadism**) due to undersecretion of
gonadotrophic hormones from the pituitary gland. Children may show defiant
behaviour. Both syndromes are rare; Prader–Willi syndrome, for example, affects
fewer than one person in 10,000 (Sadock et al. 2009), and Angelman syndrome
affects one person in 10,000 to 25,000.

The **Lissencephalic disorders** ('**lissos**' = smooth, '**encephalon**' = brain; i.e.
the 'smooth brain' disorders) include a number of **microdeletions** (very small genetic deletions), which result in a degree of mental retardation and other symptoms

(Pilz and Quarrell 1996). In these disorders, abnormal neuronal migration occurs during fetal development, resulting in a smooth cortex, i.e. a significant loss of the normal folding into sulci and gyri, together with varying changes of cortical cell layers. Neuronal migration is described in Chapter 2. A gene that is vital in the control of cortical cell structure, called the **lissencephaly gene** (**LIS1**), is now known on chromosome 17 (17p13.3). This gene is probably involved in cell signalling during fetal neuronal migration of the cerebrum. The microdeletion of this gene is a major cause of these 'smooth brain' disorders. Other genes have also been found: **LIS2** at 7q22; **LIS3** at 12q12-q14; **LISX1** at Xq22.3-q23 and **LISX2** at Xp22.13. Lissencephalic disorders are usually divided into **type I** ('**classical**'), and **type II** (**variant** or **Walker's lissencephaly**).

- Type I lissencephaly shows a smoothing of the brain surface with disruption of the cell structure (**cytoarchitecture**) causing a thick, four-layered cerebral cortex (normally, the cerebral cortex has six distinct cell layers). The cerebellum is basically normal. The clinical features are mental retardation, **diplegia** (bilateral paralysis) and fits. Type I lissencephaly is more likely to be sporadic in origin, rather than inherited. Sporadic genetic changes involve the affected individual only and are not passed on to subsequent generations through the sperm or ova. **Miller–Dieker syndrome** (**MDS**), which is caused by a microdeletion at gene locus 17p13.3 (the lissencephaly gene), results in severe mental retardation with other neurological deficits (e.g. difficulty in swallowing), and growth deficiency with **craniofacial defects** (sometimes called the '**Miller–Dieker face**') involving a prominent forehead, a short, upturned nose, protruding upper lip and small jaw. Death usually occurs within the first year of life.
- Type II lissencephaly shows a smoothing of the brain surface with disruption of the cytoarchitecture in a manner that results in no distinct cell layers. The main features of type II are severe neurological dysfunction from an early age, eye abnormalities and hydrocephalus. Type II lissencephaly is thought more likely to be genetically inherited than type I. The disorders that fall into the type II category are those that cause various forms of muscular dystrophy (muscle wasting with weakness) due to the neurological dysfunction. **Walker–Warburg syndrome** (**WWS**) is a cause of severe mental and psychomotor retardation, but is also part of this group of muscle disorders known as the **congenital muscular dystrophies** (**CMD**), where muscle weakness, losses of muscle tone and muscle contractures are predominant symptoms (Leyten et al. 1996). Walker–Warburg syndrome shows an autosomal recessive inheritance pattern and is linked to five genes at loci 14q24.3, 9q34.1, 9q31, 22q12.3-q13.1 and 19q13.3. It should not be surprising that a brain lissencephaly causes muscle problems since the main motor cortex that controls skeletal muscle movement is part of the cerebrum (Brodmann 4).

A deletion close to that seen in Miller–Dieker syndrome occurs at 17p11.2, resulting in the **Smith–Magenis syndrome**. This causes brachycephaly (short, broad skull caused by early closure of the coronal skull suture and excessive lateral skull growth), a prominent forehead, a broad face and nasal bridge, heart defects, hyperactivity and fits. Maladaptive behaviour causes problems such as self-harm and sleep pattern disturbance (Dykens and Smith 1998).

Key points

Chromosomes and genes

- The human karyotype is made up of 46 chromosomes.
- Autosomes are chromosomes 1 to 22 in the human karyotype, i.e. 22 pairs of autosomes.
- The chromosomes making up the final pair are the **sex chromosomes** – X and Y in males, X and X in females.
- Each pair consists of two chromosomes that are the same, called homologous chromosomes.
- Two alternative versions of the same gene are called alleles, one allele on each chromosome.
- Being from different parents, these alleles are of different traits.
- Whether a gene is expressed into the phenotype or not depends on whether it is dominant, recessive or codominant.
- Genes demonstrate varying degrees of penetrance, or how much each individual gene contributes to the completed body (the phenotype).
- The DNA determines what proteins will be produced, the amino acids it will contain and their sequence in the protein.
- Genes are found on the chromosome at sites called the gene locus (or gene slot), written by giving the chromosome number first, then the arm of the chromosome, 'p' for short arm and 'q' for long arm.
- Mutations are DNA errors, e.g. point mutations, translocations, deletions, frame shifts, inversions, base-sequence repeats and fragile sites.

Disorders of inheritance

- Inherited genetic disorders are often familial, i.e. found in successive generations of the same family.
- First-degree relatives of an affected person are their parents, brothers, sisters, sons or daughters; second-degree relatives are their grandparents, aunts or uncles; and third-degree relatives are those such as cousins.
- Monozygotic (MZ) twins are identical twins, i.e. most of their genes are the same; dizygotic (DZ) twins are nonidentical twins, i.e. about half of their genes are the same.

Autosomal disorders

- A genetic disorder may involve one gene or a few genes, but a chromosomal disorder involves abnormalities of the whole or part of a chromosome, adding up to perhaps several thousand genes.
- A trisomy is one extra chromosome attached to a pair; a monosomy is only one chromosome instead of a pair.

- When all the cells contain a trisomy it is known as a full trisomy, but if there is a mix of trisomy and non-trisomy cells this is called a mosaic trisomy.

Sex chromosome abnormalities

- The sex chromosomes are X and Y, where XX corresponds to female and XY to male.
- 'Maleness' requires the Y chromosome, whilst 'femaleness' occurs in the absence of the Y chromosome.
- X-linked gene disorders are more severe in males than in females.
- XXY male is Klinefelter syndrome and XXX is superwoman syndrome.
- These conditions are trisomies, i.e. three chromosomes in place of two (47 chromosomes in the karyotype).
- XYY males also occur.
- Monosomy means one chromosome in place of two (giving 45 chromosomes).
- Monosomy X is Turner's syndrome.
- The X chromosome is the source of a large variety of mental retardation syndromes, albeit that they are generally rare.
- Fragile X syndrome is a mental retardation syndrome caused by a trinucleotide repeat.

Genetic disorders

- Cri–du–chat syndrome (cry of cat syndrome) is caused by a deletion of part of the short arm of chromosome 5.
- Williams syndrome is caused by the loss of about 15 genes from 7q11.23.
- Prader–Willi and Angelman syndromes are both caused by deletion of part of chromosome 15 at the gene locus 15q11.
- Lissencephalies, the 'smooth brain' disorders, include a number microdeletions resulting in mental retardation and other symptoms.
- These disorders include Miller–Dieker and Walker–Warburg syndromes.

References

Cohen P. (2000) Shaping up. *New Scientist*, **165** (2227): 16.

Dykens E. M. and Smith A. C. M. (1998) Distinctiveness and correlates of maladaptive behaviour in children and adolescents with Smith–Magenis syndrome. *Journal of Intellectual Disability Research*, **42** (6): 481–489.

Faraone S. V., Tsuang M. T. and Tsuang D. W. (1999) *Genetics of Mental Disorder, a Guide for Students, Clinicians and Researchers*. The Guilford Press, London.

Lenhoff H. M., Wang P. P., Greenberg F. and Bellugi U. (1997) Williams syndrome and the brain. *Scientific American*, **277** (6): 42–47.

Leyten Q. H., Gabreels F. J. M., Renier W. O. and Ter Laak H. J. (1996) Congenital muscular dystrophy: a review of the literature. *Clinical Neurology and Neurosurgery*, **98** (4): 267–280.

McCance K. L., Huether S. E., Brashers V. L. and Rote N. S. (2010) *Pathophysiology, The Biological Basis of Disease in Adults and Children* (6th edition). Elsevier-Mosby, London and Oxford.

Pilz D. T. and Quarrell O. W. J. (1996) Syndromes with lissencephaly. *Journal of Medical Genetics*, **33** (4): 319–323.

Sadock B. J., Sadock V. A. and Ruiz P. (2009) *Kaplin and Sadock's Comprehensive Textbook of Psychiatry* (9th edition). Lippincott, Williams and Wilkins, Baltimore.

Visootsak J., Rosner B., Dykens E., Tartaglia N. and Graham J. M. (2007) Behavioral phenotype of sex chromosome aneuploidies: 48,XXYY, 48,XXXY, and 49,XXXXY. *American Journal of Medical Genetics Part A* **143A** (11): 1198–1203.

7 Pharmacology

- Introduction
- Pharmacokinetics
- Pharmacodynamics
- Pharmacotherapeutics
- Pharmacogenetics
- Key points

Introduction

The study of drugs is called **pharmacology** (*pharm* = drug; *ology* = study of), and involves the chemistry of the agents themselves, their passage through the body (**pharmacokinetics**), how they work in the body (**pharmacodynamics**), how they are used and administered in clinical practice (**pharmacotherapeutics**) and even how they can interact with genes and gene products (**pharmacogenetics**).

Pharmacokinetics means 'drug movement' and documents the passage of drugs through the body, from point of entry to point of exit. Pharmacodynamics studies the way drugs act in the body. A useful, if simplified distinction between pharmacokinetics and pharmacodynamics is that the former looks at *how the body handles the drug*, while the latter looks at *how the drug handles the body*.

Drugs are a major component in mental health treatment. Because nurses are responsible for the delivery of drug therapy it is vital that nurses have a good understanding of why a particular drug is prescribed, how drugs work and how they are administered safely. Henry (2007) and Katzung et al. (2009) are both good general texts on most drug groups including mental health drugs.

The major classes of drugs used in mental health are as follows (each class of drugs is covered in more detail on the pages indicated):

1. **Sedatives** (**hypnotics**) have a calming effect at standard doses, and only cause sleep at higher doses.
2. **Anxiolytics** are anti-anxiety drugs. The word *anxiolytic* means 'anxiety breaking'. *See page 184*
3. **Antipsychotics** alter behaviour without affecting consciousness. *See page 204*
4. **Antidepressants** are drugs used for the relief of depression. *See page 230*
5. **Antimanics** are mood stabilising drugs. *See page 237*
6. **Stimulants** increase brain activity.
7. **Anticonvulsants** are drugs used to prevent fits. *See page 255*

Pharmacokinetics

As noted earlier, pharmacokinetics means 'drug movement', i.e. the passage of drugs through the body, from the point of entry to the point of exit. For example, oral medication is affected by the processes of digestion, absorption, transportation by the blood, liver function, tissue storage and excretion (Sadock and Sadock 2008). These are normally considered in the four stages of pharmacokinetics: **absorption**, **distribution**, **metabolism** and **elimination**.

Absorption is the means by which drugs enter the body, and this varies according to the route of administration. The fastest absorption rate by far is by intravenous (IV) injection, where absorption into the venous blood is instantaneous.

Table 7.1 Routes of drug administration.

Route of administration	Comments
Oral	The most frequently used method of drug administration since it is easy, can be used anywhere (e.g. at home) and is not embarrassing or painful. Absorption is generally very good and within an acceptable time frame. Medication give by this route, however, is the only route subject to **first pass metabolism** (see text).
Intravenous (IV)	Involves injection directly into a vein. Absorption into the blood is therefore instantaneous, but it is often inconvenient and may be painful.
Intramuscular (IM)	Involves injection directly into a muscle. Absorption into the blood is slower than by IV since it requires the blood to collect the drug from the muscle which is acting as a temporary reservoir. **Depot** drugs are exceptionally slow in absorption because the drug is combined with an oil base that inhibits absorption, so the injections only need to be given weekly or even monthly.
Subcutaneous (SC)	Injection of drug given just under the skin into the dermis. Used for administration of slowly absorbed drugs which cannot be given by other means, e.g. insulin, which would be destroyed if given by mouth, and would act far too fast if given by IV or IM injections.
Intrathecal	Injection directly into the spinal canal during a procedure called a lumbar puncture. Not often used except to treat **meningitis** (inflammation of the meninges, the membranes covering the brain).
Rectal	Drugs incorporated into a suppository. Rectal administration is limited in use because of hygienic concerns and it can be embarrassing. It is best used for treating local conditions of the rectum, e.g. constipation. Rarely it is used to give medication for symptoms of system disease where other routes are unavailable.
Inhalation	Inhaled medication directly into the lungs. Useful for treating lung conditions such as asthma. Small quantities of the drug are absorbed into the blood, but this is less than the oral route and therefore causes fewer side-effects.
Topical	Medication rubbed into the skin in ointment or as a cream, or as patches stuck to the skin for long periods. With patches, small amounts are absorbed into circulation gradually, so they need long periods of skin exposure, e.g. over 24 hours, to have a systemic effect. As creams and ointments, topical medication has a great value in treating local skin conditions, e.g. eczema.
Sublingual	Medication given under the tongue, not swallowed. The medication is absorbed directly into the mouth mucosa. The drug usually causes a quick beneficial response via this route.

Intramuscular (IM, direct injection into a muscle) and subcutaneous (SC, an injection just under the skin), and the oral method of administration have much slower rates of absorption. Because it would be impractical to administer all drugs by injection, the oral route becomes the method of choice wherever possible. Table 7.1 considers the various routes of drug administration.

Absorption of drugs from the digestive tract (mostly from the small bowel, or **ileum**) is affected by various factors. Bowel **motility**, the movement of the bowel that pushes the contents along, may vary according to health. Increased motility (as in **diarrhoea**) may prevent most of the absorption because the contents are propelled too quickly through the bowel. The opposite is also true, poor bowel motility (as in **constipation**), may prevent absorption as drug **transit**, i.e. movement through the bowel, is slowed down. **Vomiting** prevents drug absorption since oral drugs will be expelled too quickly if vomiting occurs soon after the drug is taken. Under normal bowel conditions, different drugs get absorbed differently. Lipid (fat) based drugs absorb better than water-based drugs. The reason for this is that lipid drugs can pass through the cell membrane (which is also lipid) more easily than water based drugs. Non-lipid drugs have to find a water channel in the membrane in order to pass through, and this delays absorption. Charged particle drugs (i.e. those with positive and negative charges, called **polar** molecules) are not as well absorbed as non-polar molecules. Drugs are best absorbed at their own **pH**, thus acid drugs are mostly absorbed from the stomach, and alkaline drugs are best absorbed from alkaline areas of the bowel. Above all, oral medication must survive the digestive process. The fact that so many drugs remain unaffected by digestive enzymes is surprising, and lucky for us, otherwise all drugs would have to be given by injection. Imagine what life would be like if we had to give our painkillers by injection just to stop a headache! Sadly, insulin is one drug that does not survive digestion, and thus must be given by injection.

On absorption, oral drugs pass into the **hepatic portal vein** and are transported to the **liver**. The liver is the main site for drug metabolism, and so a percentage of the absorbed drug will be chemically changed by metabolism as it passes through the liver. This volume of drug changed by the liver occurs *before* any of this drug has reached the general circulation, and therefore *before* the drug has had the chance to do its job. This process of early metabolism by the liver is called **first pass metabolism**, and the percentage of the drug affected varies with different drugs. First pass metabolism only applies to oral medication since administration by injection does not involve the hepatic portal vein. Finally the drug gets into the general circulation from the liver via the **hepatic vein**. The amount of active drug arriving in the general circulation, either directly (by injection) or via the liver (from oral intake), is called the **bioavailability**. Because of variable amounts of first pass metabolism, the bioavailability varies from one drug to the next. The greater the extent of first pass metabolism occurring, the lower the bioavailability. Entry into general circulation is the starting point for distribution.

Distribution describes the manner by which drugs are transported around the body. Most drugs by far are transported in the general blood circulation, but a small number of drugs are transported in the lymph. When drugs arrive in the blood plasma most are rapidly bound to blood proteins. The commonest protein in the blood is **albumin**, so most drugs bind to this. A few drugs bind to specific proteins, such as **glycoproteins**, **lipoproteins** and **gammaglobulins** found in smaller quantities in the blood. A small amount of the drug remains unbound, i.e. dissolved in the plasma. Protein-bound drugs are not available for use, i.e. they are inactive, and therefore temporarily loose their bioavailability, until they are gradually released from the protein. These blood proteins are acting as a kind of drug 'bus', transporting drugs to their site of use, and also creating a drug reservoir. As drugs become detached from the protein they regain their activity, i.e. they become bioavailable (Figure 7.1).

Target tissues are those cells on which the drugs have an effect. **Non-target tissues** are those cells unaffected by the drug. So **psychoactive** drugs will have an effect on the brain (their target tissue), but have no effect on other organs, such as bones or the bowel (non-target organs). Tissues are regarded as target or non-target depending on the presence or absence of **receptors** on the cell surface that can bind the drug. If the tissue has receptors on the cell surface that bind a specific drug that tissue becomes a target for that drug.

Drugs entering the tissues from circulation may be further bound to tissue protein (e.g. muscle) or tissue fat (e.g. adipose). This binding creates another tissue reservoir and again temporarily removes the drug's bioavailability until the drug is gradually released from that reservoir. This drug reservoir storage is dependent on the amount of muscle and adipose present in the tissues, and these change slowly with age. So the elderly and children store drugs differently from the average adult.

Metabolism

Metabolism is the chemical alteration, or **biotransformation**, of drugs prior to removal from the body. This is necessary in the vast majority of cases because the drug, as administered, is not suitable for excretion as it stands. Drugs often need to be made more **hydrophilic**, i.e. more water soluble (hydrophilic means *water-liking*). The best absorbed drugs are lipid (fat-based) drugs, but we excrete water, not fat, so a change is necessary. There is also a need to make the active drug less active, so again some chemical change is necessary. The final result of these chemical changes is known as a **metabolite** (metabolite = end product of metabolic change). The metabolite is the usual product for excretion.

So the usual scenario for most drugs is:

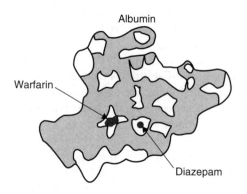

Figure 7.1 Drugs binding to albumin. This simplified and stylised albumin molecule is binding diazepam and warfarin at different sites. See also Figure 7.6.

Active drug → metabolism → inactive metabolite.

However, a few variations do occur, such as:

Active drug → metabolism → active metabolite.

Here, because the metabolite is also active, it carries on the function of the original drug until excreted. Another variation is:

Inactive drug (called a **prodrug**) → metabolism → active metabolite (often considered to be the drug).

The vast majority of drug metabolism occurs in the liver. Much smaller amounts of metabolism may occur in circulation or in the kidney. Liver metabolism uses **enzyme systems** (several enzyme working together) which, like a conveyer belt system, carry out chemical changes on the original drug. Two main phases of liver metabolism are:

- **Phase I**, the biotransformation of a drug to a more **polar** metabolite (polar meaning to give it an electrostatic charge which allows it to blend better with water: water molecules themselves being polar), which then becomes easier to excrete through the kidneys. This phase uses enzyme systems, particularly a system known as **cytochrome P-450** (**CYP**, or **P450**) which is involved in the metabolism of many drugs. In humans, these enzymes are proteins found on the inner membranes of **mitochondria** or in the **endoplasmic reticulum** (**ER**) of cells. Mitochondria and the endoplasmic reticulum are cellular components involved in metabolism. The CYP enzyme system is involved in about 75 per cent of drug metabolism.
- **Phase II**, the **conjugation** of the drug, or end product of phase I, with an endogenous substance. Conjugation means joining one substance (the drug or phase I product) with a second substance (mostly a natural product of the liver). This reduces the activity of most drugs.

Elimination of drugs is mostly through the **renal system**, i.e. the **kidneys**, where the drug metabolites become a component of urine. Far less often, some drugs may be eliminated through the bowel in faeces, or very rarely through the skin in perspiration and in breast milk. Anaesthetic gases are mostly eliminated though the lungs during exhalation.

Renal excretion requires the drug metabolites to have some specific properties. First, the metabolites must be water soluble in order to mix with the urine. Fat soluble substances cannot become a component of urine. Second, the metabolite molecular size must be small enough to pass through the holes in the **glomerular membrane** of the **nephron**. These holes are about 3nm (nanometres) in diameter, so any molecules larger than this may have problems being filtered.

The rate of metabolism and the rate of excretion are the main factors that determine a drug's **half-life**. Half-life is the standard time it takes for the body to repeatedly clear 50 per cent of the blood plasma concentration of a drug. The half-life is best explained using a diagram so consider the following example as illustrated in Figure 7.2.

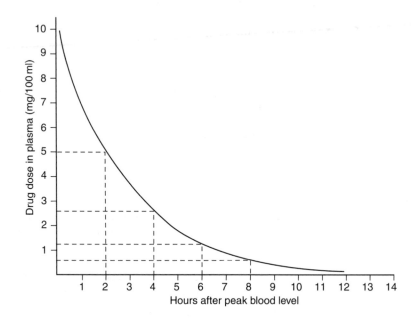

Figure 7.2 Illustration of a drug half-life. In this example, the drug half-life is two hours. By two hours after peak blood level, metabolism has removed 50 per cent of the drug from the plasma (in this case, from 10mg/100ml to 5mg/100ml). By a further two hours, 50 per cent of the remaining drug (5mg/100ml) is removed (down to 2.5mg/100ml). By another two hours again, 50 per cent of the remaining drug (2.5mg/100ml) is removed (down to 1.25mg/100ml) and so on.

Drug X has reached maximum plasma concentration (regarded as 100 per cent) a short time after consumption. Drug X has a half-life of two hours, which means that over the first two hours from this peak concentration the drug plasma concentration is reduced to half (50 per cent). Over the second period of two hours (up to four hours from peak concentration), this 50 per cent plasma concentration will be reduced by half (half of 50 per cent is 25 per cent). Over the third period of two hours (now up to six hours from the peak plasma concentration), the plasma concentration will again be reduced by half (half of 25 per cent is 12.5 per cent), and so on. The liver is removing the drug from the blood for metabolism, and the kidneys are removing the metabolites from the blood for excretion. The half-life of drugs varies widely, with some drugs having *very short* half-lives (less than one hour), or *short* half-lives (one to six hours), or *intermediate* half lives (six to twelve hours) or *long* half-lives (twelve to twenty-four hours), or *very long* half-lives (more than twenty-four hours). This has pharmacotherapeutic implications, because generally shorter half-life drugs may need to be given more often (possibly several times a day) whilst longer half-life drugs are given less frequently (possibly once daily).

If a drug metabolite cannot be excreted through the renal system into the urine, the alternative is excretion from the bowel in the faeces. The metabolite leaves the liver in the **bile**, i.e. via the bile duct into the duodenum. From here it goes through the digestive tract and gets incorporated in the faeces. However, the bowel is the organ of absorption, so some of the metabolite will be reabsorbed back into the hepatic portal vein and return to the liver. The metabolite is again put into the bile, and passes into the bowel. So a 'bowel→liver→bowel' cycle (the **enterohepatic cycle**) is set up, but with each cycle a small percentage of the metabolite is excreted (Figure 7.3). In this way the amount of drug metabolite in the body is gradually reduced with each cycle until zero or only a trace remains.

Pharmacodynamics

Pharmacodynamics is the study of the way drugs act in the body. Psychotropic drugs (i.e. those that act on the brain) work by altering the brain chemistry; mostly by acting on receptors or on ion channels.

Drugs acting on receptors

Receptors are present on brain cell surfaces to bind with the naturally produced chemicals called **neurotransmitters** and **neuromodulators**. *See page 50*

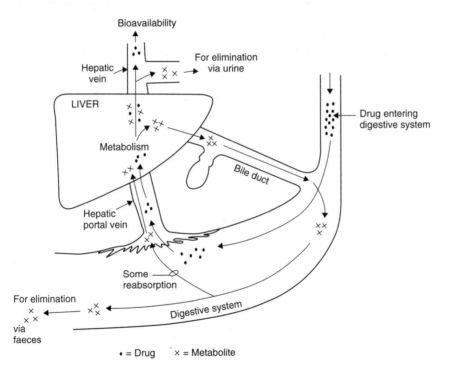

Figure 7.3 The enterohepatic cycle. Drug entering the digestive system from oral ingestion is absorbed and removed to the liver via the hepatic portal vein. First pass metabolism partly reduces this dose, producing some metabolite for excretion. Normally the metabolite would pass into general circulation and be excreted from the kidneys. Non-metabolised drug enters the general circulation, and is known as the bioavailability. Occasionally the kidneys cannot excrete the metabolite so the liver must excrete it through the bile. This is emptied into the digestive system and thus excreted in the faeces. Some reabsorption of the metabolite will take place from the bowel back to the liver, which then recycles it via the bile once again. Each bowel-liver cycle reduces the amount reabsorbed by a small quantity.

These chemicals act by binding to the receptor and then triggering a sequence of changes within the cell. These changes can be made rapidly through **ionotropic** receptors, or over a longer period of time through **metabotropic** receptors.

See page 58 The changes may also be to increase cellular activity (**excitatory**) or decrease cellular activity (**inhibitory**).

Two main types of drugs act on brain receptors, the **agonists** and the **antagonists**.

Agonist drugs (such as the dopamine agonist **bromocriptine**) bind to specific receptors (bromocriptine binds to dopamine receptors) and stimulate (or activate) these receptors, much as the natural brain chemical (called the **ligand**) does (dopamine is the natural ligand for dopamine receptors) (Figure 7.4).

These drugs are useful supplements for situations where the natural ligand is in low supply or is missing.

Antagonist drugs are sometimes called 'blockers' (e.g. the dopamine antagonist **chlorpromazine**). Antagonists bind to specific receptors (chlorpromazine binds to dopamine receptors) and blocks them without stimulating them. The ligand is prevented from binding. This reduces the activity of the ligand on the receptors significantly, and they are used when activity of these receptors is excessive and therefore causing symptoms (Figure 7.5).

Competitive antagonists are two or more drugs which compete for the same binding site. Each drug usually has a 50 per cent chance of binding, so the therapeutic outcome may be less certain. Because of this, prescribing two drugs at the same time which are competitive antagonists is usually unjustified and would be better avoided.

Partial agonists are drugs which bind to the receptor and activate the receptor but not to the full extent a full agonist or the ligand would do. A simple way

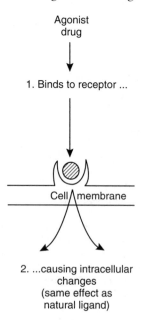

Agonist
drug

1. Binds to receptor ...

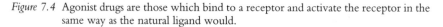

Cell membrane

2. ...causing intracellular
changes
(same effect as
natural ligand)

Figure 7.4 Agonist drugs are those which bind to a receptor and activate the receptor in the same way as the natural ligand would.

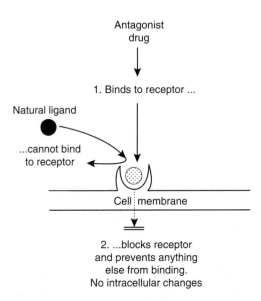

Antagonist
drug

1. Binds to receptor ...

Natural ligand

...cannot bind
to receptor

Cell membrane

2. ...blocks receptor
and prevents anything
else from binding.
No intracellular changes

Figure 7.5 Antagonist drugs are those which bind to a receptor and block it. This does
not activate the receptor and prevents the natural ligand from binding to that
receptor. They are often called 'blockers'.

of looking at this is to say that if the ligand or the full agonist drug activates the
receptor 100 per cent, the partial agonist may only activate the receptor 70 per
cent. This has the effect of not switching the receptor off totally but reducing its
activity. In some respects, partial agonists act similarly to an antagonists because by
preventing the ligand from binding they reduce ligand activity in the brain, just as
antagonists do.

Drugs acting on ion channels

Ion channels exist in nearly all neuronal membranes and when these channels
are open they allow for the passage of an ion in or out of the cell. Ion channels
(especially Na$^+$ and K$^+$ channels) are particularly important during nerve impulse *See page 45*
(**action potential**) transmission along an **axon**.

A range of drugs act on ion channels in the brain to control events such as action
potential transmission. Many of the drugs are **channel blockers**, i.e. they prevent
the passage of the ion through the channel. Typical of this kind of drug are anti- *See page 255*
convulsants such as sodium or calcium channel blockers.

Drugs acting on transport pumps

Some drugs work by blocking (or inhibiting) the action of **pumps** in the cell
membrane.

Some cell activities rely on the transportation of substances, such as neurotransmitters, across the membrane, and this process can be interrupted to change the
balance of these substances in the brain and thus affect brain cell activity. A good

example of this is the use of certain antidepressant drugs which inhibit the membrane pumps at the neuron terminus and therefore increase neurotransmitter in the synapse.

Pharmacotherapeutics

Pharmacotherapeutics is the study of how drugs are used in clinical practice, including prescription, dose calculation, means of administration, patient assessment for reactions and side-effects, drug storage and many other aspects. Those topics discussed here apply to mental health medication as much as any other branch of nursing.

Drugs come in several different forms (see also Table 7.1):

- **Tablets** and **capsules** are probably the most common form of drugs and are taken orally (Table 7.2).
- **Syrups, elixirs, solutions, colloids** and **suspensions** are liquid medications also taken by mouth (Table 7.3).
- **Injectable solutions** are either intravenous (IV), intramuscular (IM), subcutaneous (SC) or **intrathecal (**via a **lumbar puncture)**. Injectable drugs are absorbed quicker than oral drugs and are used for emergencies, and to avoid digestion and first pass metabolism.
- **Inhalations** are sprayed and inhaled directly into the lungs, mostly to treat respiratory conditions.
- **Suppositories** are lubricated and inserted into the rectum, mostly to treat **rectal conditions**.
- **Creams, lotions, ointments** and **patches** are applied directly to the skin, either for the treatment of a skin conditions (**topical** applications) or systemic conditions (e.g. patches).

Table 7.2 Different types of dry oral medication.

Tablets and **powders**	Most commonly prescribed format for medication, each tablet containing a single dose of the drug. Tablets may be **enteric coated** (a coating which allows the medication to survive gastric conditions and be absorbed further into the digestive tract and also to reduce gastric irritation). Others may be soluble in water before drinking (including **powders**). Each sachet of powder contains a single dose of the drug. **Modified-release** tablets contain special inert substances used to modify the rate, the site or the time of release of the active drug.
Capsules	Medication, often in granular format, contained within a soft dissolvable shell. Different granules may have variable time delays in absorption, so an even absorption rate is achieved over several hours (modified release).
Gum	Chewable medication in a gum, the drug is released in the mouth during chewing.
Melts	Medication made in a solid form that dissolves (melts) in the mouth, mainly for oral absorption.

Table 7.3 Different types of liquid medication.

Solutions	A **homogeneous** (i.e. uniform throughout) mixture of two or more substances. One substance is the solvent (often water) and the other is a solute (an agent dissolved in the solvent) e.g. a sodium chloride solution (used in medical practice as **normal saline**, a 0.9 per cent solution of sodium chloride in water).
Colloids	Very small solids (particles that do not dissolve) that remain dispersed in a liquid for a long time due to their small size (less than 1mm) and their electrical charges. These particles take a very long time to settle because their very small masses have extremely low gravitation force. Some colloids are given IV as **plasma expanders**, to boost plasma volume following blood loss.
Suspensions (usually for oral use) and **lotions** (for external use only)	A **heterogeneous** (i.e. made from non-uniform dissimilar components) mixture with relatively large undissolved particles dispersed throughout a liquid. Larger particle size results in settlement of the particles quickly when left to stand. Therefore suspensions must be shaken before use to disperse the particles. An example is a paediatric suspension of paracetamol, a pain-relieving drug. Lotions are aqueous preparations containing a very fine particle insoluble substance. They are for external use only. They often have 'shake well' and 'external use only' labels. An example is calamine lotion.
Elixirs and **syrups**	The active drug is mixed and dissolved in a liquid, either a concentrated sucrose solution (as in syrups) or an aromatic, sweetened hydroalcoholic solution (as in elixirs).

Therapeutic window

The therapeutic window is the dose range that exists from the lowest effective dose of a drug up to a dose where there are more harmful effects than beneficial effects. Below the lowest dose of the window the drug is ineffective and useless. Above the highest dose of the window the drug becomes a threat to health with the potential for severe side-effects and a risk of overdose. Some drugs have a narrow therapeutic window and must be prescribed and administered with caution because it would not be difficult to go above the therapeutic window and cause toxicity. *See page 138*

Drugs are normally given a dose range that falls within this window. Generally, patients are prescribed the lowest dosage within this range at first, and this can then be raised safely at a later time if necessary.

Drug names

All drugs have three types of names:

1. A **chemical name**, based on the chemical structure, used only in science, and never used in clinical practice (i.e. not used on prescriptions). An example is **7-chloro-1, 3-dihydro-1-methyl-5-phenyl-2H-1, 4-benzodiazepin-2-one.**

2. **Official, approved, generic** or **non-proprietary** name, used in clinical practice on prescriptions. Non-proprietary means there is no legal protection by means of a trademark, patent or copyright on this drug name. As such, this name identifies the drug but it does not belong to any particular drug company (see 3, below). The generic name for the example chemical in 1 (above) is **Diazepam**.

3. **Trade, brand** or **proprietary** name, given to the drug by a specific pharmaceutical company who produces it. Proprietary means the drug name is legally protected by a copyright, trademark or patent. Different companies in different countries will give the same drug different trade names. The result is a large collection of trade names worldwide for each separate agent. In the UK, the best known trade name for Diazepam is **Valium**. Trade names are not used on UK NHS prescriptions because of cost implications.

The nurse's role in drug administration

Before any drug is prescribed, a patient assessment is required. The purpose of this assessment is to determine if drugs are necessary, what drugs would be most beneficial to the patient and to check if the patient is able to comply with the treatment regime. The assessment consists of a medical and drug history (including an appraisal of the patient's current medication, if any), an examination of the main physical parameters by clinical observations (especially pulse, blood pressure and respiration), a psychological evaluation to determine the patient's ability to comply with a drug regime safely, and an assessment of the patient's social and cultural background (e.g. is the patient part of a drug addiction culture, or may they have social problems which could interfere with safe drug administration?). A treatment plan is drawn up which sets out not just the pharmacological therapy, but other therapies which are considered beneficial to the patient. The patient's family are probably in the best position to help to ensure compliance with the treatment plan, and are usually eager to help. It is therefore very important to involve the family whenever possible, with the patient's knowledge and agreement, in the planning of a treatment regime. Information on the drugs prescribed, dosage, administration routine, effects and side-effects of the drugs is shared with the patient and the family. The nurse then follows both a monitoring and an advisory role. In the community, monitoring consists of checking daily or weekly to see if the patient is taking the drugs correctly and what improvements or side-effects have occurred. Progress from there depends on what the nurse finds during the monitoring session. The family, again, can assist by giving a progress report and by reporting any problems. In hospital, with 24-hour care, it should be easier for the nurse to check drug compliance and the wanted and unwanted effects of the drugs. For patients on long-term drug regimes, the nurse maintains a liaison role with the patient and their family on all matters concerning the drug therapy. The nurse is often the first line contact for the family as the primary health care provider.

When administering drugs, nurses are expected to ensure the following:

*   That they give the correct drug, according to the prescription;
*   That they give the correct dose, according to the prescription;
*   That they give it to the correct patient;

- That they give it at the correct time, according to the prescription;
- That they give it via the correct route.

Added to this is the need to check these factors with another nurse where possible since this reduces the error risk, and to record the administration on the appropriate documentation.

Nurses are expected to keep drugs safe by:

- Preventing child and confused patients from gaining access to drugs;
- Preventing drug abusers from gaining access to prohibited drugs;
- Ensuring drugs are stored correctly according to the law (in the case of controlled drugs) and according to the instructions given with the medication to prevent deterioration;
- Keeping drugs only while in date;
- Disposing of unwanted and out-of-date drugs safely, usually by returning them to any pharmacy.

DUMP (Disposal of Unwanted Medical Preparations) campaigns are sometimes carried out to encourage people to stop the storage of unwanted drugs at home. In one such campaign, one third of a million tablets and capsules were returned to pharmacies, and over 70 per cent of these were more than a year out of date. On another occasion, in one UK city alone, two and a quarter tonnes of out-of-date medications were returned! Worse than storing these unwanted drugs is flushing them down the sink or toilet. This should never happen, especially in the case of antibiotics, which must *never* be released into the environment.

Dose calculations

It is so important to calculate the correct dosage of medications to prevent potentially dangerous drug errors. Olsen et al. (2010) state that there are four elements to calculating drug dosage accurately:

1. Common sense;
2. Ability to carry out mental arithmetic;
3. Ability to check the answers with a calculator;
4. Understanding the correct formula.

For tablets, the formula for calculation is:

Dose prescribed ÷ stock dose

Here are two simple examples:

1. Six milligrams (6mg) of the drug is prescribed, but the tablets kept in stock are 2mg each. The number of tablets to be given is: $6 \div 2 = 3$ tablets.
2. One gram (1g) of the drug is prescribed, but the tablets are 500mg each. First convert grams to milligrams (1g = 1000mg) so that you are working in the same units throughout the calculation (in this case it's milligrams). Never

work in mixed units since this makes the answer to the calculation meaning-less. The number of tablets to be given is:

$1000 \div 500 = 2$ tablets.

For liquids, the formula for calculation is:

(Dose prescribed ÷ stock dose) × stock volume

Two simple examples:

1. Fifteen milligrams (15mg) of the liquid drug is prescribed, the stock syrup is 10mg per 2 millilitres (2ml). The volume of syrup to be given is:

    $(15 \div 10) \times 2.$

    Always do the bracket part of the calculation first, which in this case is (1.5), then remove the brackets to complete the calculation, e.g.

    $1.5 \times 2 = 3ml.$

    [A quick check of accuracy is possible: in this case 2ml is too little (only 10mg), but 4ml is too much (20mg), so the answer falls between 2ml and 4ml, i.e. 3ml].
2. Prescribed: 250mg, stock dose is 100mg per 1ml. The volume of syrup to be given is:

    $(250 \div 100) \times 1$

    Doing the bracket part first gives:

    $2.5 \times 1 = 2.5ml.$

    [Quick check, 250mg to give: 1ml of syrup is 100mg (not enough), 2ml = 200mg (still not enough), 3ml = 300mg (too much); so the result must be between 2ml and 3ml, i.e. 2.5ml.]

Always state the units in the answer (i.e. mg or ml). Simply giving a number with no units is potentially confusing.

Polypharmacy and drugs in the elderly

Polypharmacy means that multiple different types of drugs are prescribed at the same time. Generally, it is better to prescribe as few types of drugs together as pos-sible, and to leave a time gap, often several days, when switching from one drug to another. This time gap allows the body an opportunity to fully excrete the first drug before starting the second. Unfortunately this is not always possible, and it is not unusual to find two or three drugs prescribed together. It should be remembered that polypharmacy also occurs when a single drug is prescribed but the patient decides to take additional drugs for themselves, such as a headache remedy or even drugs of addiction. Polypharmacy increases the risk of drug interactions and side-effects, and this is why it is better avoided when possible. Also, with polypharmacy, some patients may get drugs muddled up and start taking the wrong drug at the wrong time, increasing the risk of serious drug errors. Since the elderly are prescribed more drugs than any other age group, and they can get confused more often than younger people, they carry the biggest risk of serious drug errors, side-effects and interactions. Multiple drugs may also be stored badly, labelled poorly or not at all, and even in some cases mixed up in a single container. When this happens, multiple drugs stored together make it easier to forget individual drug administration times and also often mean drugs are kept long after their expiry dates. With some patients, drug compliance is a problem when only one drug is involved, so the problem of compliance is compounded by the prescription of several drugs together. All this turns safe administration of drugs into a nightmare.

The incidence of drug reactions and interactions, and drug-related mortalities increases with age. About 10 per cent of UK elderly admissions to hospital are due to drug reactions, and the commonest drug groups involved are cardiac drugs (e.g. digoxin) and drugs for the central nervous system (e.g. antidepressants). The elderly don't always provide an accurate drug history during examination, and rely on relatives to fill in any gaps in their memory. A confused and poor drug history makes diagnosis difficult. Confusion can be a side effect of the some drugs, so it may be prudent to stop the drugs and wait until they have been eliminated before examination, diagnosis and further prescription.

Drug reactions in the elderly are usually due to:

1. Over prescription, some patients accumulating 10 or more different drugs;
2. Inadequate review of long-term medication;
3. Inadequate clinical assessment;
4. Altered pharmacokinetics due to age and disease;
5. Complicated drug regimes leading to impaired drug compliance.

Poor compliance in the elderly is a big problem. About 75 per cent of elderly patients make mistakes in drug administration. Some 25 per cent of these mistakes are dangerous, life-threatening errors. The reasons for poor drug compliance are:

1. As symptoms improve the patient stops taking the drug as they feel it is not required anymore. This is a big problem, especially with antibiotics since they must complete the course of medication.
2. Poor eyesight means they cannot read the labels and may resort to guessing, or stopping the drug.
3. Inadequate explanation given about taking the drug when it's first prescribed (e.g. a good number of elderly patients fail to remove the wrapper from suppositories before use). It may be beneficial for this information to be written down and displayed in a prominent position.
4. Drugs may be difficult to swallow or taste bitter, or they may cause unpleasant side-effects, and these problems may cause the patient to stop taking them.
5. Some drug containers are childproof, and as a result are often elderly-proof as well, especially if they have arthritic fingers.
6. Some patients will always simply forget to take their medication.

Preplanning and discussion with the patient and their relatives is required when drugs are prescribed, to ensure the patient is fully aware of the nature of the drug and its potential side-effects. A series of drug reviews should be scheduled at regular time periods (e.g. weekly) to enable the patient to get the greatest benefit from the prescribed medication. The following is a guide to safer drug administration in the elderly:

1. Prescribe the least number of drugs possible at any one time, generally no more than three, and at the lowest effective dose. The starting dose should be kept at a minimum at first, but can be increased later if necessary when it can be confirmed that the patient is not reacting to the drug (Labbate et al. 2010).
2. Don't add any more drugs to the original prescription at a later date unless they are essential, and if another drug is required, consider which drug to stop first in order to keep to the maximum of three.
3. Monitor the drugs weekly, checking particularly for drug compliance and side-effects.
4. Patient and relatives should be aware of potential side-effects so they can check daily, and should know what to do about them.
5. Ensure the administration details are easily readable and displayed in a relevant place, e.g. in large print, and maybe fixed to the front of the drugs cabinet.

Changes in the body as we get older affect the pharmacokinetics of drugs, so these changes must be allowed for when prescribing medication. The elderly have increased gastric pH (i.e. less acid) and less gut movement (reduced **motility**) and lower blood flow to the stomach. These changes affect the absorption of drugs given by mouth. However, despite these changes the elderly generally tolerate oral drugs well. Diseases or disturbances of the gastrointestinal system, including vomiting and diarrhoea, may seriously disturb drug absorption rates. Diarrhoea often involves an increase in gut transit times, i.e. the bowel contents are propelled through the gut faster. This includes any oral medication, much of which may be eliminated before it is absorbed. Changes in the structural tissues of the body result in an overall reduction in body weight, and this also includes a reduction in the total body water content. Water-soluble drugs are eliminated quicker because of this reduced water content, and these drugs will then have a shorter half-life. Stored lipids in adipose tissue increase with age, and this changes the lean to fat ratio, and this has implications for drug storage in the tissues.

There are variations in this ratio between the sexes, with females generally storing more adipose than males. Increased storage of fat-soluble drugs in adipose delays excretion and lengthens the drug half-life. Plasma albumin falls with age and this reduces the protein binding of drugs and increases the bioavailability due to increased amounts of free drug in circulation. Lower cardiac output in the elderly slightly delays drug distribution and this favours an increase in plasma drug levels. Reduced liver mass and less blood flow through the liver with increasing age causes slower enzyme activity and reduced drug metabolism (increasing the drug half-life). The overall effect of all these changes is generally to increase the amount of active drug in the blood. These are the normal changes expected with growing old, but if you add disease states to this picture the changes become truly significant.

With increased levels of active drug in the body, taking additional doses creates a serious risk of drug accumulation in the body.

Renal elimination of drugs is reduced as renal function declines. Reduced glomerular filtration will increase the drug half-life because the drugs and metabolites are then retained in circulation. If multiple drugs are prescribed some of these drugs may compete for excretion through **tubular secretion** (the third stage of urine production) and those that lose this competition are delayed in their elimination, further lengthening their half-lives.

Drug interactions

Drug interactions are unwanted effects caused by one drug acting against another when more than one drug is administered.

See page 134

Interactions can occur not only between prescribed drugs, but when only one drug is prescribed but the patient decides also to take an *over-the-counter* medication. A typical scenario may be a patient who takes their prescribed medication then shortly after decides to take an aspirin for headache. The self-prescribed aspirin may interact with the prescribed medication. Also, drug interactions can occur between a prescribed or self-prescribed drug and substances consumed on a regular basis such as nicotine, alcohol or caffeine. It is common for patients to smoke and drink alcohol or coffee, and this introduces more drugs into the system which can then interact with the prescribed drugs. It is often the case that prescribed medication information leaflets warn patients not to drink whilst taking the medicines. In the case of drug abuse, patients run a high risk of interaction if they continue to abuse drugs whilst taking prescribed or over-the-counter medication.

Drug interactions fall into two main categories: those that occur during pharmacokinetics, and those that occur during pharmacodynamics.

Pharmacokinetic interactions occur during absorption, distribution, metabolism or elimination of drugs. During absorption, competition between drugs for absorption sites may mean that one medication is delayed in absorption, and this will affect its activity in the body. During distribution, one drug may compete for protein binding with another drug, and so one may displace the other drug from its binding site. This increases the activity of the displaced drug (because it is now free) but delays the activity of the competing drug (because it is now protein bound) (Figure 7.6).

The greatest risk is of interactions occurs during metabolism. Drugs may compete for the enzyme systems that process them.

See page 122

If the enzyme system is busy processing one drug (call it drug A), a second drug (call it drug B) may have to wait its turn to be processed. This lengthens the half-life of drug B and it will continue to perform its functions longer than expected. If then a second dose of drug B is administered, this overlap in dosage could raise the blood level to the maximum of the therapeutic window or above, and cause an accidental overdose.

Many drugs activate enzymes (a process called **enzyme induction**) or increase or reduce enzyme activity in the liver. Either way, one drug (call it drug C) may significantly influence the metabolism of another drug (call it drug D) by the process of enzyme induction, causing changes in the activity, half-life and excretion of drug D (Figure 7.7).

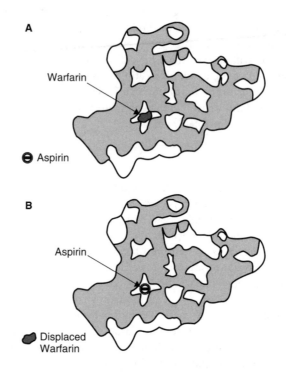

Figure 7.6 Pharmacokinetic interaction involving competitive binding during distribution. Here the stylised albumin molecule in A binds the drug warfarin. Aspirin has arrived in circulation. In B the aspirin has displaced and replaced the warfarin which is now unbound. Each free drug molecule increases the activity of the medication (in this case the warfarin), but in practice this activity increase is minimal given that free drug is excreted quickly, and that it is diluted rapidly because it is distributed throughout the circulation.

Pharmacodynamic interactions

See page 128

Drugs may compete with each other for the same receptor binding sites at the point of activity. Competitive antagonists are an example of this (Figure 7.8).

Two competing agonists would enhance each other's activity and therefore give a greater effect than expected, possibly to the point of toxicity.

Two drugs with opposite effects to each other may just cancel each other out and become ineffectual. A few pharmacodynamic drug interactions are beneficial, but by far the majority, at best, cancel each other out, and at worst can be harmful or even fatal.

Toxicology and side-effects

Toxicology is the scientific study of the effects of toxic chemical agents (poisons) on the human body. Toxicology covers not just drugs but any chemical agents taken into the body, e.g. the accidental ingestion of a detergent or bleach by children. The toxic effects of drugs are known as **pharmacotoxicology**. Drugs are most likely to cause toxic effects in the upper range of their therapeutic window

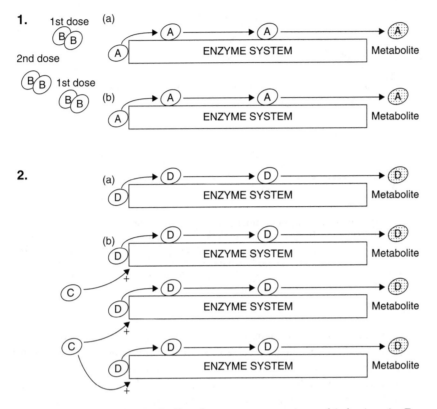

Figure 7.7 Drug interaction in the liver by enzyme occupation and induction. 1a. Drug A is being metabolised by the enzyme system, whilst drug B metabolism is delayed, which prolongs drug B's half-life. 1b. A second dose of drug B causes the potential for an overdose. In 2a, drug D is occupying a minimal amount of the enzyme system. In 2b, the arrival of drug C activates further enzyme systems which increases the metabolism of drug D, thus shortening its half-life.

and in **overdose** (dosages above the therapeutic window), but any dose of a drug can cause a rapid and unexpected toxic effect in susceptible people. The term **side-effects** would be used to describe unwanted, unpleasant adverse symptoms occurring as a result of drug consumption at normal dosage. They are usually mild and mostly cause no lasting harm, but toxic effects (or toxic reactions) are sudden, serious effects on the body, usually as a result of high dosage, which are potentially harmful or even life threatening.

Side-effects are the result of the drug acting on parts of the body it was not intended to act on. An example of this is the dopamine antagonist chlorpromazine. Ideally this should block receptors in the brain pathways known as the **mesocortical** and **mesolimbic** pathways, but unfortunately it also blocks receptors in the **nigrostriatal** pathway, and this causes unwanted side effects involving difficulties with movement.

Side-effects may be the reason for patient non-compliance and this should be considered when patients refuse to take their medication. Side-effects are often mild, and they may reduce in severity over a period of time without any need for

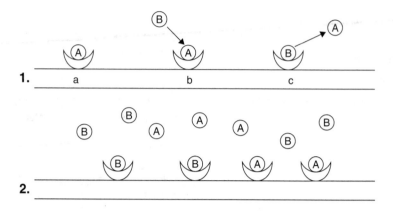

Figure 7.8 Pharmacodynamic interactions at a receptor. In 1a, drug A occupies the receptor. In 1b, drug B challenges drug A for receptor occupancy. In 1c, drug B has replaced drug A at the receptor, shortening the active period of drug A In 2a, a mix of drugs A and B, both being equal competitors for the receptors, results in some receptors being occupied with drug A, others with drug B. The result could be a doubling of the effect (if they both had similar activity) or a cancellation of the effect (if they had opposing actions).

intervention. If they are unpleasant enough, the patient should seek medical advice so the drug dose may be safely reduced, or so that another drug can be substituted. There should be no need to put up with unpleasant side-effects.

With toxic reactions the drug must be stopped immediately and urgent medical intervention obtained. Very severe reactions may require life-support measures and investigations may be necessary to determine the liver and renal function. Overdose from ingested drugs often requires measures to be taken to recover as much drug from the body as possible, e.g. a **gastric lavage**, also known as a stomach washout. The action of some drugs can be reversed by giving a second drug, e.g the effects of morphine can be reversed with the drug **naloxone**.

Tolerance, dependence, addiction and withdrawal

Tolerance means that over a period of time on a specific drug, the effects of this drug gradually diminish, and the patient finds the need to slightly increase the dosage every so often to get the same beneficial effect. Of course, increasing the dosage means a higher risk of side-effects and a step closer to achieving a toxic dose. Tolerance may be due to changes in the cell surface receptors that bind the drug. Over a period of time taking the same drug, the surface receptors decrease in number (a process called **down-regulation**), so with fewer receptors the cell binds less drug. One course of action, which may prove better than increasing the dose, is to stop the drug altogether for a few days whenever possible (sometimes known as a '**drug holiday**'). The exceptions to this are antibiotics, where it is important to complete the course. A few days without the drug encourages the cells to replace the receptors (called **up-regulation**).

Dependence occurs over a long period of time when the drug becomes an everyday part of normal life, because stopping the drug would mean that

withdrawal symptoms then occur. Withdrawal symptoms are usually very unpleasant (e.g. headache, vomiting, sometimes fits) and the drugs are taken to avoid these, i.e. taken just to feel normal. Sometimes you hear people say, 'I can't do anything in the morning until I have had my cup of coffee.' This is a form of caffeine dependence.

Addiction is when drugs are taken repeatedly for the purpose of mental pleasure and euphoria. One such experience promotes a repeat of this experience. After a number of repeated doses, failure to take the drug results in an unpleasant low state of mind, akin to depression, which the addict tries to avoid by taking more drugs. Therefore, both dependence and addiction promote legal or illegal drug-seeking behaviour but for different reasons. Occurrence of addiction varies according to different drugs (some cause addiction faster than others), but generally addiction occurs over a shorter time span than dependence.

Pharmacogenetics

This is the study of how genetic variation between people causes different responses to drugs. It has been known for many years that no two people respond alike to the same dose of the same drug, but it has always been hard to explain why. Now, recent advances in genetics have revealed that because everyone has a unique set of genes they respond to drugs in a unique manner. This applies to any one individual and to any race. There are clinical implications attached to this research because is shows that no single drug, even at identical dosage, will have the same impact on everyone. Drug treatments must be tailor made for each individual, with the drugs and dosage that are best for them. This indicates that careful assessments combined with a sound knowledge of drugs are critical prerequisites for prescribing drugs.

Key points

Pharmacokinetics

- Pharmacokinetics is the study of the way drugs pass through the body from the point of entry to the point of exit.
- First-pass metabolism reduces the dose of many drugs given by mouth but does not affect drugs given by injection.
- The bioavailablity is the amount of drugs arriving in general circulation after first-pass metabolism.
- The half-life is the time it takes to reduce the blood concentration of a drug by 50 per cent over the first half-life period, by 75 per cent over the period to the end of the second half-life, by 87.5 per cent over the period to the end of the third half-life period and so on.
- Most drugs are metabolised by the liver and excreted through the kidneys.
- Liver and renal disease will affect drug half-lives.

Pharmacodynamics

- Pharmacodynamics is the study of the way drugs act in the body.
- An agonist is a drug which binds to a receptor and activates that receptor.

- An antagonist (or 'blocker') is a drug which binds to a receptor but does not activate that receptor. Instead, it prevents the natural ligand from activating that receptor.

Pharmacotherapeutics

- It is so important to calculate the correct dosage of medications to prevent dangerous drug errors.
- Dosage may be affected by the lean-to-fat ratio which can change with age, and by liver or kidney disease.
- The therapeutic window is the dose range from the lowest effective dose of a drug up to the dose where there are more harmful effects than beneficial effects.
- Patients should be warned of the commonest side-effects and given information on what to do if side-effects occur.
- Drugs should never be kept or used after the 'use by' date, and should be disposed of safely by returning them to the pharmacy.
- Weekly or monthly drug reviews should be part of standard care.
- As few drugs as possible, and certainly no more than three drugs, should be given at a time to prevent drug interactions.

Pharmacogenetics

- This is the study of how genetic variation between people causes different responses to drugs.

References

Blows W. T. (2001) *The Biological Basis of Nursing: Clinical Observations.* Routledge, London.

Henry J. A. (Editor) (2007) *New Guide to Medicines and Drugs.* British Medical Association, Dorling Kindersley, London and New York.

Katzung B. G., Masters S. B. and Trevor A. J. (2009) *Basic and Clinical Pharmacology* (11th edition). McGraw-Hill Companies, New York and London.

Labbate L. A., Fava M., Rosenbaum J. F. and Arana G. W. (2010) *Handbook of Psychiatric Drug Therapy.* Lippincott Williams and Wilkins, Philadelphia.

Olsen J. L., Giangrasso A. P., Shrimpton D. M., Dillon P. M. and Cunningham S. (2010) *Dosage Calculations for Nurses.* Pearson Education Limited, Harlow and London.

Sadock B. J. and Sadock V. A. (2008) *Kaplan and Sadock's Concise Textbook of Clinical Psychiatry* (3rd edition). Lippincott, Williams and Wilkins, Baltimore.

8   Drug abuse

- **The reward pathways of the brain**
- **The opiate drugs**
- **Cocaine, amphetamines and other dopamine-enhancing drugs**
- **Cannabinoids**
- **Alcohol**
- **Nicotine and caffeine**
- **The hallucinogenic drugs**
- **Key points**

The reward pathways of the brain

One of the major quests in brain research over the past ten years or so has been to try to identify the neurological areas involved in euphoria and pleasure. This endeavour has met with some success and has resulted in the identification of some areas of the brain involved in drug addiction. As with many other functions of the brain, the so-called **reward centres** are not one or two isolated areas but rather appear to be several centres linked by reward pathways involving mostly dopamine as the neurotransmitter.

See page 20, Table 1.2

Important areas stand out as reward centres, in particular the **medial forebrain bundle**, which links the **ventral tegmental area** of the midbrain with the **nucleus accumbens** (Figure 8.1). This pathway forms part of a larger system called the **mesotelencephalic dopamine system** (Figure 8.1). The nuclei in the brain stem, from which the neurons of the mesotelencephalic system arise, are the ventral tegmental area and the substantia nigra. Apart from the nucleus accumbens, the system serves other nuclei, notably the **septum** and the **prefrontal cortex** and two other important areas of the brain, the **limbic cortex** and **amygdala** (see Chapter 1). This dopamine pathway is strongly implicated in many self-administered stimulatory drug effects, including those of the opiates and amphetamines, and is therefore of great importance in drug abuse research. The ventral tegmental area is involved in behavioural arousal, and activation of this centre causes dopamine to be released from the synapses of the medial forebrain bundle. This dopamine binds to receptors at the nucleus accumbens, causing further activity. One such receptor, the **A1 receptor** (a variety of dopamine 2 receptor), if present, increases the risk of addiction, especially to alcohol. Like all receptors, its presence or absence depends on inheritance: the

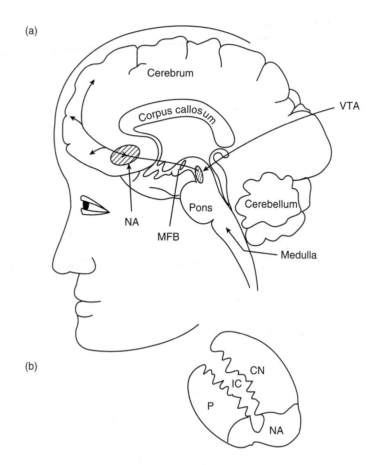

Figure 8.1 (a) Lateral view of a mid-section of the brain showing the medial forebrain bundle (MFB) extending from the ventral tegmental area (VTA) to the nucleus accumbens (NA). (b) The nucleus accumbens in association with the caudate nucleus (CN), internal capsule (IC) and the putamen (P).

gene that codes for the A1 receptor can be passed between generations of the same family, or may be absent entirely from a family. Alcoholic fathers who have the gene can pass it to their children, who may therefore develop a higher risk of alcoholism.

Other brain areas involved in the reward mechanisms, and therefore reinforcing pleasure-seeking activity, are the septum (a site of sexual pleasure, optimism, euphoria and happiness), the temporal lobes of the cerebrum and parts of the hypothalamus (Figure 8.2). The septum, as well as the nucleus accumbens, also receives input from the ventral tegmental area via the medial forebrain bundle. This bundle also carries connections linking the substantia nigra (in the midbrain) with the nucleus accumbens (Figure 8.2). All of these connections are dopaminergic and stimulation of either the ventral tegmental area or parts of the substantia nigra causes an increase in dopamine levels in the nucleus accumbens during a sensation of euphoria or pleasure. It should not be a surprise, therefore, to find that many stimulant and addictive drugs are those that cause high dopamine levels to occur in the brain and in the nucleus accumbens in particular.

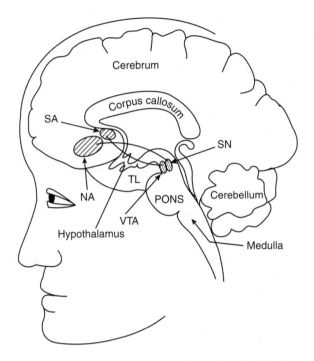

Figure 8.2 Same view as in Figure 8.1a showing the main pathways from the substantia nigra (SN) to the nucleus accumbens (NA), and from the ventral tegmental area (VTA) to the septal area (SA). TL is the temporal lobe.

Drug addiction has become the subject of increasing genetic research, especially alcoholism. Interest grew in this area mainly because of the individual variations shown by people in response to drugs, a phenomenon which is most likely to have a genetic basis. More information will become available as work continues in this new area of research.

The opiate drugs

These drugs are derived from **opium**, a resin obtained from the opium poppy. The best-known examples of the opiate derivatives are **morphine, heroin, pethidine** and **methadone**. They are all potentially addictive and dangerous; morphine and heroin together killed 754 people in the United Kingdom in 1999 and 897 people in 2008.

Opiates (the word refers to the drugs) act on specific opioid receptors (opioid = 'like opium', the word refers to the endogenous neurotransmitters), which occur mostly in the upper parts of the spinal cord and the brain stem. These receptors are called **mu** (μ), **delta** (δ) and **kappa** (κ). Opioid receptors are metabotropic, involving the activation of the secondary messenger cAMP via a G-protein coupling mechanism.

See page 59

Opiate drugs cause a number of different effects on both the body and the mind, including analgesia, euphoria, sedatory and depressant effects. The effect of most importance in drug addiction is the euphoria and the feeling of well-being these drugs induce, as this is the reason that people take them. The exact mechanism by which this effect is achieved is not fully known, but it appears to be mediated through binding primarily to the mu receptor at the ventral tegmental area (VTA). At the same time, activity on this receptor causes the classic analgesic effects and reinforces drug-seeking behaviour. This mu receptor binding at the VTA also causes release of dopamine into the nucleus accumbens. Dopaminergic neurons of the medial forebrain bundle are inhibited by a GABA-mediated system within the ventral tegmental area. Opiate drugs reduce this inhibition, allowing dopamine to be released in the nucleus accumbens (Figure 8.3). Morphine binds mostly to the mu receptor and least of all to the delta receptor, whilst pethidine also has its greatest activity on the mu receptor. Heroin (diamorphine) is made from morphine but is more lipid-soluble and more potent than its parent molecule. Long-term use of morphine and heroin causes damage to the immune system, making addicts more susceptible to infections.

Opiate addiction, as with other drugs, leads to two problems encountered by the addict. One is **withdrawal**, a set of unpleasant symptoms that occurs within hours of abstinence from the drug and can last up to three or more days. Symptoms include hot and cold flushes, loss of appetite, muscle cramps, tremor, nausea,

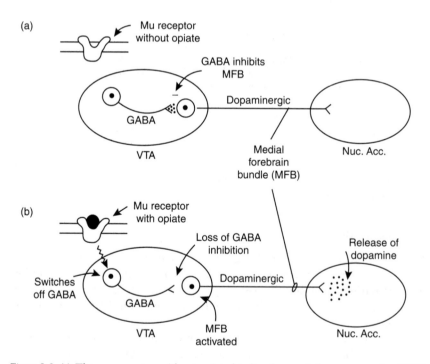

Figure 8.3 (a) The mu receptor without opiate binding has no influence over the GABA neurons of the ventral tegmental area (VTA). These neurons therefore inhibit the dopaminergic neurons of the medial forebrain bundle (MFB), which pass from the VTA to the nucleus accumbens (Nuc. Acc.). (b) Opiates binding to mu receptors switch off the GABA neurons, thus removing the GABA inhibition, and the MFB becomes activated, causing release of dopamine in the nucleus accumbens.

vomiting and insomnia. Physical changes include increased heart rate and blood pressure and raised respiration rate and body temperature. While drugs are sought and taken initially for their euphoric effect (positive symptoms), drug-seeking behaviour is reinforced by the need to avoid the unpleasant effects of withdrawal (negative symptoms). This change from *nondependent* drug seeking for pleasure to *dependent* drug seeking for prevention of withdrawal could be the result of a shift in the activation of different parts of the brain. While the neurological basis of euphoria appears to be located primarily within the mesotelencephalic dopamine system, the neurological basis of withdrawal appears to be the result of activity of another pathway, the '**extended amygdala**'. This consists of the **amygdala central medial nucleus**, part of the **stria terminalis**, part of the nucleus accumbens and the **sublenticular substantia innominata** (Figure 8.4). This system has connections with other parts of the brain through inputs (afferents) and outputs (efferents), as shown in Figure 8.4. Studies of the neurochemistry during withdrawal have indicated reduced levels of both dopamine and serotonin in the brain, i.e. *down-regulation* of these systems, and increased levels (*up-regulation*) of **corticotrophin-releasing factor** (**CRF**) (Koob 2000). CRF is probably best known as the hormone from the hypothalamus that enters the pituitary gland and controls the release of one of the anterior pituitary hormones called **adrenocorticotropic**

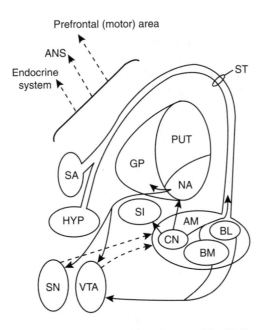

Figure 8.4 Pathways of the extended amygdala. The amygdala (AM) main nuclei are the central nucleus (CN), the basolateral nucleus (BL) and the basomedial nucleus (BM). Part of the stria terminalis (ST), which links the amygdala with the septal area (SA) and the hypothalamus (HYP), is involved, along with the sublenticular substantia innominata (SI), the nucleus accumbens (NA), the substantia nigra (SN), the ventral tegmental area (VTA) and the globus pallidus (GP). This system influences the prefrontal motor area (motor planning), the autonomic nervous system (ANS) and the endocrine system, the last two through the hypothalamus. PUT is the putamen.

hormone (ACTH). It is also, however, a neurotransmitter of the limbic system and is involved in emotions and stress (see Chapter 9), and in withdrawal from drugs (Carlson 2010). The mechanism involving CRF in drug craving during withdrawal is not fully known, but part of the withdrawal effect appears to involve the activation of CRF systems within the central medial nucleus of the amygdala, part of the 'extended amygdala' circuit (Koob 2000).

The second problem for the addict is that of **tolerance**, the state in which over time increasing doses of the drug become necessary to achieve anything like the original feelings of euphoria. It appears that the opioid receptors become less sensitive to the drug, a process of *down-regulation* of sensitivity, although the receptor numbers remain constant. This may be due in part to the action of a protein called **cyclic AMP-responsive element-binding protein (CREB)**. When opiates bind to the mu receptor, cAMP is produced, and this passes to the nucleus and interacts with CREB (Figure 8.5). The role of CREB is one of gene regulation, and the way in which the binding of cAMP influences this role is little understood. CREB is a major link in the chain from receptor to gene and evidence suggests it may be involved in opiate tolerance and the effects of drug withdrawal (Carlson 2010). Other proteins are undoubtedly important in drug addiction. A gene (the **AGPS3**, **activator of G protein signalling 3** gene) has been discovered that codes for a protein involved in euphoria. This protein is a vital component in the pathway that leads from the brain's release of beta-endorphins to the sensation of euphoria or pleasure that these endorphins produce. Blocking the gene (dubbed the *pleasure gene*), reduces the amount of protein produced, causing loss of the euphoric state. It is thought that the same mechanism will probably also be effective in reducing the euphoric (and thus addictive) effects of opiate drugs like morphine and heroin. In the future, drugs designed to block the production of the protein

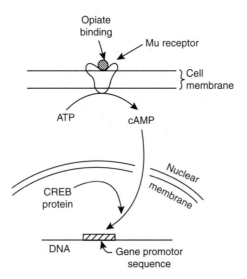

Figure 8.5 Opiate binding to the mu receptor. This creates cyclic adenosine monophosphate (cAMP) from adenosine triphosphate (ATP) inside the cell. cAMP influences gene expression inside the chromosomes of the nucleus by binding with CREB (cyclic AMP-responsive element-binding) protein.

may help heroin addicts to withdraw from their addiction more easily, with fewer or less intense side-effects. The analgesic qualities of these drugs do not appear be affected when this gene is blocked.

Some important *drug interactions* involving opiates with other drugs occur and are shown in Tables 8.1 and 8.2.

An important drug used as a treatment of abuse of the so-called hard drugs (usually heroin and pethidine) is **methadone**. Although methadone itself is addictive and harmful, it is considered to cause fewer problems than the 'hard' drugs and for this reason has been used as a substitute for them for many years. It is hoped that by replacing heroin and pethidine with methadone not only will the need for the 'hard' drug be removed, but at the same time the effects of its withdrawal will be reduced. However, the potential dangers of methadone are demonstrated by the 298 deaths it caused in the United Kingdom in 1999, and 378 deaths in 2008.

Table 8.1 Drug interactions with opiates.

Other drug	Opiate drug interaction and notes
Chlorpromazine	May react with heroin, giving uncontrolled limb jerks
Clozapine (antipsychotic)	May react with heroin, causing drowsiness
Fluoxetine (antidepressant)	May react with heroin, causing fits
MAOI (antidepressant)	Reacts with pethidine, potentially fatal
Barbiturates	Increases the metabolism of all opiate drugs

Table 8.2 Drug interactions with methadone.

Other drug	Methadone interaction and notes
Phenobarbitone	Phenobarbitone blocks the action of methadone causing opioid withdrawal symptoms
Diazepam, and other benzodiazepine drugs	Inhibits methadone metabolism causing increased methadone blood levels
Tricyclic antidepressants	Methadone blocks the metabolism of the antidepressant, increasing the blood level of the antidepressant
Hypnotics (e.g. zopiclone and chlormethiazole)	Increased sedative effect with methadone
SSRI antidepressants	Increased levels of methadone in the blood
Disulfiram (anti-alcohol drug)	Some methadone products contain alcohol; a reaction with these products can be alarming and unpleasant
Other opiate drugs	Increased sedation and respiratory depression
Naloxone (opiate antagonist)	Blocks methadone action causing withdrawal
Alcohol	Increase sedation and respiratory depression; increased liver toxicity
Nevirapine, zidovudine and ritonavir (anti-HIV drugs)	Nevirapine causes increased methadone metabolism, i.e. lower blood methadone levels. Methadone raises blood level of zidovudine. Ritonavir may raise blood methadone levels by blocking methadone metabolism

Because of methadone's place in therapy, a separate drug interaction table for methadone is given in Table 8.2. Anti–HIV drugs are included in Table 8.2 because of the increased risks of HIV infection due to the dangerous habit of needle sharing by drug-abusing patients.

Cocaine, amphetamines and other dopamine-enhancing drugs

Cocaine is produced from the leaf of the coca bush and has been used for many years as a local anaesthetic. When injected intravenously or inhaled (e.g. as *crack cocaine*, a very potent form), cocaine will reach the brain quickly, causing a sense of well-being, euphoria, alertness and increased energy; the person taking it becomes extraverted, restless and talkative. It also causes a reduction in food intake. Cocaine is extremely addictive, partly owing to its rapid transportation to the brain and fast onset of effects, and at high dosages the user becomes unable to sleep and has tremors, nausea and psychotic outbursts (hallucinations, delusions, mood disturbance and bizarre behaviour; the so-called *cocaine psychosis*). Fits and unconsciousness may follow, with a corresponding risk of death.

Cocaine blocks the re-uptake of monoamines, especially dopamine and noradrenaline, into the presynaptic bulb by inhibiting the pumps (or transporters) in the presynaptic membrane (Figure 8.6). These neurotransmitters then accumulate in the cleft, exerting a greater than normal effect on the receptors. Areas of the brain affected include the basal ganglia (putamen and caudate nucleus), the amygdala and the cerebral cortex. However, the nucleus accumbens is particularly affected, with long-term changes in this area occurring following exposure to the drug. These

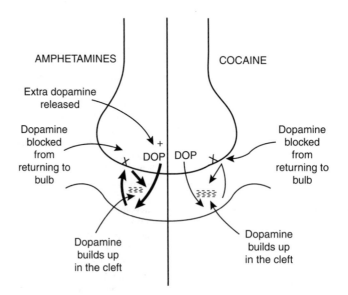

Figure 8.6 The action of amphetamines (left) and cocaine (right) at the dopaminergic synapse. Dopamine (DOP) is blocked from reabsorption back into the presynaptic bulb by both drugs, thus increasing the quantity of dopamine within the synaptic cleft. In addition, amphetamines increase the quantity of dopamine released from the bulb.

changes involve an increase in the density of dopamine receptors, notably D_3, and can cause a rapid return to psychotic symptoms on re-exposure to the drug even after quite some time without it.

A single dose of cocaine has been shown to cause major changes in the brain resulting in memory loss and addiction, due to its prolonged neuroleptic action of about a week's duration (Ungless et al. 2001). This action interferes with the normal process of memory and renders the brain vulnerable to successive doses, leading to rapid addiction. Users 'remember' the euphoria and this reinforces further drug abuse. Cocaine is also responsible for a quarter of the non-fatal heart attacks found in those younger than 45 years of age. The drug causes cardiac spasms and induces the immune system to destroy cardiac muscle cells. Deaths from cocaine use in the United Kingdom increased sevenfold in the six years from 1993 to 1999, i.e. 12 deaths in 1993 compared to 87 deaths in 1999. The deaths continued to rise, the drug causing 235 deaths in 2008.

One possible way of treating cocaine addiction in the future may be with a cocaine vaccine. The vaccine stimulates production of antibodies which lock onto cocaine, forming a complex which is too large to cross the blood–brain barrier and thus preventing cocaine from entering the brain.

Some important *drug interactions* involving cocaine with other drugs occur and are shown in Table 8.3.

Amphetamines act in a way similar to cocaine, i.e. they increase dopamine (and noradrenaline) levels within the synapses by blocking their re-uptake, but they also have the additional effect of increasing dopamine release from the presynaptic bulb (Figure 8.6). Amphetamines were responsible for 79 deaths in the United Kingdom during the year 1999 and 99 deaths in 2008.

Ecstasy (3,4-methylenedioxymethamphetamine, or MDMA) is one of a group of related amphetamine-associated drugs. MDMA is converted in the body to the active metabolite **4-hydroxy-3-methoxymethamphetamine (HMMA)**. Ecstasy increases the release of serotonin into the synapses of the serotonergic diffuse modulatory system by causing the transporters that normally facilitate serotonin re-uptake to reverse the flow into the synapse. The larger amounts of serotonin released in this way increase the 'high' that users experience (Concar 2002). HMMA is associated with an increased release of the pituitary hormone **ADH** (**antidiuretic hormone, or vasopressin**) (Figure 8.7). This hormone causes

Table 8.3 Drug interactions with cocaine.

Other drug	Interaction with cocaine
Alcohol	Increased euphoric effect. Increased heart rate and blood cortisol levels
Heroin	Increased euphoria
Lithium	Decreases the effect of the cocaine
MAOI antidepressant	High temperature, muscle rigidity and tremor, coma
Antipsychotics	Increase in the positive (psychotic) symptoms of cocaine (see *cocaine psychosis*)
Calcium channel blockers (anti-epileptic)	Reduce the cardiac effects of cocaine, but may increase the risk of fits
Beta-adrenergic blockers (cardiac drugs)	Increased risk of cocaine-induced constriction of the coronary artery (i.e. risk of myocardial ischaemia)

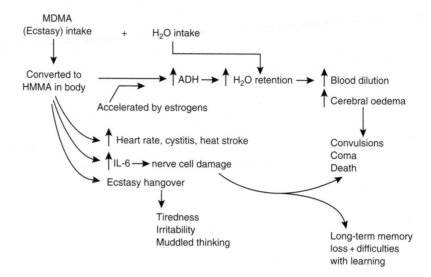

Figure 8.7 Ecstasy intake and the events that follow. ADH = antidiuretic hormone, H₂O = water, IL-6 = interleukin-6.

retention of water in the blood from the kidney, preventing its loss in the urine. The extra water in the blood dilutes the plasma electrolytes, especially sodium, causing low plasma sodium due to the blood dilution (a **hyponatraemia**). The change in plasma salts level affects neurons, which are sensitive to electrolyte levels in their extracellular fluid. The increased water content of the blood puts a strain on the heart which then risks failure (called **cardiac failure**). The brain becomes swollen with water (called **cerebral oedema**), and drinking more water accelerates the harmful effects. Women are particularly vulnerable to this effect since the female hormone oestrogen speeds up the process. High levels of circulating oestrogen occur just prior to ovulation, about midway through the ovarian cycle, and women at this point may already be suffering some disturbance in cerebral sodium levels, putting them more at risk from the effects of Ecstasy. They also risk increasing the body temperature (**hyperthermia**) leading to **heatstroke** (a state of collapse due to uncontrolled body temperature above 40°C). If Ecstasy is taken at a party, the risk of hyperthermia is increased by dancing in a crowd. The brain reacts to the MDMA-induced excess water and hyperthermia with convulsions and coma, possibly leading to death within a few hours or days. Deaths from MDMA in the whole of the United Kingdom total 202 from 1996 to 2002, from 5 in 1998 rising to 44 in 2008. However, there was a worrying sharp increase in deaths reported for 2001 (England and Wales alone recorded 43 deaths) despite media coverage highlighting the dangers. The deaths occur mostly in the under-30 age range. The causes of death were mainly **hyperthermia**, **hyponatraemia** and **cardiac failure**. The risks vary between individuals because of sexual and genetic differences (see oestrogen above).

See page 141

For the majority of Ecstasy takers who survive, other physical changes take place, including increased heart rate, cystitis and heavy periods in women, heatstroke (Blows 1998; Concar 2002) and possible **cerebral infarcts** if blood capillaries become blocked in the brain. MDMA also interferes with the immune system by raising the level of a chemical called **interleukin-6** (**IL-6**), which at the new higher levels can damage nerve cells, particularly the serotonergic neurons. This puts the user at higher risk of infections. In the brain, MDMA initially gives a sense of euphoria, but it seriously affects the serotonin pathways, causing damage to areas of the cerebral cortex and hippocampus. This damage can occur quickly, within four days of Ecstasy use, and the damage is permanent, causing memory losses and difficulties with learning for years. Long-term widespread use of the drug could result in a whole generation of people with memory problems who will have difficulty in carrying out simple mental tasks. As many as 500,000 Ecstasy users in the United Kingdom and 20 million people worldwide could be affected in this way. It has been estimated that between 2.5 and 5 million Ecstasy tablets are taken in the UK every month! After use, Ecstasy can cause a hangover effect similar to that induced by alcohol (the **Ecstasy hangover**) with tiredness, irritability and muddled thinking, due to the decline in levels of serotonin.

Some important *drug interactions* involving amphetamines with other drugs occur and are shown in Table 8.4.

Cannabinoids

Marijuana comes from the dried leaves of the Indian hemp plant called **Cannabis sativa**. The active ingredients consist of more than 80 **cannabinoids**, many of which are probably psychoactive. The most potent of these is **delta-9-tetrahydrocannabinol** (**delta-9-THC** or **Δ9-THC**, now usually called **THC**). After absorption, this substance binds to cannabinoid receptors in several parts of the brain, notably the basal ganglia, the hippocampus, the cerebellum and the frontal lobe of the cerebrum. The effects of taking cannabinoids in sufficient dosage are alterations in cognition, euphoria and other mood and emotional changes. A sense of unreality with sensory distortion, slurred speech, analgesia (without respiratory depression), sedation and suppression of the immune system have all been reported. The reason for taking the drug – that is, the euphoric effect produced – is probably due to its ability to raise dopamine levels within the nucleus accumbens. The mood changes and loss of short-term memory linked to the use of marijuana are probably due to hippocampal involvement. The hippocampus has particularly high numbers of cannabinoid receptors and therefore the drug may act especially here, resulting not only in impairment of short-term memory but also in disruption of the release of cortisol, a hormone involved in

Table 8.4 Drug interactions with amphetamines.

Other drug	Interaction with amphetamines
MAOI antidepressants	Dangerous interaction: risk of hypertensive crisis due to raised sympathetic nervous system activity (i.e. sympathomimetic); plus nausea, cardiac arrhythmias and chest pain
Opiates	Increased analgesic effect of the opiate
Chlorpromazine (antipsychotic)	Both drugs are reduced in their efficiency causing an increase in psychotic symptoms
Lithium	Reduces the amphetamine euphoria

mood regulation. An important function of the hippocampus is regulation of some hormones, including cortisol.

Cannabinoid receptors occur in at least two known subtypes, **CB₁** and **CB₂**. CB₁ is the major cannabinoid receptor subtype of the central nervous system (CNS), with CB₂ in the brain limited to possibly only the cerebellum (it occurs more in other organs). Apart from the hippocampal effects, the drugs acting on CB₁ receptors in the basal ganglia can cause loss of control of voluntary movements, the addition of involuntary movements and **akinesia** (a loss of initiating a movement). CB₁ receptors are especially predominant in the **globus pallidus**, the **substantia nigra** (**pars reticulata**) and the **caudate** and **putamen**. In the **limbic system**, there are significant levels of CB₁ receptors in the **amygdala**, an area central to the control of emotional responses, and in the **hypothalamus**, the control centre of body temperature. The **cerebellum** has some areas with dense levels of CB₁ receptors, enough to cause disturbance to motor function and balance given sufficient dosage of the drug. Levels of CB₁ receptors in the **brain stem** and **spinal cord** are lower than in these previously mentioned areas.

Some evidence has emerged that cannabinoids have effects similar to those of the so-called hard drugs (heroin in particular), not only causing the dopamine release in the nucleus accumbens noted above but also causing high levels of CRF release during withdrawal (see opiates) (Wiedemann 2010). This has led to further speculation and controversy about whether the use of cannabis can lead to addiction to hard drugs like heroin. The risk of addiction to cannabis itself has always been considered to be low, usually because it is only used occasionally and because users give up smoking the drug in their thirties or forties. Recently, however, there have been indications that cannabis is as potentially addictive as heroin or morphine (Wiedemann 2010). The number of recorded deaths from cannabis in the UK for 2008 was 19.

The presence of natural receptors for cannabinoids suggests that the nervous system must produce its own endogenous cannabinoid substance, and the discovery of **anandamide**, an unsaturated fatty acid, confirmed this. Anandamide, produced by neurons of the cortex and parts of the basal ganglia, binds to CB₁ receptors, producing analgesia, reduced levels of movement and hypothermia (a hypothalamic effect). Its duration of action is short owing to rapid breakdown to arachidonic acid in neurons and astrocytes.

Some medical uses of cannabinoids are becoming better recognised. Their antiemetic quality has been used for some time in the drug **nabilone** to prevent nausea and sickness in patients having chemotherapy in cancer treatment. Some cannabinoids have been shown to reduce fits, dilate the bronchus in **asthma** and improve the eye disease **glaucoma**. Now the beneficial analgesic qualities of cannabinoids may become available to **multiple sclerosis** sufferers if the legal issues surrounding marijuana can be resolved.

Some important *drug interactions* involving cannabinoids with other drugs occur and are shown in Table 8.5.

Alcohol

Alcohol (ethyl alcohol or ethanol) is a psychoactive drug with a small molecular size and therefore reaches all parts of the body quickly after absorption. In a low

Table 8.5 Drug interactions with cannabinoids.

Other drugs	Interactions with cannabinoids
Fluoxetine (SSRI antidepressant)	Increased energy and sexuality
Tricyclic antidepressant	Tachycardia and restlessness, orthostatic hypotension, sedation and unstable body temperature
Lithium	Increased blood levels of lithium, which in turn may reduce the effect of the cannabinoid
Opiates	Increased heart rate and respiratory depression
Cocaine	Raised blood levels of cocaine, causing increased cocaine activity
Amphetamines	Increased and sustained heart rate
Propranolol (cardiac drug)	Blocks the increased heart rate and blood pressure associated with cannabinoids

dose it acts as a *mild stimulant*, giving a feeling of well-being, due to the release of small amounts of dopamine into the nucleus accumbens. This is the reason for the *social* drinking of alcohol. However, if too much alcohol is taken it becomes a *depressant*, shutting down many areas of brain activity. The problem is that this depressant level of alcohol can be quickly and easily reached. Such depressive effects include cognitive impairment (i.e. distorted thinking, judgement and reasoning), slowed reaction times (one good reason for not driving after drinking), verbal impairment (slurring of speech) and motor impairment (inability to stand up or walk in a straight line). Very high doses (i.e. a blood level greater than 0.5 per cent or 5 mg/dl) can cause unconsciousness and a risk of death from respiratory suppression. One in every eight young male deaths in the United Kingdom each year is caused by alcohol, either directly or indirectly, through alcohol-related accidents, violence and inhalation of vomit. In 2007, recorded alcohol-related deaths reached 8,724 in the UK. Some 12.8 per cent of British men aged 15–29 years, and 8.3 per cent of British women of equivalent age die from alcohol-related causes each year (Harrington-Dobinson and Blows 2006, 2007a and 2007b).

Alcohol also has a dilatory effect on peripheral blood vessels, taking blood from the core towards the skin (the red nose effect). Blood flushing the skin makes the skin *feel* warmer, but actually this blood moves more heat from the body's core and that actually cools down the body temperature. It seems at odds with the way they *feel* to say that alcohol makes the person colder. However, in this situation, the brandy barrel carried by the rescue dog is not the best thing for a very cold person trapped in snow. Alcohol abuse over time causes both tolerance (the individual can consume more and more without undue effect) and dependence (the person needs alcohol in order to get through the day). Quick withdrawal from a long-term drinking habit causes nausea, vomiting, headache and tremors, as well as **delirium tremens** (known as the **DTs**), a collection of symptoms including agitation, confusion, tachycardia, hallucinations and delusions. The person in withdrawal can also become **hyperthermic** (raised body temperature) because alcohol is no longer available to promote heat loss.

Korsakoff syndrome is a chronic state of **amnesia** (memory loss) and **Wernicke's encephalopathy** is a state of intellectual impairment; these often occur together in a patient with long-term alcohol abuse. Both syndromes are thought to be due to a combination of factors, notably the deficiency of the vitamin called **thiamine** (vitamin B₁), alcohol neurotoxicity and hepatic dysfunction (Nolen-Hoeksema 2007). Distinguishing one syndrome from the other in chronic alcoholic patients is not always easy. Many alcoholics lack nutrients as they tend not to eat properly, and chronic alcohol abuse results in gastric damage which impedes the absorption of vitamins, particularly thiamine. These factors lead to a degeneration of the brain stem (**periaquaductal grey**), the hypothalamus (**mammillary bodies**) and the thalamus (**dorsomedial nucleus**). Korsakoff syndrome is characterised by a loss of short-term memory, inability to learn new skills, disorientation and confabulation to fill in missing gaps in knowledge. The features of Wernicke's encephalopathy are rapid eye movements with double vision (**diplopia**), reduced muscle coordination and a decline in mental ability that may be of any degree from mild to severe. Some recovery may be possible provided the damage is not severe and the patient abstains from alcohol for at least six months and ensures an adequate *See page 37* intake of thiamine.

Alcohol acts at the **GABA**$_A$ receptor site and promotes GABA to open the chloride channels (Figure 4.13). This increases the inhibitory effect of the GABA synapses and shuts down brain activity by reducing the firing rate of neurons. People have varying responses to alcohol and not every drinker is equally at risk of becoming alcoholic. Two basic types of drinkers have been identified: the *steady drinker* and the *binger*. Steady drinking has a strong genetic basis, a case of 'like father like son'. If the father has a history of alcohol abuse as a steady drinker, the son has a seven times greater risk of abusing alcohol than the son of a non-drinker. They also have a greater than average risk of developing a personality disorder. The daughters of steady drinking fathers do not show the same degree of slide into alcoholism as the sons, but they do tend to complain more about physical symptoms for which pathology cannot be found; a condition known as **somatisation disorder**. The offspring of alcoholic mothers also show three to five times more risk of developing a psychopathology, e.g. depression, anxiety, misconduct or **attention deficit hyperactivity disorder** (**ADHD**), compared to age-matched, low-risk children from non-alcoholic mothers.

Steady drinking starts early in life and is associated with many kinds of antisocial behaviour, such as fighting, impulsive actions and lack of remorse. Bingeing alcohol abuse has a greater environmental than genetic cause. The father-to-child hereditary pattern is only activated in an environment where the child is exposed to bouts of heavy drinking. Bingers start drinking later in life and can be of either sex. They show increased emotional states and anxiety, become rigid in their outlook, fearful of any changes, cautious and sensitive to social cues.

The genetic basis of alcoholism has become the subject of greater interest with the sequencing of the human genome. It became particularly important with the discovery of the *A1* allele on chromosome 11. This particular allele is a variation of the gene that codes for the dopamine receptor known as D₂, and its presence increases the risk of alcohol abuse. Of all severe alcoholics, 56.3 per cent have the *A1* allele compared with only 25.7 per cent of a control population. Given that dopamine is involved in the reward pathways of the brain, it may be that the *A1* *See page 143* allele is also linked to increased risk of abuse of other drugs.

Some important *drug interactions* involving alcohol with other drugs occur and are shown in Table 8.6. Nurses need to be aware of these interactions because of the common social nature of alcohol consumption, but particularly in the known alcoholic patient who may be taking other medication.

Table 8.6 Drug interactions with alcohol.

Other drug	Interaction with alcohol
Barbiturates; warfarin; phenytoin; rifampicin	Interaction varies according to how much alcohol is consumed. Heavy drinking increases at least one liver enzyme activity, withdrawal decreases that activity.
Paracetamol	Alcohol increases activity of the liver enzyme that acts on paracetamol, causing increased toxicity of paracetamol at normally nontoxic dose. Overdose of paracetamol with alcohol can cause lethal liver failure.
Opiates; benzodiazepines	Alcohol adds to the depressive effect of the drugs on the brain.
Tricyclic antidepressants	Unexpected reactions and behavioural changes. Lower blood levels of the tricyclic reduces clinical effects.
SSRI antidepressants	No known interaction.
MAOI antidepressants	Risk of hypertension, especially if tyromine is present in the alcoholic drink. Modern reversible MAOI may not be such a problem.
Antipsychotics	Poor psychomotor skills and impaired nervous system function.
Disulfiram (anti-alcohol)	Flushing, hypotension, nausea, increased heart rate; some reactions could be fatal.
Nonsteroidal anti-inflammatory drugs	Increased risk of gastrointestinal bleeds since alcohol is a gastric irritant.
Insulin	Too much alcohol causes severe and prolonged hypoglycaemia in diabetic patients, following lowering of stored liver glycogen.
Antihypertensive drugs	Increased risk of postural hypotension.

Nicotine and caffeine

The two biggest health problems of this century are the **human immunodeficiency virus** (**HIV**, the causative agent of **acquired immunodeficiency syndrome**, or **AIDS**) and **tobacco smoking**. Both problems are increasing globally. Any individual in the Western world who can avoid both HIV and tobacco has a life expectancy of 70 years at least, and often more. Both these problems are relevant to this chapter because HIV infection is a major risk to intravenous drug abusers who share contaminated needles, and tobacco contains the addictive drug nicotine. Nicotine addiction is a major hazard, causing the deaths of about *300 people per day* in the United Kingdom alone from smoking-related diseases. In 2008, diseases caused by smoking claimed the lives of more than 100,000 people in the UK. It's a massive death toll, but one that is entirely avoidable, simply by choosing not to smoke. Unfortunately, however, the health message is not reaching young people as more and more take up the habit. Smoking in young women in particular is increasing at alarming rates. Nicotine addiction must not be underestimated. Addiction to this drug prevents many people who want to give up smoking from doing so. Only about 20 per cent of people attempting to stop smoking are still non-smokers two years after abstaining from cigarettes, and this 80 per cent failure rate still occurs even when they are faced with serious health problems or even death. Nicotine is probably the worst addiction problem facing society today. A vaccine against nicotine, now in an advanced stage of development, may be instrumental in the treatment of nicotine addiction and in prevention.

Nicotine binds to nicotinic acetylcholine receptors on the ventral tegmental area (VTA), and this increases the level of dopamine in the nucleus accumbens, but also raises the activity levels of many dopaminergic neurons. By binding to nicotinic receptors, nicotine also causes the opening of sodium channels and increases cellular excitation. Another (as yet unidentified) substance in tobacco smoke causes inhibition of the enzyme **monamine oxidase B (MAO-B)** which normally breaks down dopamine. Inhibition of this enzyme results in accumulation of dopamine in the nucleus accumbens. Smokers have between 30 per cent and 40 per cent less MAO-B in their brain. Nicotine peaks in the blood within ten minutes of inhalation, but it wears off quickly, therefore requiring further inhalations of the drug.

Evidence is now pointing towards smoking tobacco as an important cause of anxiety states, depression and perhaps other mental health disorders, due in part to the increased dopaminergic activity that nicotine causes in the brain (Petit-Zeman 2002). Table 8.7 demonstrates the effects of inhaling nicotine on both non-smokers and smokers. Given these differences, it becomes obvious how tolerance to nicotine changes a person's perception of the drug and how intolerable passive smoking is to the non-smoker.

Very few known *drug interactions* involving nicotine with other drugs occur (Table 8.8). Other interactions probably do occur but they remain unstudied. Smoking is a common habit, not least amongst those under treatment for mental health disorders. Combinations of prescribed drugs with nicotine may be a problem that nurses should be aware of.

Caffeine is another drug that causes release of dopamine in the nucleus accumbens, thus promoting a state of well-being. But caffeine is best known as a drug that promotes wakefulness. This it achieved by binding to **adenosine receptors** in the brain. Adenosine is a central nervous system modulator, and by binding to adenosine receptors it slows neural activity and induces sleep. Caffeine is an adenosine receptor antagonist, and by blocking the receptor it prevents adenosine from binding. This causes wakefulness and alertness. Caffeine has another role, that of increasing the release of adrenaline from the adrenal cortex. Adrenaline can also increase the alertness of the brain by as much as 40 per cent.

The hallucinogenic drugs

One of the most potent hallucinogenic agents is **lysergic acid diethylamide (LSD)**, which produces a dream-like state with heightened senses and a strange

Table 8.7 The effects of inhaling nicotine on non-smokers and smokers.

Non-smokers	Smokers
Various combinations of nausea, vomiting, coughing, sweating, dizziness, flushing of the face, even abdominal cramps and diarrhoea	Relaxation, alertness, reduced hunger

Table 8.8 Drug interactions with nicotine.

Other drugs	Interactions with nicotine
Benzodiazepines	Increased activity of the liver enzymes that metabolise the benzodiazepines, causing reduced efficiency of these drugs

blending of those senses such that, for example, visual images can cause sounds or weird smells. During the early stages of LSD administration the effect is of witnessing abstract coloured geometric shapes, such as parallel stripes, hexagons and checkers. This is followed by the appearance of four specific forms: tunnels, spirals, cobwebs and honeycomb patterns. This phenomenon is akin to **hallucinations**, i.e. sensing something that is not real, and the study of these effects may give clues to the origin of psychotic hallucinations. Under the influence of LSD, neurons in the visual sensory area of the brain (area VI, Brodmann 17, in the occipital lobe) fire even when there is nothing on the retina to see (Mackenzie 2001).

See page 6

The chemical structure of LSD is very similar to that of serotonin and this means it probably works on the serotonergic pathways of the brain stem. It certainly causes less serotonin to be secreted in the raphe nucleus of the brain stem. Serotonin usually has an inhibitory function on other brain areas and the LSD-induced lower secretion removes this inhibition, so the brain become more active.

Phencyclidine (PCP) is another hallucinogen, causing excitement, agitation, delirium and mixed, disorganised perception. It is an NMDA receptor antagonist and causes the release of dopamine. Another less potent NMDA receptor antagonist is the anaesthetic **ketamine**, which can also cause brief dream-like states and psychotic symptoms. The brain pathways along which these drugs act are speculative, but may lie in the prefrontal cortex of the cerebrum.

Solvents also have hallucinatory and intoxicating effects. These are **volatile hydrocarbons** based on petroleum and natural gas, or **ketones**. As a liquid they evaporate rapidly at room temperature and are used as a range of glue solvents, paint thinners, nail polish remover and various gases. Inhalation of these gases and vapours causes a drunk-like state with the possibility of hallucinations, emotional disturbance and distortions of perception. They enter the blood and move quickly to the brain and liver. In the brain they have an initial euphoric effect, causing a 'high' which is probably due to dopamine release. However, this is followed by disorientation, possible fits, nausea and vomiting, and a depressant effect which slows respiration and heart rate, and reduces mental activity. These agents are slow to be excreted from the body and therefore the effects can last for days. Death can occur from **asphyxia** (failure of breathing) or heart failure. Solvent abuse caused 50 deaths in the UK during 2008, mostly young people of secondary-school age. Solvents also cause tolerance and addiction, and withdrawal causes symptoms similar to alcohol withdrawal.

Key points

The reward pathways

- The medial forebrain bundle links the ventral tegmental area of the midbrain with the nucleus accumbens of the cerebral frontal lobe. This pathway forms part of the mesotelencephalic dopamine system.
- This dopamine pathway is strongly implicated in the activities of many self-administered stimulatory drugs.
- Many stimulant and addictive drugs are those that cause high dopamine levels to occur in the brain, and in the nucleus accumbens in particular.

Opiate drugs

- Opiate drugs cause analgesia, euphoria, sedatory and depressant effects.
- The mechanism that leads to euphoria and the feeling of well-being appears to be mediated through the mu (μ) receptor, which also reinforces drug-seeking behaviour.
- Withdrawal from drugs is associated with reduced levels of both dopamine and serotonin in the brain, and increased levels of corticotropin-releasing factor (CRF).
- Tolerance appears to result from receptors becoming less sensitive to the drug, which may involve a protein called cyclic AMP-responsive element-binding protein (CREB).

Cocaine and amphetamines

- Cocaine and amphetamines block the re-uptake of dopamine into the presynaptic bulb by inhibiting dopamine pumps in the synaptic membrane.
- Amphetamines also increase dopamine and noradrenaline levels within the synapses by increasing dopamine release from the presynaptic bulb.
- Ecstasy (MDMA) is converted in the body to an active metabolite (HMMA), which causes increased antidiuretic hormone (ADH or vasopressin).
- ADH increases water in the blood, and this extra water dilutes the electrolytes around the neurons. The brain becomes swollen and suffers convulsions, coma with a potential to cause death.

Cannabinoids

- Marijuana comes from the dried leaves of the Indian hemp plant called *Cannabis sativa*.
- The psychoactive ingredients are cannabinoids.
- The most potent is delta-9-tetrahydrocannabinol (THC), which binds to cannabinoid receptors in the brain, notably the basal ganglia, the hippocampus, the cerebellum and the frontal lobe of the cerebrum.
- Cannabinoids cause not only dopamine release in the nucleus accumbens but also high levels of CRF release during withdrawal.

Alcohol

- Alcohol is a psychoactive drug which in low dosage acts as a mild stimulant, giving a feeling of well-being.
- In higher doses, alcohol is a depressant to many parts of the brain. Depressive effects include cognitive impairment, slowed reaction times, and verbal and motor impairment.
- Very high doses can cause unconsciousness and death.
- Rapid withdrawal from alcohol causes nausea, vomiting, headache and tremors, as well as delirium tremens (DTs), i.e. agitation, confusion, tachycardia, hallucinations and delusions.
- Korsakoff syndrome is a chronic state of amnesia with confabulation and Wernicke's encephalopathy is a state of intellectual impairment; these occur often together in a patient with long-term alcohol abuse.

- There are two basic types of drinkers: the steady drinkers and the bingers.
- Steady drinking has a strong genetic basis, starting early in life, and is associated with antisocial behaviour.
- Bingeing alcohol abuse is more environmental than genetic in origin. It starts later in life and affects both sexes.

Nicotine and caffeine

- Nicotine causes major problems of addiction, and tobacco smoking causes about 300 deaths per day in the United Kingdom alone.
- Nicotine and caffeine both increase the level of dopamine in the nucleus accumbens.

References

Blows W. T. (1998) Crowd physiology: the 'penguin effect'. *Accident and Emergency Nursing*, **6** (3): 126–129.

Carlson N. (2010) *Physiology of Behaviour* (10th edition). Allyn and Bacon, Boston.

Coffey M. (1999) Psychosis and medication: strategies for improving adherence. *British Journal of Nursing*, **8** (4): 225–230.

Concar D. (2002) Ecstasy on the brain. *New Scientist*, **174** (2339; 20 April): 26–33.

Harrington-Dobinson A. and Blows W. T. (2006) Part 1: nurses' guide to alcohol and promoting healthy lifestyle changes. *British Journal of Nursing*, **15** (22): 1217–1219 (14th Dec. 2006).

Harrington-Dobinson A. and Blows W. T. (2007a) Part 2: nurses' guide to the impact of alcohol on health and wellbeing. *British Journal of Nursing*, **16** (1): 47–51 (11th Jan. 2007).

Harrington-Dobinson A. and Blows W. T. (2007b) Part 3: nurses' guide to alcohol and promoting healthy lifestyle changes. *British Journal of Nursing*, **16** (2): 106–110 (25th Jan. 2007).

Koob G. F. (2000) Opiate tolerance and dependence. *Science and Medicine*, **7** (2): 28–37.

MacKenzie D. (2001) Secrets of an acid head. *New Scientist*, **170** (2296; 23 June): 26–30.

NPF/BNF (1999) *Nurse Prescriber's Formulary and British National Formulary 1999–2001*. British Medical Association and the Royal Pharmaceutical Society of Great Britain.

Nolen-Heoksema S. (2007) *Abnormal Psychology*. McGraw-Hill, Boston.

Petit-Zeman S. (2002) Smoke gets in your mind. *New Scientist*, **174** (2338; 13 April): 30–33.

Ungless M. A., Whistler J. L., Malenka R. C. and Bonci A. (2001) Single cocaine exposure *in vivo* induces long-term potentiation in dopamine neurons. *Nature*, **411** (31 May): 583–587.

Wiedemann C. (2010) Addiction: Cannabis against heroin? *Nature Reviews Neuroscience*, **11**: 3.

Wolf C. R., Smith G. and Smith R. L. (2000) Pharmacogenetics. *British Medical Journal*, **320**: 987–990.

9 Anxiety, fear and emotions

- **The limbic system and the biology of emotions**
- **The biology of stress**
- **The emotions of life experiences**
- **Anxiety disorders**
- **Fear**
- **Phobias and obsessive-compulsive disorder**
- **Eating disorders**
- **The anxiolytic drugs**
- **Anxiety-related personality disorders**
- **Key points**

The limbic system and the biology of emotions

The limbic system is a series of centres collectively involved in *preservation of the individual* (i.e. *self-preservation*) and *preservation of the species*. It governs behaviour essential to the survival of the individual, ensuring, for example, that we seek food or respond to threats, and also promotes reproductive behaviour (see Chapter 1) to ensure survival of the species. The major components of the limbic system (Figure 9.1) are the amygdala; the mammillary bodies of the hypothalamus; the anterior and dorsal nuclei of the thalamus; several deep nuclei and the septal area. The orbitofrontal cortex of the cerebrum, several other areas of the cortex, such as the hippocampus; the parahippocampal gyrus and parts of the temporal lobe are together known as the **limbic cortex** because of their close association with the functions of the limbic system.

The limbic system has the following functions:

- It is the centre for the control of emotions, including fear and aggression.
- It controls reproductive and other survival behaviours.
- It influences memory because the hippocampus stores short-term memory.
- Through the hypothalamus, it influences hormonal release and the autonomic nervous system.

See page 18

See page 61 The whole system is set in a ring structure (limbic = bordering, fringeing or ringing) deep in the brain (see Chapter 1, and Figures 1.4, 1.5, and 9.1).

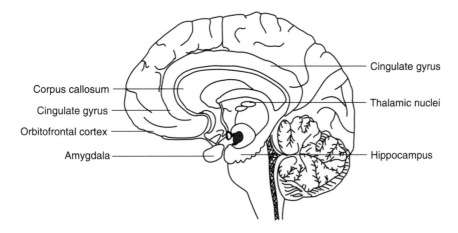

Figure 9.1 The main components of the limbic system.

The **amygdala** (Figure 9.2) is a pea-sized collection of nuclei situated within the limbic system inside the temporal lobes, below the level of the cortex. It sits at the end of the tail of the caudate nucleus (Figure 1.4). The important nuclei of the amygdala and their functions are listed below.

See page 9

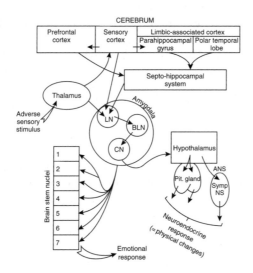

Figure 9.2 Inputs and outputs of the amygdala. Sensory information coming into the thalamus is passed to the sensory cortex, but also directly to the lateral nucleus (LN) of the amygdala. The sensory cortex passes the information to the prefrontal cortex to produce an action plan, which is passed to the septo-hippocampal system. Information identifying the sensory information passes through the limbic-associated cortex to the septo-hippocampal system. From here, input to the amygdala is via the lateral nucleus, to the basolateral nucleus (BLN) and on to the central nucleus (CN). The central nucleus has outputs to the brain stem nuclei (for emotional response), and the hypothalamus (for physical response).

1   The *corticomedial* group is very small and not well defined in humans. It plays a role in inhibiting aggressive behaviour.

2   The *basolateral* group relays sensory information from the primary sensory cortex of the cerebrum (Brodmann 1, 2 and 3), the sensory association cortex (Brodmann 40) and the thalamus to the central nucleus.

3   The central nucleus receives the information from the basolateral group and has its output to the brain stem and the hypothalamus (see Figure 9.3). The output to the brain stem is to various nuclei which carry out different functions in relation to emotional reactions. The output to the hypothalamus causes physical responses by influencing hypothalamic control of both the sympathetic nervous system and the pituitary hormones (collectively known as a **neuroendocrine response**).

The amygdala receives input from several sources, as listed at (2) above, with slightly delayed time intervals. The following text should be read in conjunction with Figure 9.2.

Primary amygdala input. The primary input to the amygdala is the direct automatic input of unconscious sensory stimuli from the thalamus, just as they are received from the environment. This unprocessed (or *raw*) data is the first to arrive at the amygdala and for a brief moment it is all the structure has to work on to determine the emotional response. As a result there is a rapid but not always appropriate response. The amygdala simply gives the individual the best option for survival, responding in a protective manner that may turn out to be unnecessary. Impulsive reactions and behaviour can be seen as *acting without thinking* or, in the case of the amygdala, acting on unconscious and unconsidered, and therefore unprocessed, stimuli (note here an interesting correlation with murderers; see later text). It should not be surprising that impulsive behaviour of this kind is often seen in children, since a child's limbic system is immature. The processing and consideration of sensory stimuli requires sophisticated and complex neural systems, coupled with extensive memory stores, both of which the young brain has not had time to develop fully.

Not only has the sensory stimulus gone from the thalamus to the amygdala, but the thalamus has also passed the raw stimulus on to the primary sensory cortex of the cerebrum (if the stimulus comes from the body) or to one of the specialist sensory areas such as hearing or vision. Here the task of interpretation takes place to determine what the stimulus actually is. This involves comparing the new stimulus with memories of previous stimuli to find a match. The cerebrum adds a conscious element to the stimulus, so the individual is aware of the stimulus and can add a degree of reason to the response.

Secondary amygdala input. The secondary input to the amygdala comes from the cerebral cortex. This cerebral output also passes to the **limbic-associated cortex**, which is made up of the **parahippocampal gyrus** and the **polar temporal lobe cortex**. The limbic-associated cortex consists of those areas of the cerebral cortex which work with the limbic system in the determination of stimuli. It should not be surprising to find the cerebrum and limbic system working together on emotions, since the limbic system does not have extensive memory banks to use in the identification and evaluation of stimuli. Most of the memory banks for this are found in the sensory association areas of the cerebrum. Thus it is in the limbic association cortex that interpretations and evaluation of the stimulus are mostly made: the polar temporal lobe cortex evaluates the stimulus for potential danger to the individual. The sensory cortex also sends the stimulus to the **prefrontal cortex**, where an action plan is formulated in response to the stimulus. The prefrontal cortex is close to the main motor cortex that activates skeletal muscle, so any action plan, such as running away or fighting, can be rapidly implemented. The outputs from the prefrontal cortex and the limbic-associated cortex are passed to the **septo-hippocampal system**, consisting of the **septum** and the **hippocampus**. Here integration of the action plan with the interpretation and evaluation of danger can take place, with input from short-term memory and perhaps aggression control if needed, since these are both functions of the hippocampus.

Tertiary amygdala input. The tertiary input to the amygdala is the final output from the septo-hippocampal system. The amygdala now has all the relevant information necessary to determine an appropriate emotional response.

We can put all this together in a simple scenario. Your friend decides to play a joke on you. She hides behind the door with the intention of jumping out and surprising you. As you enter the room she does just that, springing out and making a loud noise. The *primary and secondary amygdala inputs* would occur so close together that they would appear to be simultaneous. You would become aware of the sudden appearance of someone jumping out at the same time as hearing a loud noise. This could be anyone or anything, a potential threat to safety. In a purely automatic defensive strategy, you are likely to attempt to move out of danger and perhaps lash out physically. This may be coupled with a scream, or some brisk language, and very rapid changes in physiology – for example, the cardiovascular system would show a dramatic rise in the pulse rate and blood pressure. But very quickly the *tertiary amygdala input*, hot on the heels of the previous two inputs, will allow some recognition of who this person is and what their intentions were. Your response to the outburst would then be modified once this tertiary input has established the true nature of the surprise.

The outputs from the amygdala (Figure 9.3) can activate:

1   Various nuclei of the **brain stem** which are responsible for the following *emotional reactions*:

   • the **trigeminal** (cranial nerve V) and **facial** (cranial nerve VII) nuclei, which control the muscles of facial expression during emotions such as fear;
   • the nuclei of the **periaqueductal grey** (**PAG**) area, which cause four main responses, those of *freeze reaction* (i.e. behavioural arrest), *defensive* and *predatory aggression* and *flight from danger*, depending on which part is stimulated;
   • the **nucleus reticularis pontis caudalis**, which causes a startled response;
   • the **dorsal lateral tegmental** nucleus, which activates the higher centres of the cortex onto full alert;
   • the **locus coeruleus** nucleus, which increases cortical vigilance through noradrenergic pathways;

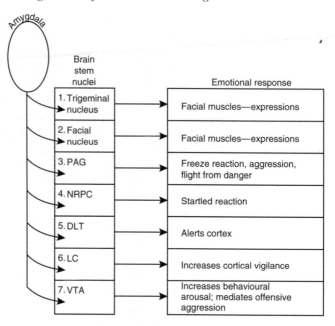

Figure 9.3 The brain stem nuclei are influenced by the amygdala to achieve various emotional responses, depending on which nucleus is activated. PAG = periaqueductal grey; NRPC = nucleus reticularis pontis caudalis; DLT = dorsal lateral tegmental nucleus; LC = locus coeruleus; VTA = ventral tegmental area.

See page 61

- the nuclei of the **ventral tegmental area**, which increases behavioural arousal through dopaminergic pathways and mediates for offensive aggression.

2   Various nuclei of the **hypothalamus**, which are responsible for the following *physical responses*:

- the **periventricular group** of nuclei, which causes increased *sympathetic nervous system* activity;
- various nuclei which together influence the release of stress-related *hormones* into the blood.

The neurobiology of emotions is now becoming clearer as research unpicks the delicate nerve networks that link the various components of the brain.

The biology of stress

As a subject, stress is assuming much importance in everyday life, with many articles being published on aspects such as stress in the workplace and **post-traumatic stress disorder**. Stress is both a physical and a mental phenomenon, and an examination of the physiological processes it causes emphasises the harm that excessive or long-term stress can do.

Stressors – adverse environmental factors causing stress – cause undesirable stimuli to enter the thalamus of the brain via the sensory nervous system. Using the emotional pathways shown in Figures 9.2 and 9.3, the stress stimuli pass through the amygdala and on to the hypothalamus. The hypothalamic **neuroendocrine response** (Figure 9.4) occurs, causing a number of physical changes:

- The autonomic nervous system switches to *sympathetic* activation and this causes the heart rate, blood pressure and blood sugar to rise. The hormone **adrenaline** is secreted into the blood from the **adrenal medulla** by direct stimulation from the sympathetic nervous system. This has the effect of augmenting the sympathetic activity, pushing up the blood pressure and heart rate further. The other hormone released into the blood from the adrenal medulla is **noradrenaline**, which diverts blood away from the skin to supply to the brain and muscles. This may be essential for a quick retreat from the stressor.
- The endocrine component of the hypothalamus releases **corticotropin-releasing factor** or hormone (**CRF** or **CRH**), which causes the release of **adrenocorticotropic hormone** (**ACTH**) from the anterior lobe of the pituitary gland into the general circulation. This in turn causes the release of **cortisol** from the adrenal cortex. The blood level of cortisol then rises, a well-known physical response to stress. In fact, the rise in blood cortisol level is so significant in stress that measuring cortisol levels has been suggested as a way of measuring stress itself.

Cortisol binds to receptors in the cytoplasm of many neurons and causes **gene transcription** (activation of genes) leading to **protein synthesis**. The production of proteins is, in the short term, protective to nerve cells. One effect is to increase

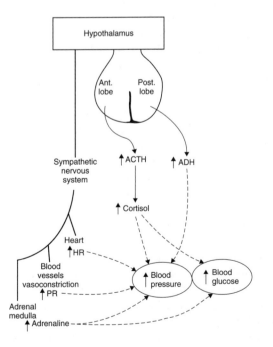

Figure 9.4 The neuroendocrine response to stress.

the influx of calcium (Ca^{2+}) into the neurons and this improves neuronal function. Cortisol also activates the brain so that it can cope better with new experiences in the short-term. It causes increased blood glucose levels by counteracting the action of **insulin**. In the long-term, as in chronic stress, high cortisol level appears to inhibit **GLUT3**, one of several **glucose transport molecules** found in cells, GLUT3 being widely found in neurons. GLUT3 is responsible for the passage of glucose into the neuron, and long-term inhibition may cause cellular damage due to reduced glucose energy supply. The hippocampus (and thus short-term memory) is particularly affected in this way. High levels of cortisol in stressed children can damage their mental ability, causing withdrawn, shy behaviour associated with increased physical ill health, while the child becomes more easily upset.

CRF is itself generating a lot of interest amongst researchers because high or low CRF levels are now implicated in a number of neuropsychiatric conditions, including anorexia nervosa, anxiety and depression (see Chapter 11). A low CRF level is also involved in neurodegerative disorders such as Alzheimer's disease. Two CRF metabotropic receptors have been isolated, CRF1 and CRF2, which bind the hormone in the pituitary gland, in several parts of the brain and, somewhat surprisingly, in the gut and spleen. Stress normally causes a down-regulation of the number of CRF receptors in the anterior pituitary. In chronic stress, this down-regulation may be insufficient or simply fail, and a future generation of drugs designed to block CRF receptors is under development to help relieve the symptoms of chronic stress.

Components of the immune system become involved in the stress response, a process studied under the title **psychoneuroimmunology** (meaning *mind, nervous system and immune system*). Stress causes changes to the immune system, in particular **immunosuppression**, a reduction in the immune response which increases the risk of infection. **Natural killer (NK) cells** (those that kill virally infected and malignant cells), **lymphocytes** (the main cells of the immune system) and an antibody called **immunoglobulin A (IgA)** are all significantly reduced in stress. These responses suggest that brain neuromodulators released during stress have a wide influence over body functions both inside and outside of the nervous system (Kaye et al. 2000).

The symptoms of stress are pallor, raised pulse rate and blood pressure, deeper respiration, sweating, raised blood sugar levels, dilated pupils, nausea, frequency of urination and restlessness. Many of these can be recognised as 'side-effects' of the neuroendocrine response; the sweating, for example, is due to increased sympathetic activity, and the sympathetic activity combined with adrenaline also drives up the blood pressure and increases the heart rate. The release of cortisol helps to drive up the blood glucose levels. These **compensatory mechanisms** are brought into play by the body to correct the initial physiological changes, which would otherwise cause the body harm during the period of stress.

In the long term, when stress is persistent for months or years, the result is different. The body tries to compensate for the effects of stress for as long as possible, but will eventually fail. When this happens, the individual will suffer symptoms of ill-health, both physically and mentally. Three distinct phases are recognised as the **General Adaptation Syndrome (GAS)** (Figure 9.5) (Nolen-Hoeksema 2007). Phase 1 (**alarm phase**) occurs soon after exposure to the stressor. Physiological factors such as blood pressure and blood glucose levels fall, but the neuroendocrine

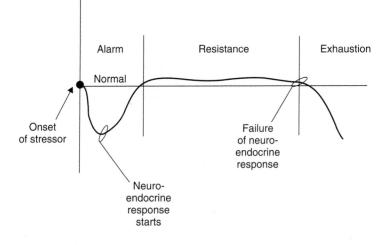

Figure 9.5 The general adaptation syndrome (GAS) with phase 1 (Alarm), phase 2 (Resistance) and phase 3 (Exhaustion). See text for explanation.

response then compensates. Phase 2 (**resistance phase**) is the period during which compensation is able to continue. How long this lasts depends on the severity of the stressor and the length of the time period involved. Phase 3 (**exhaustion phase**) is marked by the collapse of the neuroendocrine response and the return of symptoms. If the exhaustion phase is prolonged, or the stressor is great, ill-health will follow. Chronic stress causes many complications, including possible premature ageing of the brain with neuronal losses. The hippocampus is the most likely candidate for cellular losses due to chronic stress. Other long-term effects of chronic cortisol release during stress include **hypertension** (high blood pressure), **peptic ulceration** (ulcers of the stomach and duodenum), depression, substance abuse and anxiety.

Stress and child abuse

Stress occurring during childhood causes 'a cascade of molecular and neuro-biological effects that irreversibly alter neural development' (Teicher 2002). Such stress is the result of child abuse, either active (physical beatings or sexual abuse) or passive (neglect or isolation). In each case the brain is exposed to extensive fear, and permanent damage often results from this type of stress. The damage includes:

- irregularities in the function of the left frontal and temporal lobes of the cerebrum;
- reduced size of the hippocampus and amygdala, again most often seen on the left side of the brain;
- abnormalities within the cerebellar vermis.

The hippocampus continues its development beyond birth, well into childhood, and is one of the few areas of the brain where neurons continue to grow after birth.

New neurons form new synaptic connections, and it is these neurons and their connections that are disrupted permanently when subjected to the extreme fear of abuse. In the amygdala, the $GABA_A$ receptor is significantly altered by the severe fear accompanying abuse, causing a loss of its inhibitory function. The result is excessive stimulation of the limbic system (called **limbic irritability**), i.e. abnormal excessive function of the area that governs emotions.

The cerebellar vermis (the central ridge between the cerebellar hemispheres, see Figure 15.3) is another area that continues growing and developing new neurons after birth. The vermis has some control over noradrenaline and dopamine release within the brain stem. Vermis abnormalities (now being linked to several mental disorders including depression, schizophrenia and autism) may push these neurotransmitters into imbalance. Activation and dominance of the dopamine system is linked with increased attention in the *left* hemisphere; activation and dominance of the noradrenaline system is linked with increased attention in the *right* hemisphere. Developmental abnormalities occurring in the vermis after birth as a result of the stress of child abuse may be the cause of the left lateral defects observed in the cerebral and limbic areas. The results of such damage are depression, withdrawal, suicidal tendencies, anxiety, anger, aggression, delinquency, unstable relationships and personality disorders, any of which can occur at any point later in life. Teicher (2002) summarised the studies by saying:

> Society reaps what it sows in the way it nurtures its children. Stress sculpts the brain to exhibit various antisocial . . . behaviours. . . . Stress can permanently wire a child's brain to cope with a malevolent world. . . . Our stark conclusion is that we see the need to do much more to ensure that child abuse does not happen in the first place, because once these key brain alterations occur, there may be no going back.
>
> (Teicher 2002)

Rather bizarrely, some children become emotionally attached to their abusers, rather than do everything they can to leave the relationship. This situation is akin to **Stockholm syndrome** where hostages become emotionally attached to their kidnappers and do what they can to help them, rather than punish them for their crime. In the case of abused children, the 'emotional' attachment to the abuser is thought to be an adaptive response caused by the child's need for care, despite the poor quality of that care. Neurobiologists have pinned down this phenomenon to low levels of dopamine in the child's amygdala (Westly 2010).

The emotions of life experiences

The neuroanatomy and physiology of the many possible human emotions have fascinated neuroscientists for a long time. Here, we consider some of these emotions and what little we know of their neurological basis.

Humour is both a pleasant emotion and one that is said to be beneficial to our health and well-being. Imaging techniques have highlighted several areas of the brain involved in understanding a joke and responding to it with laughter. The areas most active in this process are the **left posterior temporal gyrus**, the **left inferior frontal gyrus** and the **temporoparietal junction**. Humour requires language appreciation, learning and decision-making skills, and these areas are involved in these functions. Activity also takes place in the **ventral striatum** of the limbic system, the emotional area of the brain. Here, the level of activity corresponds well with our recognition of how funny the humour is. Variations between the sexes also occur, e.g. women show greater activity in the prefrontal cortex and a greater response to funny situations from the limbic system than men do. This suggests that women undergo more in-depth executive and language processing than males when getting to grips with a joke, although the reasons for these differences are not clear. So-called extroverts appear to have greater activity in their reward circuits of the brain, including the ventral striatum, during humorous situations than do 'neurotic' or 'introverted' individuals (Elkan 2010).

Religious experiences occur when a subject becomes aware of a sense of an almighty power in their presence, which they usually call God, and may experience what they call Heaven. In some people this has changed their lives and they have become ministers of various churches and preached or administered healing powers to others. Neuroscientists go to some lengths to point out that while they have no wish to attempt to disprove the existence of God, they have found that specific types of stimulation of the **temporal lobes** of the cerebrum (especially the right temporal lobe) and the limbic system can generate what can be an overwhelming religious feeling. This is usually coupled with a release of endogenous opiates, which intensifies the experience. It is interesting that some people suffer overwhelming religious feelings when first visiting the holy city of Jerusalem. So-called **Jerusalem syndrome** causes previously normal individuals to re-enact scenes from the bible, in full biblical dress, at the sites in Jerusalem where they originally took place. During this time they are overwhelmed with emotion, bordering on psychosis. This sounds like a joke, but in 1999 more than 50 people with no previous mental health problems needed emergency psychiatric care whilst visiting the city.

Love is an experience most people go through at some point in their lives. Scans of the brains of volunteers taken during the intensified mental emotions of love reveal four main areas of increased brain activity: the **anterior cingulate cortex** (see Figures 9.6, 10.1), the **medial insula** (part of the cerebral cortex hidden from the surface), and two areas of the **corpus striatum** (part of the basal ganglia) (Figure 9.6) (Phillips 2000a). But love is not confined to the emotions experienced between two people. It is common to love abstract concepts such as music or art, or to express love of a place of great beauty. **Stendhal syndrome** (also known as **Florence syndrome**) is a feeling of palpitations, dizziness, fainting, confusion and even hallucinations when coming face to face with a piece of great art, or overwhelming amounts of great art. Florence syndrome is named after the city of Florence in Italy where substantial numbers of visitors have become overwhelmed by the city's beautiful architecture, and have needed treatment. There have been discussions concerning the possibility of stationing ambulances at regular intervals in the streets of Florence because of the number of visitors falling emotionally ill when confronted with the beauty of the city!

Music has attracted much interest from neuroscientists for several reasons. Notably, musical ability is often associated with being a genius and what makes a genius is of great interest to many people. Music has therapeutic properties and

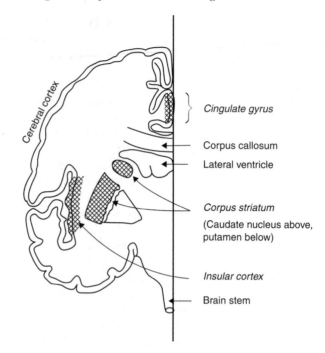

Figure 9.6 The brain areas of love. The areas shaded are activated during the emotional feelings of love.

for many years has been used as a psychological therapy (*music therapy*). More research needs to be done before we can fully explain why music therapy is good for the disturbed mind. Also, music generates some of the most intense emotions in some people, anything from excitement to depression, and the question is *why*?

This question remains unanswered, but some interesting concepts point the way. Music has a lot to do with *motion*, and motion has a lot to do with *emotion* (the two words have a common origin, i.e. *motum* = movement). Indeed, the separate sections of a symphony are called movements, and when experiencing emotion from the music the listener may describe the experience as 'moving'. Specific emotions, such as love or fear, have definite signs which we can identify in each other and can respond to and take forward. Tonal music also has specific signatures that we can pick out and relate to, like a rhythm or a tune, and music is rarely static, it is constantly driving forward. So music and emotions have very similar components. Just as one angry or laughing person can make others angry or laugh, so music performed by one person can engender emotional moods in an audience.

The parts of the brain involved in music appreciation are slowly being revealed. Scans have shown a distinct response from the right temporal lobe of the cerebrum when exposed to tonal music. This is part of the conscious brain and its activation should be no surprise, since the temporal lobe is involved in both hearing and personality. But below this level of the brain, the subconscious areas involved in emotion are also contributing to the response to music. Since sound is one of the earliest experiences we have, even while still in the uterus, the sounds of pitch and rhythm affect our neurological development from the start of life. Neuroscientists believe that the corpus callosum is involved in the mother–child relationship, of which sound is a major part, and the corpus callosum, along with the limbic system, is associated with emotion. Another unusual observation is the appearance of bizarre musical hallucinations in patients who have had damage to the dorsal part of the **pons** (part of the brain stem). The music they hear is in keeping with the style of music that is already familiar to them, as though a musical memory is unlocked and floods out into the conscious brain. Perhaps the damage has removed certain inhibitory pathways, allowing the music to be heard.

A lot of speculation revolves around whether musical ability is genetic, and therefore runs in families. The composer Mozart was taught by a musical father and had a highly talented musical older sister, and other famous composers such as Bach and Johann Strauss also had musical offspring. Now scientists have identified genes that are involved in the musical ability of both parents and their offspring. An association between the variations of the **arginine vasopressin receptor 1A (*AVPR1A*)** gene and music has been found. Vasopressin is also known as **antidiuretic hormone**, and is produced in the hypothalamus (and is released from the posterior pituitary gland) and part of the amygdala. Vasopressin binding sites are found in the septum, thalamus, amygdala and brainstem, all areas associated, in one way or another, with emotion. The AVPR1A gene had previously been linked to emotion and various social behaviours.

One or several genes are thought to control the function of several sites in the brain that determine **pitch perception**, i.e. the ability to recognise different notes when played. Pitch and rhythm are reported as left hemisphere functions, while the right hemisphere works on melody and timbre (the tone quality of an instrument). Indeed, a part of the temporal lobe called the **planus temporale** (see also Williams syndrome) is normally bigger on the left than the right, but is bigger still on the left in those persons with perfect pitch (Figure 15.2). Children with pitch control genes that are active from an early age can progress quickly with music, while others without these genes may progress more slowly or abandon music in favour of other pursuits.

Ghosts, phantoms and doppelgangers may have a neurological basis. The phenomenon of **phantom limb** (i.e. the feeling that an amputated limb is still present) has been a problem for years. Certain cells in the somatic sensory cortex that receive sensations from that limb find they no longer have an input because the limb is gone. They are redundant cells, but they are still alive and may generate their own random impulses which then trick the brain into thinking that the limb is still present.

Perhaps doppelgangers (identical copies of a person, often called 'doubles'), which are seen by that same person or by someone else, have a similar cause; i.e. the phantom limb phenomenon may be elaborated to become the entire body. 'Out of body' experiences and ghosts could also be phantom copies of the body generated by the cerebral cortex, 'seen' by the *mind* rather than the eye and interpreted as an external image (Phillips 2000b). One good example of this is the case of a man driving his van to work who passed *himself* driving exactly the same van in the opposite direction. Both *he* and *himself* stared at each other in amazement as they drove past. For such an event to occur in reality is impossible, and a mental image of himself, generated by his own brain and 'seen' by the mind as an external image, is the best explanation we have at present. The fact that neither 'person' stopped, got out or spoke to the other (i.e. the obvious thing to do) suggests that physical evidence of the other person being real was probably unobtainable, indirectly supporting the brain image theory.

Other cases of '**out of body experiences**' (also called **depersonalisation**), such as the patient who felt as though *he* (his conscious self) was about one meter in front of *himself* (his physical body) all the time, can cause a great deal of distress and may require some form of 'therapy' and very sensitive nursing care. Out of body experiences are **dissociative disorders** and are related to a similar phenomenon called '**near death experiences**' (Kotler 2005) where some people have 'died' for several minutes and then been revived. Some tell of an out-of-body experience during this time, during which they floated above their dead body. Mild stimulation of the right temporal pole, just above the right ear, sometimes causes out-of-body experiences, hearing heavenly music, intense religious feelings and hallucinations. Right temporal lobe epilepsy induces similar symptoms. EEG (electroencephalogram) studies show that those claiming near-death experiences entered REM (rapid-eye movement sleep) later (110 minutes into sleep) than normal (60 minutes into sleep) and they needed less sleep than normal. The significance of this is not yet established.

See page 7

A related phenomenon is **derealisation syndrome**, another form of dissociative disorder. Here the individual sees the world around them as a film playing, with all the people being the actors in this film. It affects 1 or 2 per cent of the population, although many more people are thought to experience it very briefly in their lifetime.

Anxiety disorders

Anxiety is a major psychological problem to which there is no easy solution. Drugs can alleviate the symptoms (see *anxiolytic drugs*) and make life more tolerable for the patient, but they are not a cure. Anxiety appears to involve the amygdala, where cholecystokinin (CCK) receptors are found, and an increase in the level of this hormone in the amygdala will generate a bout of anxiety. The psychological symptoms of anxiety include a sense of fear or apprehension, restlessness and irritability, loss of concentration and disturbed sleep. The physical symptoms include sweating, pallor, palpitations, dry mouth, numbness, dizziness and fainting, frequency of micturition, difficulty in swallowing, shortness of breath and tightness of the chest, perhaps with chest pain. There are four categories of anxiety disorder: **general anxiety disorder** (a category of patients who fail to meet the criteria for any of the other three disorders in this group), **panic attacks**, **phobias** and **obsessive-compulsive disorder** (Nolen-Hoeksema 2007).

See page 177

Fear

Fear is potentially a useful attribute since its presence is a warning that something is hazardous and should be avoided, and this can save lives. But fear is a double-edged sword, a phenomenon that can be either exciting or destructive in people's lives. As an excitement, people seek fear for recreational purposes (roller-coaster rides or horror movies); but as a destructive mechanism, fear keeps people at home and prevents them from getting on with their lives. Neuroscientists are keen to understand the anatomy and physiology of fear so as to be able to unlock the prison in which so many frightened people spend their lives.

Fear can be stored as memories (called *emotional memories*) in the brain in a form unlike all other memories. These emotional memories amount to 'learned fear', i.e. fear learnt from previous adverse experiences, and can, in susceptible people, short-circuit rational thinking and block normal behaviour even in non-fearful situations. As with other memories, an often harmless trigger is enough to cause uncontrollable outbursts of irrational behaviour. In anxiety, emotional fear appears to dominate the personality, and emotional memories are often life-long.

Three brain components appear to be communicating during periods of fear brought about by a potentially threatening environmental stimulus, either real or imaginary:

- The prefrontal cortex of the frontal lobe, which, along with the tip of the temporal lobe, assesses the stimulus for its life-threatening potential. These two areas are often collectively called the **neocortex**. Part of the prefrontal cortex, known as the **ventromedial prefrontal cortex (vmPFC)**, acts to switch off fear by reducing the activity of the amygdala, a function sometimes called 'fear extinction'.
- The amygdala, which adds the emotional dimension to the experience of fear, and is the centre of emotional memories. The amygdala has been called 'the driver of fear' as it has outputs to the brain stem and hypothalamus which generate all the emotional and physical symptoms of fear under amygdala control.
- The hypothalamus, which sets in motion the **hypathalamo–pituitary–adrenal axis** (i.e. **HPA axis**, the CRF → ACTH → cortisol route) and autonomic nervous system (sympathetic) responses. *See page 223*

The importance of the temporal lobe and amygdala in the creation of fear is illustrated in the **Kluver–Bucy syndrome**. This condition is caused by a lesion of the temporal lobes, apparently extending into the amygdala below. Such a lesion may be the result of a stroke or a head injury or may be associated with epilepsy or dementia, and brings about a general blunting of emotions coupled with a profound loss of fear. Five distinct behavioural symptoms are characteristic of the disorder:

- **Psychic blindness**, an inability to recognise common objects and what they represent, despite normal vision. This means that patients cannot recognise objects that are a potential threat.
- Oral tendencies, where all such objects are 'tested' by being put in the mouth. This leads to the notion that these patients eat everything, but more probably they are using the mouth as a mechanism of sensory input to aid recognition.
- **Hypermetamorphosis**, an overwhelming compulsion to explore everything in the immediate environment, despite any hazards.
- Increased sexual tendencies, including making inappropriate sexual advances to others, even inanimate objects.

• Emotional blunting (known as **flattening of affect**), with a profound loss of all sense of fear.

The mechanism by which the amygdala becomes overactive, and thus triggers fear and anxiety, is related to the level of GABA within circuits built into the organ's lateral nucleus (Figure 9.7). GABA (gamma amino butyric acid) is a major inhibitory neurotransmitter which is vital for reduction of excessive brain activity. With low GABA in the amygdala emotional memories can surface and generate the symptoms of acute anxiety and fear responses. Two genetic errors may be involved:

1. The gene that codes for **gastrin-releasing peptide (GRP)**, a protein which binds to GRP receptors found on GABA neurons in the lateral nucleus of the amygdala. On binding to the receptors, GRP promotes GABA release which then inhibits the amygdala. Failure of the gene causes low GRP and therefore low GABA response.
2. The gene that codes for GRP receptors. Errors in this gene could cause low numbers of receptors, or receptors that do not bind GRP, and therefore failure to bind adequate amounts of GRP leads to low GABA levels.

The hormones released during fear are basically **adrenaline** (released into the blood and circulated to all parts of the body) and **endorphins** (released into the central nervous system). These help the brain to cope with the stress that accompanies the fear; adrenaline promotes the sympathetic response and endorphins help to

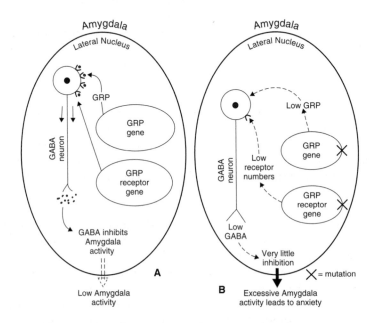

Figure 9.7 The genetic basis of fear within the amygdala. Either one gene mutation causes low GRP, or another causes few GRP receptors. Either way, the result is low inhibitory GABA, and the amygdala becomes excessively active leading to acute anxiety or fear.

protect the brain from excessive stress stimuli. After the experience of fear is over, the hormone **dopamine** is released into the brain, giving the mind a sense of joy, well-being and the satisfaction of achievement (similar to the feelings achieved by increased dopamine as a consequence of drug abuse; see Chapters 5 and 8). The *feel-good factor* created by dopamine is probably the reason some people seek out excitement. The dopamine receptor known as D_4 appears to be involved, and this receptor is coded for by a gene on chromosome 11 (the **D4DR** gene). However, there appear to be two forms of this gene: *long* and *short*. Those who have inherited the slightly longer form of the gene are more resistant to dopamine, and therefore need additional dopamine to have the feel-good effect that they call a *buzz*. These people have to take extra risks to obtain more dopamine, and therefore they seek out adventurous and risky activities. For those with the shorter version of the gene the dopamine binds much better, and so less dopamine is required, making risk-taking activities unnecessary and apparently foolhardy.

Phobias and obsessive-compulsive disorder

A **phobia** is an irrational and pathological fear centred on a specific situation or object, which dominates the lifestyle of the sufferer. There are many common phobias, e.g. fear of an *object* such as a spider (**arachnophobia**) or fear of a *situation* such as an enclosed space (**claustrophobia**), but there are many less common phobias, e.g. fear of phobias (**phobophobia**), and some very rare and rather bizarre phobias, e.g. the fear of becoming ill (**nosophobia** or **nosemaphobia**) and ironically, the word for 'fear of long words' is (**hippopotomonstrosesquipedaliophobia**)! **Agoraphobia** sufferers avoid public and unfamiliar places, especially large, open spaces where there are no hiding places. This particular disorder is responsible for keeping some sufferers 'trapped' in their homes for 40 years or more. This is the way the patient copes with their fear, by staying in their home. The person concerned avoids the cause of the phobia as much as possible, and this allows them to continue a 'normal' life, albeit a poorer quality of life. Pathological phobic states incapacitate the patient and require medical intervention to re-establish a reasonable quality of life.

Obsessions are repeated thoughts, ideas or phrases, and **compulsions** are irresistible repetitive activities, such as repeated hand-washing, which the patient must go through in order to prevent some degree of fear and anxiety. Both of these together in the same patient make up **obsessive-compulsive disorder (OCD)**. If these activities are stopped or prevented in some way, the person concerned may quickly go into a **panic attack**.

There is some evidence to suggest that both *panic attacks* and *obsessive-compulsive disorder* carry a genetic susceptibility, as a higher than average incidence of such attacks can be demonstrated in some families. Relatives of those with OCD have a six-times greater risk of developing OCD than relatives of those without OCD. People with OCD also have a higher risk of depression and anxiety than the general population. It has also been found that an injection of **lactic acid** will cause some individuals to have a panic attack whereas the same injection has no such effect on others, and this suggests that some individuals are genetically more susceptible to panic attacks than others (Maier 1999). The **catecholamine-O-methyl-transferase (COMT)** gene codes for the enzyme that breaks down the neurotransmitters dopamine, adrenaline and noradrenaline, and *COMT* gene errors are suspected as part of the cause since it was discovered that this gene is underexpressed in OCD.

Temporal lobe abnormalities have been found in association with anxiety states and panic attacks. It seems that the greater the abnormality, the younger the age of onset of the anxiety (Rosenzweig et al. 1999). Reduced frontal lobe activity is also implicated in panic attacks. In the case of both frontal and temporal lobes, a diminished level of activity causes the attack, suggesting that the role of these lobes in understanding and rationalising sensory stimuli is reduced, leaving the limbic system to respond independently. There may be some gene variants involved in the serotonin (5-HT) system of the brain although exactly how this influences the condition is not fully known. Abnormal levels of **cholecystokinin (CCK)** appear

See page 71 to be involved, in particular CCK-4 which is also known to induce panic.

Obsessive-compulsive disorder is associated with increased activity of several brain areas, notably a loop extending from the orbitofrontal cortex, through the caudate nucleus and the thalamus, then back to the cortex (Insel 2010). Two pathways connect the caudate nucleus with the thalamus, an excitatory pathway and an inhibitory pathway (Figure 9.8). The former is said to facilitate previously learned and automatic behaviour, while the latter reduces it, thereby allowing the individual to move on to new behaviours. Brain scan evidence shows that in OCD this

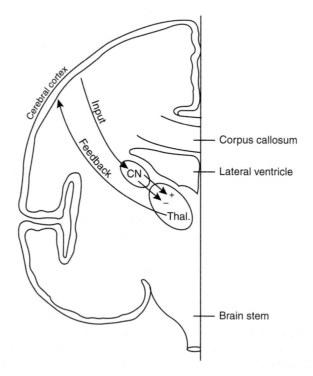

Figure 9.8 The loop extending from the cerebral cortex through the caudate nucleus (CN) to the thalamus (Thal.), either excitatory or inhibitory, and back to the cortex, influences learning and automatic behaviour.

loop and the excitatory pathway in particular are overactive, causing an imbalance that keeps the patient locked in a cycle of repetitive behaviour (Carlson 2010).

An alternative view is that the link between the thalamus and the cortex, including the reciprocal feedback from the cortex to the thalamus, has become inhibited, i.e. deactivated, for some unknown reason (Clayton 2000). This problem may also be implicated in the cause of depression and the hallucinations suffered in schizophrenia. The cause of this disturbance of loop function remains unknown, but a reduction of serotonin and an increase in noradrenaline in the diffuse modulatory systems may be responsible (see Chapter 11 for these systems). Together the modulatory systems help to control the loop function, but an imbalance between serotonin and noradrenaline could cause an increase in loop activity. The standard treatment of OCD involves the use of antidepressant drugs called **SSRI (selective serotonin re-uptake inhibitors)** which improve the level of serotonin in the brain (see Chapter 11) and this helps to reduce the symptoms. Neurosurgery has been used successfully to reduce the symptoms of OCD in cases which fail to respond to drugs. This involves cutting through some of the pathways that pass from the frontal lobe to the limbic parts of the brain (Ron 1999).

Post-traumatic stress disorder

Post-traumatic stress disorder (**PTSD**) is a stress condition that occurs in some people exposed to a severe traumatic incident, such as a train crash, either as a survivor or as a rescuer. It affects children and adults subjected to abuse, casualties or witnesses of traumatic events, soldiers in battle situations (it was originally called 'shell shock', 'battle fatigue' or 'combat neurosis' during the First World War), victims of violent crime, those subjected to long periods of incarceration and those receiving bad news, such as the loss of a family member or being told about a poor prognosis. The incident that triggers the stress clearly has some major effect on brain function, involving changes in the neurochemistry. Neuroimaging has established the major problem as abnormal activity of the ventromedial prefrontal cortex (vmPFC) which, as noted previously, reduces fear by inhibiting the fear response from the amygdala. The vmPKC is part of a loop linking the dorsolateral prefrontal cortex with the amygdala and hippocampus (Insel 2010). The dorsolateral prefrontal cortex is important in learning to tolerate and overcome fear. Each time the vmPFC decreases its function, the link between the dorsolateral prefrontal cortex and the amygdala is diminished (or broken) and the fear shutdown activity is lost. As a result, fear response levels increase in the amygdala. This causes the sudden manifestation of symptoms of PTSD, such as **flashbacks**, in which the original events of the incident, e.g. the sights, sounds and smells, are relived, often many times, for months or years after the event. The vmPFC in PTSD sufferers is also smaller than normal, and this directly reduces this areas ability to switch off fear (Insel 2010). The pathway that links the hypothalamus to the pituitary, and on to the adrenal gland (known as the **HPA axis**; the hormones being CRF → ACTH → cortisol, Figure 11.5) is severely affected, resulting in low cortisol release into the blood (the opposite of acute stress) and therefore causing a compensatory increase in cortisol receptor sensitivity. In the brain, serotonin and noradrenaline activities are increased, both of which are involved in memory retrieval, and the hippocampus is enlarged. Since the hippocampus is a site of memory function, these changes may account for the number and frequency of flashbacks these people suffer. This constant re-enactment of the incident is a trauma in itself, seriously disturbing the lifestyle of those who suffer from it. It may require several years of therapy and sensitive understanding on the part of nurses to achieve an outcome that improves the quality of life for those who suffer from this problem.

Breedlove *et al.* (2010) reported studies done on American Vietnam war veterans with PTSD who suffered from memory changes (e.g. **amnesia** of some traumatic events), flashbacks and problems with short-term memory. They showed an 8 per cent reduction in the size of the hippocampus, but no other structural abnormality. There also appeared to be a genetic susceptibility involved, making some more vulnerable to the effects of trauma than others.

Eating disorders

Several stress-related disorders which result in disturbance of normal eating patterns sometimes need psychological support and therapy. The most important of these are **obesity** (excess weight), **anorexia nervosa** (inadequate eating) and **bulimia nervosa** (loss of control of food intake). The sufferer of anorexia nervosa will eat very little, leading to severe weight loss and starvation to the point of death. In contrast, the patient with bulimia nervosa will periodically go on an eating 'binge'. They will eat lots of high-calorie food and then, feeling guilty, cause vomiting and use laxatives to get rid of it. The biological mechanism of normal food control is very complex and as yet not fully understood. Not until recently has there been any clear idea of what is going wrong in these disorders.

Adipose tissue (stored fat under the skin and around internal organs) releases a hormone called **leptin** into the blood (Figure 9.9). This hormone binds to **leptin receptors** in the **arcuate nucleus**, one of the nuclei of the hypothalamus. The binding of leptin to its receptor causes a shutdown of neurons which normally secrete a combination of two proteins, **neuropeptide Y** (**NPY**) and **agouti-related protein** (**ARP**). Together, these two proteins normally act by binding to, and inhibiting, another receptor, the **melanocortin-4 receptor** (**MC-4**). Inhibition of the MC-4 by NYP and ARP in the hypothalamus causes feeding activity, so the blocking of NYP + ARP by leptin stops the individual from feeding. This makes sense when you consider that the greater the mass of adipose tissue the larger the release of leptin; and in circumstances of large adipose mass the need for food should be less. To reinforce this effect, leptin receptors activated by the binding of leptin also stimulate other arcuate neurons, which then release two other proteins called **cocaine and amphetamine regulated transcript** (**CART**) and α**-MSH** (**alpha-melanocyte stimulating hormone**). Together these two neuromodulators act on MC-4 receptors to inhibit feeding. So leptin causes *inhibition* of feeding behaviour by *increasing* CART+α-MSH and *decreasing* NYP + ARP (Figure 9.9). It appears that short-term acute stress causes the normal neuroendocrine response, resulting in raising the blood adrenaline and cortisol levels. This change in hormone levels acts to switch off ARP, just as leptin does, and therefore inhibits feeding. However, once the acute stress is over, the cortisol and adrenaline levels fall to normal, and ARP is activated again with feeding behaviour restored. In anorexia nervosa, the stress is retained in a chronic form (although it may not be recognised as such by the patient or their family), so that high levels of adrenaline and cortisol

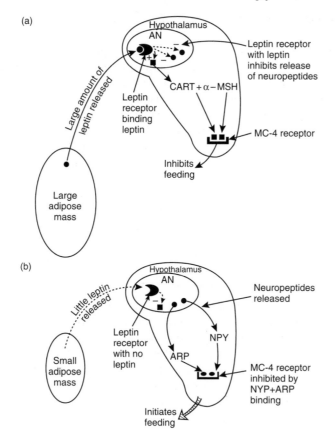

Figure 9.9 Adipose feedback to the brain. (a) With large adipose volume, more leptin is released, which binds to leptin receptors in the arcuate nucleus (AN) of the hypothalamus. This causes inhibition of neuropeptide release, but promotes the release of the cocaine and amphetamine regulated transcript (CART) and the alpha-melanocyte stimulating hormone (α-MSH). These bind to MC-4 receptors and inhibit feeding. (b) Little adipose volume releases low levels of leptin; the empty leptin receptor then inhibits the CART/α-MSH release but causes release of neuropeptides. When these bind to MC-4 receptors, feeding is initiated. NPY = neuropeptide Y; ARP = agouti-related protein.

are retained in the blood. In this way, ARP is continually inhibited, feeding behaviour may be chronically suppressed and the individual will starve. One of the long-term effects of persistent starvation is that the hippocampus shrinks, causing a permanent reduction in the hippocampal role in regulating appetite. Long-term anorexia may cause the type of brain damage that is both irreparable and perpetuates the problem.

In **bulimia nervosa (BN)**, the pathophysiology is poorly understood. Three types of bulimia have been described:

1. **Simple** bulimia nervosa starts in girls under 18 who were regarded as normal before they started showing symptoms. It may be triggered by an emotional

upset, and dieting in this bizarre manner may be seen by the sufferer as a way of restoring self-esteem.

2. **Anorexic** bulimia nervosa, which starts with a period of anorexia first. This recovers and there is a brief time of normality before the bulimia begins. The food binging intensifies, with vomiting being introduced at part of the process. These girls often have a disturbed family background.

3. **Multi-impulsive** bulimia nervosa is a severe variation than starts similarly to simple BN. The girls lack control over their emotions and their eating habits, and they succumb to impulsive behavioural problems. There is often a highly disturbed family background which offers little or no support to the patient.

Bulimia may involve disturbed serotonin levels in the brain, and even recovered bulimia patients show abnormal brain levels of serotonin. However, there are clearly huge environmental and social causes that contribute towards this disorder.

Obesity may be due to a reduction in the brain's *sensitivity* to leptin, rather than a reduction in the amount of leptin production. This is possible through several mechanisms:

*   The gene for leptin (the **OB** gene at 7q31.3) mutates, the changed gene coding for a form of leptin that does not bind to its receptor.
*   The gene for the leptin receptor (the **Db** gene at 1p31) mutates, the changed gene coding for a form of receptor that cannot accept leptin.
*   The transporter system that is essential for leptin to cross the blood–brain barrier becomes faulty and less leptin reaches the brain.
*   The gene for the MC-4 receptor may develop errors and therefore MC-4 does not function normally.

Some of these mechanisms have been found in humans, often occurring in families as an inherited trait.

The neurophysiology of eating is further complicated by other control mechanisms. For example, the liver detects levels of blood glucose and fatty acids and signals the brain about these via the vagus nerve (cranial nerve X) (Figure 9.10). The signals arrive at the **nucleus of the solitary tract** (**NST**) in the brain stem. This nucleus, in turn, relays the information to the hypothalamus. In this way the liver keeps the hypothalamus informed of nutrient levels in circulation. The **lateral hypothalamus** is a major player in the generation of hunger which would be activated through this route if the blood nutrients arriving at the liver are low. The **ventromedial hypothalamus** initiates the sensation of **satiety**, i.e. the feeling of fullness, which would be activated if the blood nutrients arriving at the liver were high, as would be the case shortly after a meal. However, most researchers in this subject also acknowledge the important regulatory role played by other brain areas, notably the amygdala, the frontal cortex, the substantia nigra and the hippocampus. **Orexins** (**hypocretins**) are two neuropeptide hormones, **orexin A** and **B**. They promote food intake and wakefulness. They are products of the lateral hypothalamus (Carlson 2010). Orexin is also active in the sleep–wake cycle. They bind to two excitatory metabotropic receptors, OX_1 and OX_2. Leptin appears to inhibit orexin production, whilst **ghrelin**, another hormone from the stomach, promotes food intake by activating orexin production.

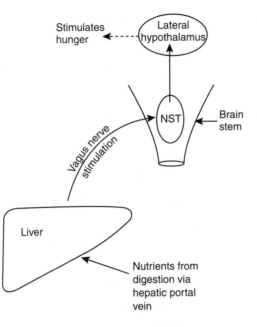

Figure 9.10 The liver control of hunger. Vagus nerve stimulation by the liver informs the hypothalamus, via the nucleus of the solitary tract (NST) in the brain stem, about the condition of nutrients in storage. Low nutrient levels may stimulate hunger.

Anorexia nervosa has been associated with abnormally low levels of some immune chemicals called **interleukins** (**Il**) (in particular **Il-6**), and **tumour necrosing factors** (**TNF**)(in particular **TNF-1β**). This may increase the risk of infection. Anorexia has also been linked to disturbance of **haematopoiesis** (blood forming), a bone marrow function which normally produces the circulating red and white blood cells. Disturbance of this function leads to abnormal blood cell counts.

One idea is that anorexia nervosa is a *fat phobia*, and *compulsive eating* is a major cause of obesity, in which case these may be a distinct subset of anxiety-related disorders. In any case, control of body weight is important for health; being either too thin or too fat causes severe problems for the cardiovascular system and can result in death. The **body mass index** (**BMI**) is a standard method of recording if a person is under or over weight. The BMI is:

Weight (in kilograms; kg) ÷ height (in m²)

An adult female should have a BMI between 20 and 25 kgm². Above this level constitutes varying degrees of obesity, and below constitutes underweight. It is not uncommon for anorexic women to have a BMI of less than 17.5 kgm².

The anxiolytic drugs

The **benzodiazepines** are a major group of anxiolytic drugs (anxio = anxiety, lytic = dissolving), typified by **diazepam, alprazolam, chlordiazepoxide, lorazepam** and **oxazepam**. They are used widely to reduce levels of acute anxiety. These drugs bind to the **GABA$_A$** receptor (Figure 4.13) and promote the function of GABA to open the chloride channel that runs through the receptor. In this respect they have a similar action to that of barbiturates and alcohol. The subsequent increase in the influx of chloride into the neuronal postsynaptic membrane causes a greater degree of *resting membrane potential* and blocks any chance of an action potential in that cell. On a widely distributed basis throughout the brain, this drug group has a sedatory effect, i.e. it calms the brain but without inducing sleep (except in high dosages). **Benzodiazepines** are best used as a short-term management of severe anxiety, for no longer than about six weeks. Long-term use is associated with dependence and should be avoided. These drugs are well absorbed from the digestive system and well tolerated when given orally. Diazepam has a long half-life (20 to 100 hours) due to active metabolites, and therefore has a sustained effect.

See page 65 The non-barbiburate **Buspirone** is thought to act at specific serotonin (5HT$_{1A}$) receptors. Relief of symptoms may take up to two weeks.

Anxiety-related personality disorders

Several anxiety-related personality disorders have been identified, although the underlying biology is not understood in most of these disorders:

1. **Avoidant personality disorder** occurs when individuals avoid interactions with others because they fear criticism. They become hypersensitive, nervous and self-restrained when interaction with others is essential. They are very anxious about being embarrassed and tend to lead solitary lives. They may get depressed or feel inadequate when in social settings. It probably affects anything from 1 to 7 per cent of the population. **Social phobia** is a similar problem, the difference being that those with social phobia want to enjoy others' company but may fear specific social functions, while in avoidant personality disorder they do not want company with others because that would aggravate their feels of inadequacy causing an anxiety state.
2. **Dependent personalities** are those people who depend entirely on others for many aspects of their lives. These aspects include decision-making and affection, as well as personal care and guidance. They thrive only in close relationships and they fear the break-up of those relationships, which would require them to take more control of their lives. This disorder makes the sufferer vulnerable to exploitation and abuse. It can affect up to 6 per cent of the population and involves more women than men.
3. **Obsessive-compulsive personality** has features in common with OCD, but differs by the individual being rigid and dogmatic, with blunted emotions. They work continuously, finding little or no time to maintain friendships or indulge in leisure. Obsession with perfectionism and following rules dominates their activities. They may be seen as dominating and authoritarian to their subordinates. As many as 7 per cent of the population may have obsessive-compulsive personality, with more men than women affected.
4. **Histrionic personality** involves individuals with rapidly shifting, intense and flamboyant emotions. They are often overdependent on others and form rather unstable relationships. Their dramatic approach to life makes them the centre

of attention, and this can result in a higher than average number of medical consultations. Up to 22 per cent of the population may show evidence of histrionic personality, with the majority of affected individuals being female.

5. **Narcissistic personalities** are people with dramatic, grandiose behaviour, the purpose of which is to gain admiration and affection from others. They indulge in their own self-importance, and they see themselves as superior to others. Beneath this facade, they have shallow emotions and are poor at establishing relationships. Less than 1 per cent of the population demonstrate narcissism, and these are largely males.

6. **Borderline personalities** are unstable people with a loss of control of emotions. They form very strong attachments to others, fearing abandonment. They suffer from instability of mood, which can result in depression or anxiety, and they may act impulsively, or commit self-harm. They may describe having transient **dissociative states**, which are periods of detachment from reality, during which the individual sees the world as one would see a film, i.e. they are not actually part of it. Borderline personality affects 1 or 2 per cent of the population, women more than men. Families with some members diagnosed as borderline personality disorder often show increased rates of mood disorder, suggesting a possible genetic origin for this problem. There is sometimes an increase in the activity of the amygdala when the individual is shown pictures of faces demonstrating emotions. There is low serotonin activity (which is linked to impulsiveness) and reduced metabolism within the prefrontal cortex.

Key points

The limbic system

*   The limbic system is a series of centres involved in self-preservation and preservation of the species.
*   The major components of the limbic system are the amygdala, the mammillary bodies of the hypothalamus, the anterior and dorsal nuclei of the thalamus, several deep nuclei, the septal area, the orbitofrontal cortex of the cerebrum, the hippocampus and parahippocampal gyrus and parts of the temporal lobe.
*   The amygdala is the main site for emotions, although emotional states are moderated through several other brain areas as well, notably the frontal and temporal cortex, the hypothalamus and the hippocampus.
*   The neuroendocrine response is a normal mechanism adopted by the hypothalamus to combat the effects of stress. It consists of a neurological response via the sympathetic nervous system, and an endocrine response via certain pituitary hormones.

Stress

*   Post-traumatic stress disorder (PTSD) is a stress condition that occurs in some people exposed to a severe traumatic incident. It causes flashbacks, which appear to be due to reduced activity of the vmPFC which normally switches off fear.

Anxiety disorders

- Anxiety appears to involve the amygdala, where increased cholecystokinin (CCK) can cause anxiety.
- There are four categories of anxiety disorder: general anxiety disorder, panic attacks, phobias and obsessive-compulsive disorder.

Fear

- Three brain components appear to be communicating during periods of fear, the prefrontal and temporal cortex, the amygdala and the hypothalamus, involving the hypathalamo–pituitary–adrenal axis.
- The hormones released during fear are adrenaline and endorphins and, after the experience of fear, dopamine is released.

Phobias and obsessive-compulsive disorder

- A phobia is an irrational fear centred on a specific situation or object.
- Obsessions are repeated thoughts, ideas or phrases; compulsions are irresistible repetitive activities.
- Reduced frontal lobe activity is implicated in panic attacks.
- Obsessive-compulsive disorder is associated with increased activity of a loop consisting of the orbitofrontal cortex, the caudate nucleus and the thalamus.

Eating disorders

- The lateral hypothalamus is the main component that causes hunger, the ventromedial hypothalamus initiating the sensation of satiety.
- The most important of the eating disorders are obesity, anorexia nervosa and bulimia nervosa.
- In anorexia nervosa, chronic stress may cause high adrenaline and cortisol to remain in the blood, inhibiting ARP and feeding, leading to starvation.
- Obesity may be due to a reduction in the brain's sensitivity to leptin.

The anxiolytic drugs

- The anxiolytics bind to the $GABA_A$ receptor and promote GABA to open the chloride channel, causing inhibition of action potentials and calming of the brain.
- They should be used in the short-term only, for no longer than six weeks.
- The non-barbiburate Buspirone is thought to act at specific serotonin ($5HT_{1A}$) receptors.

References

Breedlove S. M., Watson N. V. and Rosenzweig M. R. (2010) *Biological Psychology: An Introduction to Behavioral, Cognitive and Clinical Neuroscience* (6th edition). Sinauer Associates, Massachusetts.

Carlson N. R. (2010) *Physiology of Behavior* (10th edition). Allyn and Bacon, Boston.

Clayton J. (2000) Caught napping. *New Scientist*, **165** (2227): 42–45.

Elkan D. (2010) The comedy circuit. *New Scientist*, **205** (2745): 40–43.

Insel T. R. (2010) Faulty circuits. *Scientific American*, **302** (4): 28–35.

Jenkins J. and Murray C. S. (2001) Mozart 'can cut epilepsy'. http://news.bbc.co.uk/hi/english/health/newsid_1251000/1251839.stm.

Kaye J., Morton J., Bowcutt M. and Maupin D. (2000) Stress, depression and psychneuroimmunology. *Journal of Neuroscience Nursing*, **32** (2): 93–100.

Kliewer G. (1999) The Mozart effect. *New Scientist*, **164** (2211; 6 Nov): 34–37.

Kotler S. (2005) Extreme states. *Discover*, July, 61–66.

Maier M. (1999) Magnetic resonance spectroscopy in neuropsychiatry, in Ron M. A. and David A. S. (eds), *Disorders of Brain and Mind*. Cambridge University Press, Cambridge.

McKie R. (1998) The people eaters. *New Scientist*, **157** (2125): 43–46.

Nolen-Hoeksema S. (2007) *Abnormal Psychology* (4th edition). McGraw-Hill, Boston.

Phillips H. (2000a) So you think you're in love? *New Scientist*, 8 July: 11.

Phillips H. (2000b) Mind phantoms. *New Scientist*, 8 July: 11.

Ron M. A. (1999) Psychiatric manifestations of demonstrable brain disease, in Ron M. A. and David A. S. (eds), *Disorders of Brain and Mind*. Cambridge University Press, Cambridge.

Teicher M. H. (2002) The neurobiology of child abuse. *Scientific American*, **286** (3; March): 54–61.

Westly E. (2010) Abuse and attachment. *Scientific American Mind*, **21** (1): 10.

10 Schizophrenia

- Introduction
- The genetic influence in schizophrenia
- Brain pathology
- Neurodevelopment as a factor
- The biochemical changes in schizophrenia
- The possible role of environmental factors
- Schizoaffective disorder and schizoid-related personality disorders
- The antipsychotic drugs
- Key points

Introduction

A student of psychiatric nursing in the 1960s would have had a classroom session on schizophrenia possibly consisting of a description of the symptoms and types of the disease, with mention of the drugs used at the time to treat the condition. Hardly anything would have been said about what was happening in the brain, simply because very little was known then about the biology of the disease. Much progress had been made by the 1960s, of course, to dispel the pre-Victorian notion that this disorder was due to devils in the brain, but the emphasis was placed on the psychology of the condition rather than any physical disorder. Now, however, the evidence is mounting that there is an organic cause for schizophrenia, and much intense research is now being conducted in a major effort to solve this mind-destroying problem.

Schizophrenia is a major psychotic illness causing a series of symptoms that rob the patient of their cognitive thought, their socialisation skills and ultimately their personality. These symptoms fall into two categories, positive and negative (Table 10.1). These two groups of symptoms may indicate that the term 'schizophrenia' is being used to describe an amalgamation of two distinct syndromes, one demonstrating a predominance of positive symptoms (**Type I**), the other a predominance of negative symptoms (**Type II**) (Nolen-Hoeksema 2007). The relationship between the two syndromes is interesting. Delays in the early neurodevelopment of an individual have been correlated with negative symptoms, disturbance of language and attention, and poor social adjustment later in life. The

Table 10.1 The symptoms of schizophrenia.

Symptom	Types	Explanation, examples
Positive symptoms		
(Type I)		
Those unwanted aspects that the patient would prefer to do without, caused by increased dopamine activity. Usually associated with abrupt onset of the disease.		
Thought disorder *includes* **Delusions** (disorder of thought content) (Holland et al. 1999)	Ideas of reference	Ordinary items have special meaning for the patient, e.g. 'Three milk bottles delivered today means I have three days to live.'
	Concrete thinking	Everything is literal, no abstract thinking, e.g. 'I must fly' means to the patient you will grow wings and take to the air.
	Flights of ideas	Rapid, uncontrolled thoughts passing quickly from one to another.
	Grandeur	False belief of great status or importance, e.g. 'I own the hospital.'
	Paranoia	False belief that harm is directed at the patient, e.g. 'Next door's TV is beaming death rays at me.'
	Persecution	False belief that people are against the patient, e.g. 'The doctor is killing me with drugs.'
	Body	False belief that the body is changed in some way, e.g. 'My head is made of plastic.'
Hallucinations (Holland et al. 1999)	Tactile	Feeling things that are not there, e.g. worms crawling over the skin.
	Aural	Hearing things that are not there, notably voices talking to them.
	Visual	Seeing things that are not there, notably little people.
Bizarre behaviour	e.g. catatonia or inappropriate aggression	Long periods of no visible movement.
		Violent outbursts.
Negative symptoms		
(Type II)		
Those attributes taken away from the patient that they would prefer to keep, caused by neuron losses. Usually associated with gradual onset of the disease.		
Withdrawal from reality	Isolation from the real world into an inner world of the mind	Profound loss of self-care.
Loss of volition (or motivation)	The willingness to do things is lost	Remains seated all day if not motivated.
Loss (or blunting) of affect	Mood and emotions are lost or inappropriate	Remains emotionless or cries (or laughs) without reason.
Loss of speech (or speech content)	Speaks very little	Remains quiet all day.

negative symptoms are usually resistant to all attempts to prevent them as they may be the consequence of irreversible brain damage (see brain cell losses) (Carlson 2010) and, in young people, this indicates a poor outcome. Positive symptoms such as hallucinations and delusions, on the other hand, tend to occur a little later in life, as the disorder becomes more advanced. They are probably due to increased activity in the dopamine and possibly the noradrenaline brain circuits (Carlson 2010). It seems that negative symptoms, language plus attention problems and social maladjustment are also symptoms of **affective disorder** (see Chapter 11), but if you add positive symptoms to this scenario it becomes schizophrenia. If this *two-syndrome hypothesis* turns out to be correct, it will have implications for the treatment and management of schizophrenia. The management of schizophrenic symptoms provides a major challenge for nurses caring for these clients. Symptoms such as hallucinations and delusions are hard to comprehend and manage successfully (Holland et al. 1999).

Although at the moment the cause of schizophrenia is still unknown, there is a huge and growing volume of biological data concerning the disease. It does now appear, however, that a number of factors act together to influence the onset of schizophrenia.

The genetic influence in schizophrenia

The risk of developing schizophrenia is about 1 per cent for the population of the world as a whole; that is, 1 in 100 persons will develop the disease on average. The age of onset of symptoms is mostly later in women than in men; males usually begin showing evidence of the disease in their teens or early twenties (around 15–25 years).

The evidence strongly implicates a genetic component in the cause of schizophrenia (Taylor 1999), and some specific genes have been found that may play a part in the cause. The disease is probably **polygenic** (i.e. several genes are involved, interacting with environmental factors). The suggestion of gene involvement is based on studies of **monozygotic (identical) twins**, who have about 98 per cent of their genes in common, and other family groups involved in schizophrenia. Table 10.2 shows the concordance rate, i.e. the percentage chance of related members of the family developing the disease.

If one of a set of monozygotic twins develops schizophrenia, the other twin has a 40 to 50 per cent chance of having the disease, which is clearly much higher than the 1 per cent general population rate. However, given that nearly all their genes are the same, it might be expected that the concordance rate would be close to

Table 10.2 Risk of developing schizophrenia.

Family relationship	Genetic risk concordance rate
Monozygotic twins	40–50%
Dizygotic twins	15–17%
A sibling affected	10%
One parent affected	15%
Both parents affected	35%
One parent and one sibling affected	17%

Table 10.3 The major genes examined in schizophrenia research. See text for explanations of terms.

Gene	Gene locus	Function (if known)	Gene error (if known)	Possible role in schizophrenia
KCNN3 (SK3)	1q21–q22	Calcium-activated potassium channel	CAG repeats	The longer gene may code for a potassium channel with subtle abnormal changes in function, altering neuron activity.
DRD3	3q13.3	Codes for dopamine receptor D_3	Polymorphism	Dopamine receptors implicated in the biochemical cause of psychosis.
Multiple genetic variants*	6p21.3–22.1	Major Histocompatibility Complex (MHC)	Single nucleotide polymorphisms (SNPs)	Increase risk of schizophrenia.
ATX1 (ATX = ataxin)	6p23	Codes for the protein ataxin 1		Possibly associated with severity of symptoms.
DRD4	11p15.5	Codes for dopamine receptor D_4		Dopamine receptors implicated in the biochemical cause of psychosis.
DRD2	11q23	Codes for dopamine receptor D_2	Polymorphism	Dopamine receptors implicated in the biochemical cause of psychosis.
DISC1 (DISC = disrupted in schizophrenia)	1q42.1	Codes for protein that interacts with others in neurone development	Translocation t(1;11) (q42.1;q14.3)	Disruption by translocation causes failure of protein product.
5-HT 2A receptor	13q14–q21	Codes for serotonin receptor 2A	Polymorphism	Receptor variation may disturb serotonin pathways from the raphe nucleus.
CHRNA7	15q14	Codes for the alpha-7 subunit of the nicotinic acetylcholine receptor	Polymorphism	Nicotinic receptors are involved in the inhibition of sensory stimuli that may be reduced in schizophrenia leading to hallucinations.
GNAL	18p	Codes for the G-protein alpha subunit coupled to the D_1 dopamine receptor	Nucleotide repeat sequence	Dopamine receptors implicated in the biochemical cause of psychosis.
SCZD4 (SCZ = schizophrenia)	22q11–q13		Deletions within 22q11	Increases susceptibility to schizophrenia.
DXYS14	X telomere		Shared alleles in affected siblings	Schizophrenic patients often have excess X chromosomes.

5-HT 1A receptor gene	5q11.2–q13	Codes for serotonin receptor		Receptor variation may disturb serotonin pathways from the raphe nucleus.
cPLA2 (phospholipase gene)	Chromosome 19	Controls the production of the enzyme cytosolic phospholipase	Diamorphic site	Excess enzyme may cause neuronal phospholipid breakdown in schizophrenia.
Type 1 sigma receptor gene	19p13.3	Codes for sigma receptor	Polymorphism	The drug haloperidol binds to sigma receptors.

★ Multiple genetic variants within the MHC at gene loci 6p21.3–22.1 have been shown, from pooling the results of three major studies, to significantly increase the risk of schizophrenia (Stefansson H. et al. 2009, see text for more information).

100 per cent if it were purely genetic, such that if one twin acquired the disease the other definitely would. But this difference is the result of environmental factors influencing the course of events, the environment being an important part of all polygenic disorders. Table 10.3 identifies the most important genes thought to influence schizophrenia and what we understand of their function. This list is not exhaustive; other genes appear in the literature from time to time, and no doubt will continue to do so.

The type of **gene errors** involved are varied (see Table 10.3). Examples include **fragile sites, nucleotide repeat sequences** and **translocations**. Fragile sites are points where the DNA is particularly prone to breakage (fragile sites are especially involved in several mental health disorders, see **fragile X syndrome**). Nucleotide repeat sequences are abnormal multiple copies of three nucleotide bases along the DNA, e.g. **CAG** or **CGG repeats**, in this case **cytosine–adenine–guanine** and **cytosine–guanine–guanine**, respectively. Repeat sequences are sometimes the cause of disorders of the brain (see Huntington's disease). Translocations involve swapping genetic material with another chromosome. **Dimorphism** and **polymorphism** are the existence of two (di-) and multiple (poly-) variants of the gene respectively. A **single nucleotide polymorphism** (**SNP**) is a number of variants (or changes) of just one base (the bases being adenine, thymine, cytosine or guanine) within the DNA sequence of a gene.   *See page 99*

The discovery of various SNPs within the **major histocompatability complex** (**MHC**) region of chromosome 6 which are linked to schizophrenia raises the prospect of the cause of schizophrenia being linked to infection. MHC proteins are cell-surface proteins involved in the immune response to foreign infective agents (called **antigens**). MHC proteins are crucial for the correct and adequate response to antigens. SNPs in this gene region would alter these proteins sufficiently to prevent a proper response, and an infective agent could then survive and infect body tissues, including the brain. This links in well with the growing evidence that viral infections, particularly the flu virus, may be involved in the cause of this disorder.   *See page 202*

The discovery of the **DISC1** gene (DISC means 'disrupted in schizophrenia') on chromosome 1 is an important breakthrough since the protein product of this gene is part of a vital signalling pathway which gets corrupted in this disorder and which may be available as a target for drug therapy (Ross and Margolis 2009).

Brain pathology

The pathological changes seen in the schizophrenic patient's brain when compared to normal brains at post mortem are not gross, but some distinct abnormalities have been consistently reported. These include mostly enlarged ventricles, a reduction in brain weight of about 5 per cent and a shortening of the length of the brain. Enlarged ventricles occur in some schizophrenia and bipolar depressed patients. Enlargement of the lateral ventricles requires loss of some brain tissue around the ventricle, and variations in this loss may account for the variations in the types of schizophrenia seen. Those with enlarged ventricles show social, emotional and behavioural problems for some years before the onset of the major symptoms. They also have abnormal connections between the amygdala, hypothalamus and the prefrontal cortex.

On close study, it can be seen that there are some reductions in the volume (i.e. neuronal losses) within the prefrontal cortex, the insula cortex (part of the cerebrum hidden from view deep at the bottom of the lateral fissure), the entorhinal cortex, the hippocampus and the temporal lobe grey matter. The entorhinal cortex and the anterior hippocampus both suffer losses of about 20 per cent of their neurons. These areas of the brain also apparently show a change in the **cytoarchitecture**, i.e. alterations in the tissue *structure*, not just numbers of cells lost.

The frontal cortex has two large areas that show changes in schizophrenia, these areas are known as Brodmann 10 and Brodmann 4 (the primary motor cortex). Brodmann 10 shows significant losses of neurons in cell layer vi, and lower than normal density of the interneurons in layer ii. Brodmann 4 shows significant cell losses in layer vi. In addition, the cingulate gyrus (Brodmann 24) shows notable numbers of neuronal losses in cell layer v (Figure 10.1).

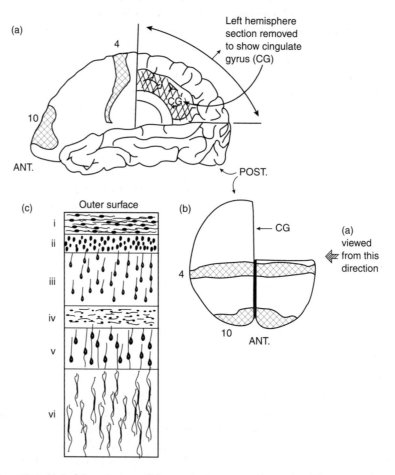

Figure 10.1 (a) Left lateral view of the cerebral cortex with much of the parietal lobe re-moved back to the midline to show the cingulate gyrus (CG), also showing Brodmann areas 4 and 10. (b) Superior view of the same as (a). (c) Section through the cerebral cortex to show the cell layers. The areas identified in (a) and (b) all suffer a loss of cells in schizophrenia. Brodmann 4 and 10 both show cell losses in layer vi, with Brodmann 10 also showing reduced cell density in layer ii. The cingulate gyrus shows cell losses in layer v. ANT. = anterior, POST. = posterior.

Cell losses in early onset schizophrenia have also been seen on brain scans (Thompson et al. 2001). Over the five-year period from 13 to 18 years of age, 12 schizophrenic patients who were scanned showed brain cell losses progressing from the parietal lobes to many other parts of the brain. This event occurring in the teens coincides with the onset of symptoms at that time, probably triggered by an environmental agent. Those with the greatest losses of cells suffered the worst symptoms.

Much of the research on brain pathology in schizophrenia has been centred on the **entorhinal cortex** (Brodmann areas 28 and 34) and the hippocampus. These are both next to the **parahippocampal gyrus**, which in turn is part of the temporal lobe cortex (Figures 10.2, 10.3). The **subiculum**, which blends directly into **Ammon's horn** of the hippocampus, is sometimes included as part of the hippocampus.

The entorhinal cortex receives input from all the **sensory association areas** of the cortex (i.e. those areas of the cerebrum that process and store sensory informa-tion), the **neocortex** and **amygdala**. This is the start of a major pathway passing through the entorhinal cortex and hippocampus (Figure 10.4). This pathway is vital

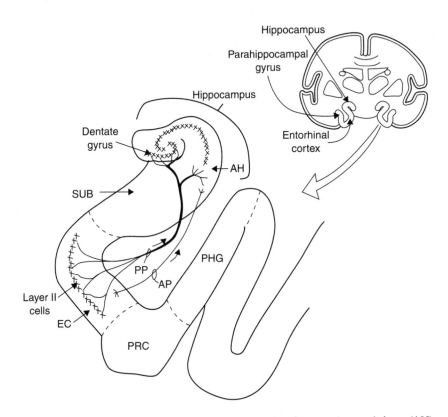

Figure 10.2 Schematic view of the hippocampal complex showing Ammon's horn (AH), subiculum (SUB), entorhinal cortex (EC), perirhinal cortex (PRC) and the parahippocampal gyrus (PHG). PP is the perforant pathway running from layer ii cells of the EC to the AH and dentate gyrus. AP is the alvear pathway run-ning from the EC to the AH. The inset shows a section through the brain with the area involved labelled.

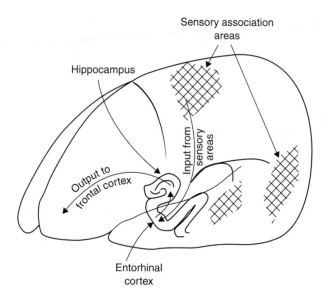

Figure 10.3 The hippocampal complex shown within the brain (left side shown) with inputs from the sensory association areas and output to the prefrontal area.

in the production of memory, in particular recognition memory (i.e. both memorising recognised objects, people etc., and using recognition memory to identify new sensory stimuli). Two main pathways link the entorhinal cortex with the hippocampus: the **alvear** pathway which goes to **Ammon's horn**, and the **perforant** pathway which also terminates in Ammon's horn and the **dentate gyrus** (Ammon's horn and dentate gyrus are both parts of the hippocampal complex) (Figure 10.2). Sensory information from the sensory association areas is therefore channelled through the entorhinal cortex, where some sensory integration may take place, a process necessary in order to make sense of the world. It is then passed on to the hippocampus, enabling it to carry out the major functions of short-term memory, and influencing thought, via pathways to the prefrontal cortex. A triple synaptic pathway, the '**trisynaptic circuit**' exists within the hippocampus (Figure 10.4), and although the functions of this pathway are unclear, they may be related to short-term memory processing. The hippocampus does not store a lot of memory as such; its powers to do so are limited to small amounts of information for a very limited time period. But it does seem to be essential for the formation of long-term memory, i.e. any information required to be remembered on a long-term basis must be processed through the hippocampus first. In this context, the hippocampus has been called the 'gateway to memory'. The entorhinal cortex, sometimes called the 'gateway to the hippocampus', appears to be a vital link in the chain of events that leads from the arrival of sensory impulses in the brain to the development of a thought or idea, i.e. the *cortical sensory association areas* → *entorhinal cortex* → *hippocampus* → *cerebral cortex* pathway (Figures 10.3 and 10.4).

Much of our thinking is centred on our responses to sensory stimuli, e.g. answering questions such as What shall I eat? or What shall I wear? and so on, so correct interpretation of these stimuli are critical to normal thought processing. But new

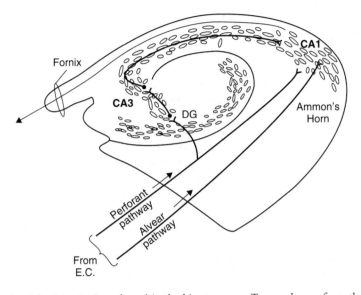

Figure 10.4 The 'trisynaptic pathway' in the hippocampus. Two pathways from the entorhinal cortex (EC) pass into the hippocampus. The perforant pathway connects
with cells of the dentate gyrus (DG) (synapse 1), which connect with cells of
CA3 (synapse 2), then on to cells of CA1 (synapse 3). The alvear pathway connects directly to CA1 cells. The CA1 cells connect to other areas via the fornix.
This concept of three synapses forming a circuit through the hippocampus is
now recognised as being more complex than this simple model suggests.

environmental stimuli are encountered daily, so it becomes necessary for the hippocampus to be able to cope with these new experiences. The hippocampus is one
of the very few parts of the brain known so far to have the ability to produce new
neurons after birth and throughout life. The reason is unknown, but is possibly
to do with improving the brain's ability to constantly adapt to new and changing
information coming in from the environment.

The entorhinal cortex is normally composed of six distinct cell layers, like the
remaining cerebral cortex, but unlike the hippocampus which has three cell layers. In schizophrenia, however, the entorhinal cortex, in particular, shows a loss of
some **layer ii** cells (Figure 10.2) and abnormal changes in the cytoarchitecture of
the remaining cells of layer ii. This kind of structural cellular disruption can only
occur during the embryological development of the brain, not later, and therefore
the individual is born with these cellular malformations already in place. It might be
expected, therefore, that the individual would show the symptoms of malfunction
from birth. However, the age of onset of symptoms in schizophrenia is usually in
the late teens or early twenties, apparently caused by a loss of neurons at that time
(Thompson et al. 2001; Carlson 2010). The question is, however, whether there
are any signs during childhood. Some of those who develop schizophrenia later
in life do show disturbed patterns of behaviour as young children, such as poor
abilities to mix and socialise with friends, and are likely to underachieve at school
(Carlson 2010). This is a form of **preschizophrenia**, and lends weight to the notion that schizophrenia is a neurodevelopmental disorder. It would appear that

in preschizophrenia the preference for social isolation, which is a major negative symptom of the fully developed disease, is present to a lesser degree, while attention and language problems are more frequent. The commonest early symptoms of the onset of psychosis are depression and anxiety (Iver et al. 2008).

Because the hippocampus is an important area for short-term memory, schizophrenic patients often perform poorly on memory-related tasks, further supporting the theory of a disruption in the hippocampal → prefrontal cortex integration (Fletcher 1998). Such a disruption is also indicated by the presence of a **hypofrontality** found in schizophrenic patients, i.e. a reduction in frontal lobe activity during thinking and task-related functions. The frontal lobe is a major part of the cerebral cortex innervated by the **mesocortical pathway** (which is reviewed later in this chapter). Low dopamine in this pathway is thought to be responsible for the negative symptoms of schizophrenia, and this ties in well with the concept of hypofrontality. Further evidence for this is indicated by a reduction in the level of **phosphomonoesters** (**PMEs**) in the frontal lobe. PMEs are precursors of phospholipids, the molecular component of cell membranes. In addition, **phosphodiesters** (**PDEs**) are the breakdown products of phospholipids. A change in the PME/PDE ratio, showing a reduction in PME and a rise in PDE, is an indication of neuronal breakdown and losses and is seen in both dementia and schizophrenia. In fact, PME reduction correlates well with negative symptoms: the lower the PME, the more profound the negative symptoms in schizophrenia (Maier 1999).

The positive symptoms are also intensively investigated, particularly hallucinations. Visual hallucinations may be due to a **disinhibition** effect caused by a reduction in the sensory input to the cortex. This allows the cortex to generate and release its own false *endogenous* sensory stimuli which are then interpreted by the visual cortex as real visual stimuli. It is thought that the normal input of stimuli may have an *inhibitory* effect on the cortex, preventing any such false signals from being produced. An alternative view is that of **cerebral irritation**, such that abnormally high cerebral excitation of the visual memory banks generates the false image (David and Busatto 1999). Given the integrating role of the entorhinal cortex and the hippocampus over a wide range of sensory stimuli, and the disruption of the cells in these areas in schizophrenia, it should not be difficult to see a situation where genuine external sensory stimuli are distorted by the brain.

Auditory hallucinations appear to be the combined result of a reduction of left superior temporal lobe gyrus function with increased right middle temporal lobe gyrus function, combined with prefrontal cortex activation. The temporal lobes have the sensory area for hearing (called the **auditory area**, Brodmann 41 and 42), and the left temporal lobe in particular specialises in language and speech. It is not surprising that hallucinations that involve hearing voices activate areas of the brain that process hearing. Clearly, memory is also involved in hallucinations, as indicated by the highly personal nature of most hallucinatory experiences, and therefore the hippocampus must be part of the aetiology.

The involvement of the left temporal lobe in auditory hallucinations is consistent with the fact that the left hemisphere of the brain bears most of the pathology in this disease. This has been termed a **lateralisation**, where one side of the brain is more dominant than the other in the cause of the symptoms (David and Busatto 1999). However, pathology has also been demonstrated in the right hemisphere, although to a lesser extent. Hence schizophrenia is a disorder that is predominantly, but not exclusively, of the left side of the brain. The reason for lateralisation is possibly to do with the way the brain is put together during fetal life, i.e. its neurodevelopment.

Neurodevelopment as a factor

The findings that the entorhinal cortex layer ii cell disruption is involved in the symptoms of schizophrenia are consistent with the theories related to the cause of thought disorder and hallucinations. Layer ii cell disruption of the entorhinal cortex could only have happened during the early development of the brain in embryo, i.e. during neuronal development. This process is described in Chapter 2. *See page 27*

It would appear that in schizophrenia, for reasons still unknown, neurons of several parts of the brain, and cells of the entorhinal cortex and the hippocampus in particular, take the wrong route during migration and end up in the wrong place (therefore making wrong synaptic connections) or die (causing neuronal losses). The result is disruption of the functions of the *cortical sensory association areas → entorhinal cortex → hippocampus → cerebral cortex* pathway (Figure 10.3). The malfunction of this pathway may be the cause of the thought disorder associated with schizophrenia; the hippocampus is unable to make its normal vital input into thought conception, which is therefore distorted and disrupted.

It is interesting that the migration of neuronal cells is accompanied at the same time by a similar migration of cells destined to become skin. It is these cells that form the skin patterns we recognise as fingerprints. Perhaps the disturbance of neuronal migration in the very early preschizophrenic brain is mirrored by similar disturbances in skin-cell migration. Twins were used to investigate this idea, so that their finger and palm prints could be compared. In those pairs of twins in which both twins developed schizophrenia, they had identical skin patterns. However, where only one twin of the pair developed the disease, each twin had a different skin pattern. It now appears that amongst monozygotic (identical) twins the 48 per cent risk of one twin developing schizophrenia if the other already has the disease is only an average figure. A closer look at these twins has identified a range of risks from 10.7 per cent for monozygotic twins who had their own separate placentas (i.e. **dichorionic**) to 60 per cent for monozygotic twins who shared the same placenta (i.e. **monochorionic**). The monochorionic group of twins had not only identical genes but also a virtually identical uterine environment, including the same products delivered through a common placenta. This is powerful evidence for gene and environmental interaction in the causation of schizophrenia.

The biochemical changes in schizophrenia

For many years now it has been recognised that dopamine is, in some way, involved in the production of some of the symptoms of schizophrenia. The *dopamine hypothesis* of schizophrenia was based on observations that drugs like cocaine and the amphetamines caused schizophrenic-like psychotic events, with hallucinations and bizarre behaviour. These drugs were known to increase dopamine levels in the brain. In addition, it was noticed that the **phenothiazine** drugs, some of which were first used as anti-emetics, reduced psychotic symptoms in schizophrenic patients. Since these drugs block the dopamine receptors, it was postulated that excess dopaminergic transmission and receptor stimulation was involved the cause of the positive psychotic symptoms (especially involving the D_2-like receptors, i.e. D_2, D_3 and D_4 receptors), and reduced dopamine was involved in the cause of the negative symptoms.

See page 61

Dopamine is the neurotransmitter within four major types of pathway in the brain (Figure 10.5) (Blows 2000):

1   The **mesocortical tracts**, passing from the brain stem to the cerebral cortex (possibly involved in the production of the *negative symptoms* of schizophrenia);

2   The **mesolimbic tracts**, passing from the brain stem to the limbic system (the system most likely to be involved in producing the *positive symptoms* of schizophrenia);

3   The **tuberoinfundibular tract**, passing between several nuclei within the hypothalamus and the pituitary stalk. This tract is not thought to be involved in schizophrenia but is involved in some drug side-effects where pituitary hormones are disturbed;

4   The **nigrostriatal tract**, passing from the substantia nigra (midbrain) to the corpus striatum (basal ganglia). This pathway produces and uses the largest amount of dopamine in the brain, but appears not to be involved in schizophrenia. It is involved in the production of extra-pyramidal side-effects (EPS) of the drugs used to treat the disorder.

The mesolimbic system, thought to be the pathway most involved in positive symptoms, originates in the brain stem, i.e. the **ventral tegmental area** of the midbrain, and terminates in the limbic system, i.e. the **nucleus accumbens** and

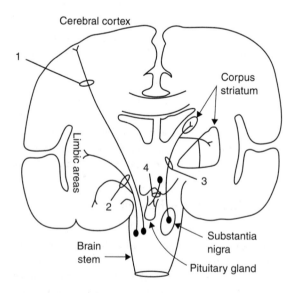

Figure 10.5 The four main types of dopaminergic pathway: (1) the mesocortical pathway (brain stem to cortex); (2) the mesolimbic pathway (brain stem to limbic system); (3) the nigrostriatal pathway (substantia nigra to corpus striatum); (4) the tuberoinfundibular pathway (hypothalamus to pituitary stalk).

the **amygdala** and other associated parts (Blows 2000). This pathway and the mesocortical pathways normally use less dopamine than the other dopaminergic tracts, but can sometimes produce excess dopamine. The nucleus accumbens has D_4 receptors, but is especially rich in D_3 receptors, and both receptor types have been found to be raised in some schizophrenics who were drug-free prior to measurement (Carlson 2010). In fact, various studies of dopamine and dopamine receptor levels in patients with schizophrenia have proved to be somewhat ambiguous, with relatively normal levels found in some patients, but disturbed levels found in other patients (Carlson 2010). One way of measuring dopamine is to measure the level of the dopamine metabolite called **homovanillic acid** (**HVA**, the waste product of dopamine) excreted via the cerebrospinal fluid (CSF). HVA has been found to be raised in schizophrenic patients, indicating a higher than normal rate of dopamine turnover, and in post-mortem studies this raised level of HVA has been found localised to the mesocortical and mesolimbic pathways.

The dopamine hypothesis has its difficulties, indicating that a more complex picture exists. Although excessive dopamine stimulation of D_2, D_3 and possibly D_4 receptors may be the cause of *some* symptoms, especially the positive symptoms, it is clear that dopamine disturbance is not the *cause* of the disease. There has to be, for example, a cause for the disturbed dopamine levels. This is further illustrated by the fact that the phenothiazine drugs do not cure schizophrenia; patients must usually continue on medication for life, otherwise the symptoms will return. Unlike the psychoses seen in cocaine or amphetamine use, the symptoms of schizophrenia are not simply the result of dopamine excess but are part of a much wider biochemical disturbance and associated pathology. The dopamine hypothesis, therefore, has lost ground as a main cause of the psychoses, and is now seen as just one more small piece of a much larger jigsaw. Other neurotransmitters are involved in this disorder, in particular **serotonin**, **glutamate** and **cholecystokinin**. Serotonin has a controlling effect on dopamine release, and 5-HT receptors are a target for atypical antipsychotic drugs (see page 207). Glutamate and cholecystokinin are both active in layer ii of the entorhinal cortex and are thought to have an important part to play in brain cortical development. Both glutamate and cholecystokinin neurons seem to have a direct dopaminergic innervation in the human brain, suggesting that dopamine disturbance could have a knock-on effect on glutamate and cholecystokinin levels.

The possible role of environmental factors

We saw that schizophrenia is considered to be polygenic in origin and, if this is so, it should be possible to identify some environmental factors at work in its aetiology. Two particular environmental factors stand out as significant: a history of birth trauma and maternal influenza during pregnancy. *See page 202*

Schizophrenia shows a higher incidence in those who have a history of cerebral birth trauma, such as prolonged periods of cerebral hypoxia during labour, or who have mothers who had problems during pregnancy, such as **pre-eclampsia** (high blood pressure caused by pregnancy). Preterm infants subjected to perinatal trauma have a tendency to acquire enlarged ventricles (as seen in schizophrenic patients), identified by brain scanning before and after birth. There is a link between perinatal complications and neurological abnormalities, and male infants seem to be more prone to lateral ventricular enlargement than female infants as a result of obstetric trauma. The reason is unknown; perhaps it is linked to differences in the male and female brains making the male brain more vulnerable. Such trauma may also permanently change some neural connections within the brain which do not show *See page 197* symptoms until maturity.

There is also generally a 10 per cent increase in the number of infants destined to develop schizophrenia who were born during the late winter and early spring (February or March in the Northern hemisphere). This is a period during which viruses are particularly active (e.g. colds and influenza) and when days are short and sunlight levels are low. This lack of **ultraviolet (UV) light** can result in low **vitamin D** levels during a winter pregnancy (Furlow 2001). Low vitamin D levels during the perinatal period are now linked with schizophrenia, although the mechanism is not known. A virus may be involved in this disorder, as indicated by some studies showing a threefold increase in the risk of schizophrenia in infants born to mothers who caught influenza during their pregnancy (a 3 per cent risk compared to 1 per cent for the general population). These findings have led to calls for all pregnant mothers to vaccinated against influenza. The role of the virus in this disease is the subject of much debate and research. The virus may cross the placenta as a **teratogen** (a harmful substance that passes from the maternal to fetal circulation) and then enter the child's brain and interfere with neuronal development in genetically susceptible children. The viral connection could be one more environmental insult in a chain of neurological insults that starts with some abnormal genes and ends with the fully developed disease.

However, this chain of events is far from clear. The problem facing neurobiologists now is piecing the jigsaw together (Figure 10.6). It is not clear how the genes and environmental factors interact, or how they in turn affect the embryonic neuronal migration, or how this disturbs the biochemistry, or how these go together

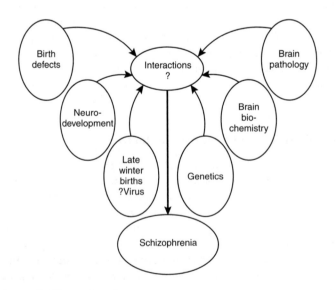

Figure 10.6 The factors affecting the cause of schizophrenia. Somehow they all contribute towards the disease, but their exact interactions, leading to the disease, are unknown.

to cause the symptoms. There is much still to learn, but we have come a long way since the 1960s when hardly any of the possibilities described above were known. With the advances being made in both neurobiology and understanding of the human genome, the prospects of solving this particular jigsaw puzzle are better now than they ever were.

Schizoaffective disorder and schizoid-related personality disorders

Schizoaffective disorder is the term used for those patients who suffer psychotic symptoms more or less continuously with occasional bouts of severe depression with or without mania. It has been known for many years that very severe bipolar disorder can result in loss of contact with reality, hallucinations and delusions, and that the two conditions, bipolar depression and schizophrenia, share some common ground. It would appear that bipolar depression and schizophrenia are closer to each other in cause and effect than bipolar depression is to unipolar depression.

Various types of this disorder are seen, some more akin to schizophrenia, others more akin to depression. This has led to some suggestions that it represents a **comorbid** state, i.e. two disorders occurring together within the same individual.

Some rare syndromes have been linked to schizophrenia:

1. **Cotard's syndrome** is where the patient believes they have lost all their internal organs, with the most severely affected believing they are dead;
2. **Capgras's syndrome** causes the patient to believe their friends and family are not the original people but are *dopplegangers*, i.e. exact replicas of the originals. Even the patient's own reflection is seen as a replica of the real thing.
3. **Fregoli syndrome** is similar to Capgras's syndrome in that the patient believes that different people are all one person taking on various disguises.
4. **Ekbom's syndrome** sufferers believe that their skin is infested with invisible parasites, which are not really there. They may even take an empty matchbox to the doctor to show captured examples of the parasites.

These four syndromes appear to be different manifestations of delusions and hallucinations, i.e. false believes coupled with hallucinatory episodes.

Schizoid-related personality disorders fall into three types:

1. **Paranoid personality**: These individuals trust no-one; they are suspicious to the point where it disrupts their normal life. They are convinced that others are trying to harm, deceive or exploit them in some way. Paranoid personality affects about 0.5 to 5.6 per cent of the population, with three times as many male as female sufferers.
2. **Schizoid personality**: These people are emotionally cold towards others; they prefer isolation and resist forming relationships. As with paranoid personality, it affects three times as many men as women, about 0.4 to 1.7 per cent of the population.
3. **Schizotypal personality**: These people seek social isolation, have odd behaviour and are very sensitive to criticism. They have restricted emotions and show poor memory, learning skills and recall. Their thought processes are

bizarre, known as 'oddities of cognition', e.g. they have strange beliefs, ideas of reference and paranoia. Their speech may be vague and overelaborate. Schizotypal personality affects 0.6 to 5.2 per cent of the population, with twice as many males as females affected. Genetics appears to be involved and there is evidence to suggest an increase in dopamine occurs in the brain.

The antipsychotic drugs

Drugs are used to control the symptoms of schizophrenia and thereby improve the quality of life of the patient, but schizophrenia as a disease remains incurable. The antipsychotic drugs (Table 10.4, Figure 10.7) fall into several groups: the

Table 10.4 The effects and side-effects of the phenothiazine antipsychotic drugs.

Drug	Desired effect	Main side-effects
Aliphatics		
Chlorpromazine	Strong sedation, antipsychotic	Extrapyramidal, hypotension, hypothermia, hormonal disturbances
Promazine		
Piperidines		
Pericyazine	Moderate sedation, antipsychotic	Few extrapyramidal
Piperazines		
Trifluoperazine	Weak sedation, variable anti-emetic, antipsychotic	Pronounced extrapyramidal
Perphenazine		
Prochlorperazine		

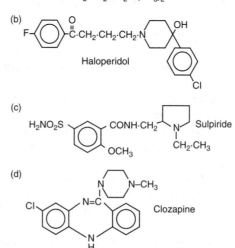

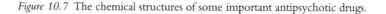

Figure 10.7 The chemical structures of some important antipsychotic drugs.

typical antipsychotics, i.e. the phenothiazines (which are further divided into three subgroups), the butyrophenones, the diphenylbutylpiperidines, the thioxanthenes and the substituted benzamides, and the newer *atypical* antipsychotics. The main effects of these drugs are to reduce the positive symptoms of psychosis, to calm the effects of bizarre behaviour and to improve the patient's ability to interact with their environment.

Phenothiazines

One of the early uses for phenothiazines was as a sedative and anti-histamine, but it was soon recognised that in schizophrenic patients they also resulted in a reduction of positive symptoms. A principal member of this drug group is **chlorpromazine**, which has been said by some to have played a key role in enabling the closure of the big Victorian psychiatric hospitals in favour of community care.

Chlorpromazine (Figure 10.7a) and the other antipsychotics are dopamine receptor **antagonists**; that is, they bind to and block the dopamine receptor sites, preventing dopamine from binding and having its effect. This dopamine blockade has for years been thought to be the mechanism of symptom prevention, lending further support to the dopamine hypothesis. However, this is not the full story of the activity of these drugs. Blocking of the dopamine receptors also has the effect of increasing the metabolism of dopamine, i.e. altering the production and destruction of dopamine, as noted by a measurable increase in dopamine metabolites (or waste products). This may have a longer-term effect on the brain chemistry of the patient, an effect that persists beyond the duration of the drug's activity, including prolonged changes to dopamine receptor activity and sensitivity. Chlorpromazine and the other phenothiazines are tricyclic (three-ringed) compounds (Figure 10.7a), with two outer carbon rings and a central pyridine ring. Each member of this group of drugs has different side branches in place of the chlorine (Cl) and the $CH_2.CH_2.$ $CH_2.N(CH_3)_2$ chain found in chlorpromazine. Three subgroups of phenothiazines are recognised: the **aliphatics** (e.g. chlorpromazine and promazine), the **piperidines** (e.g. pericyazine) and the **piperazines** (e.g. prochlorperazine, trifluoperazine and perphenazine). The inclusion of prochlorperazine (Stemetil, a valued anti-emetic medication) in this last group is a measure of the continuing importance of some of these drugs as anti-emetics as well as antipsychotics. In terms of sedatory effects (i.e. calming the patient without any loss of consciousness), the aliphatics are the most potent and the piperazines are the weakest. The main effects and side-effects of the phenothiazine drugs are listed in Table 10.4.

As dopamine antagonists, the phenothiazine drugs prevent the direct effect of dopamine on its receptors within the four main dopamine pathways of the brain. In schizophrenia, the most important pathway in which to block dopamine is generally accepted to be the *mesolimbic* tract, but the activity of these drugs is not exclusive to this tract. They block dopamine receptors also in the other tracts, and such a blockade results in unwanted effects, notably the **extrapyramidal side-effects** (**EPS**) known as **parkinsonism** (tremor, stiffness of limbs and walking difficulties), **dystonia** (abnormal movements of the face and body), **akathisia** (motor system restlessness) and late onset **tardive dyskinesia** (abnormal repeated oral and facial movements such as lip sucking or smacking, lateral jaw movements and flicking of the tongue, which may be irreversible). These are associated with dopamine blockade of the *nigrostriatal* pathway within the basal ganglia (Blows 2000). Parkinsonism is so named because it resembles Parkinson's disease but, unlike the disease, parkinsonism is reversible by reducing or changing the medication, or by adding anti-Parkinson drugs to the prescription. Other side-effects include **hypotension** (low blood pressure), due to a depressive effect on the **vasomotor centres** of the brain stem that regulate blood pressure, and **hypothermia** (low body temperature), especially in the elderly, due to the drugs' activity on the temperature control centre within the **hypothalamus**. Some of these drugs, such as chlorpromazine, can interfere with the balance of some hormones, causing increased **prolactin** production (which can stimulate breast milk production in either sex), decreased **growth hormone** and **gonadotrophins** (those hormones affecting the ovaries or testes), and variations in the levels of **adrenocorticotropic hormone (ACTH)** released, depending on the drug dosage. ACTH regulates the release of cortisol from the adrenal cortex, a hormone particularly important in stress. These hormonal effects are caused by the drug interfering with the tuberoinfundibular tract.

See page 200

Butyrophenones

Drugs more specific to one of the subtypes of dopamine receptor, especially D_2, would be more efficient, causing fewer side-effects for the patient than the phenothiazines. A selective D_2 receptor inhibitor would, at least, avoid the complications of blocking the other receptors (especially D_1) (Blows 2000) as the phenothiazines appear to do. Such a drug is **haloperidol** (Figure 10.7b), a member of another group, the butyrophenones, which also includes **benperidol**. These are all potent antipsychotics with few sedative properties, but they can produce extrapyramidal side-effects by D_2 blockade in the nigrostriatal pathway. They have a different chemical structure from the phenothiazines, in that they are not tricyclic (see haloperidol structure, Figure 10.7b). Haloperidol has a one-hundred times greater affinity for the D_2 receptor than for the D_1 receptor and is therefore a more selective D_2 receptor antagonist than any of the phenothiazines. As a potent antipsychotic, haloperidol is very useful as a treatment for acute psychotic states as it causes a quick recovery of normal behaviour.

Thioxanthenes

The thioxanthenes group contains two main drugs: **flupenthixol**, which is useful in the treatment of withdrawn and apathetic patients, and **zuclopenthixol**, which should not be used in patients with predominantly negative symptoms but is a suitable treatment for agitation and aggression in schizophrenia.

Diphenylbutylpiperidines

The diphenylbutylpiperidines, of which the only member is **pimozide**, is similar in action to the butyrophenones, being potent antipsychotics, but with extrapyramidal and potential cardiac side-effects. It is not often used since there are antipsychotics without the risk to cardiac function.

Substituted benzamide

The only drug in this category is **sulpiride** (Figure 10.7c), which can control severe positive symptoms when given in high dosage or improve activity in those affected by dominant negative symptoms if given in lower dose. Sulpiride appears to have a greater affinity for the D_2 receptor than for any of the other dopamine receptors.

Atypicals

The newer atypical antipsychotics include the drugs **clozapine** (Figure 10.7d), **risperidone, olanzapine, quetiapine** and **amisulpride**. Studies have suggested that these drugs appear to have three mechanisms of action that are distinct from the typical drugs, as follows:

1. They have significant 5-HT2_A serotonin receptor as well as dopamine receptor antagonist properties.
2. They produce fewer side-effects generally, but especially fewer extrapyramidal side-effects (EPS).
3. They appear to have a different 'hit and run' profile to that of the typical drugs.

The inclusion of the serotonin 5-HT2_A receptor subtype within the antagonistic properties is a feature of all the atypical drugs but not the typical drugs. This is thought to be significant because serotonin has a regulatory role in dopamine release; i.e. serotonin limits dopamine release from the presynaptic bulb. By blocking the 5-HT2_A receptor, the atypical drugs promote additional dopamine release. At first, this may sound counterproductive in a system where excess dopamine is thought to cause the symptoms of psychosis. The rationale suggested as to why this is helpful needs to be explained in the context of the four separate dopaminergic pathways:

- In the *mesolimbic pathway* (the main pathway involved in *positive* symptoms) the atypical drugs block the dopamine receptors and reduce the symptoms. Serotonin blockade in this pathway is restricted because there are lower numbers of 5-HT2_A receptors in this pathway, so the increased dopamine produced is not enough to overcome the dopamine blockade (Figure 10.8).
- In the *mesocortical pathway* (the main pathway involved in *negative* symptoms) the dopamine blockade is reversed by the considerable amount of dopamine released by the blockade of 5-HT2_A receptors which are present in much higher numbers. The cerebral cortex is also served by the diffuse modulatory systems (see depression, Chapter 11) which involve a serotonergic component, so the cortex is rich in serotonin receptors. Releasing dopamine in larger quantities provides significant improvement in the negative symptoms (Figure 10.8).
- In the *tuberoinfundibular pathway* (the pathway involved in the hormonal side-effects), a reciprocal relationship exists between dopamine and serotonin receptor activity in the control of prolactin release from the pituitary. Blockade

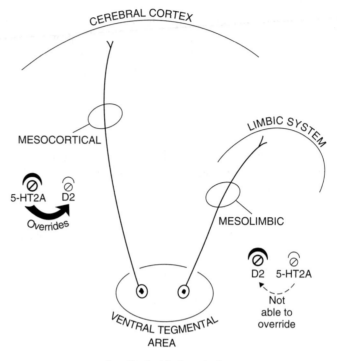

CEREBRAL CORTEX

MESOCORTICAL

5-HT2A   D2

Overrides

LIMBIC SYSTEM

MESOLIMBIC

D2   5-HT2A

Not
able to
override

VENTRAL TEGMENTAL
AREA

⊘ = Atypical Antipsychotic

Figure 10.8 The atypical antipsychotic effects on the mesocortical and mesolimbic systems. Low dopamine activity in the mesocortical system is thought to be the cause of the negative symptoms in schizophrenia, but high dopamine activity in the mesolimbic system is thought to cause the positive (psychotic) symptoms. In the mesocortical system there are more 5-HT2A serotonin receptors than D2 dopamine receptors. The serotonin blockade by the atypical drugs reverses the blockade on dopamine receptors, thus causing increased dopamine activity which improves the negative symptoms. In the mesolimbic system there are more D2 receptors than serotonin, so dopamine blockade dominates, relieving the positive symptoms.

of the 5-HT2_A serotonin receptors increases dopamine release which then prevents the excessive prolactin release seen in treatment with the typical drugs.

- In the *nigrostriatal pathway* (the main pathway involved in extrapyramidal side-effects), the blockade of 5-HT2_A receptors causes increased dopamine release which is enough to reverse the blockage of dopamine receptors and allows the dopamine to bind to these receptors. This prevents the onset of extrapyramidal side-effects (EPS). This is very effective, as seen with the drug quetiapine which has virtually no EPS.

In addition, the atypical drugs are said to have a different 'hit and run' profile to that of the typical drugs. This means that the mechanism of the atypical drug action on the dopamine receptors is different to that for the typical drugs (Figure 10.9). Typical drugs bind and block dopamine receptors (the 'hit') more tightly and for

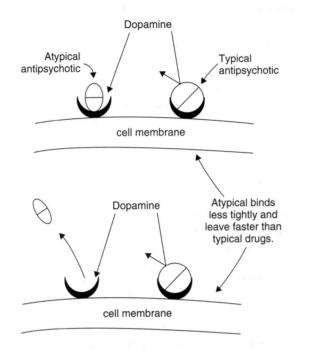

Figure 10.9 The 'hit and run' theory of atypical antipsychotic activity. Atypical drugs bind and block dopamine receptors (the 'hit') less tightly and for a shorter period than typical drugs. Atypical drugs release and go quicker from the receptors (the 'run') than typical drugs. Atypical drugs therefore reduce side-effects by shortening the blockade time span so that dopamine can return to the receptor quicker than with the typical drugs.

longer than atypical drugs. Atypical drugs release from the receptors and leave sooner (the 'run') than the typical drugs. This means the atypical drugs shorten the blockade time span and allow dopamine to return to the receptor quicker than is the case with typical drugs, thus reducing the side-effects caused by blockade.

Clozapine

Clozapine is an excellent atypical antipsychotic drug, probably the best currently available, with low side-effects and high efficacy. However, it is used only for schizophrenic patients who do not respond to other drug treatments. This is because it can cause blood **dyscrasia** (a serious disturbance of the number of blood cells in circulation, sometimes causing dangerous falls in the leukocyte count). As a result, patients prescribed this drug must be treated by a specialist and registered on a special monitoring service.

Clozapine metabolites have been found to inhibit the growth of the **human immunodeficiency virus (HIV**, the known cause of **acquired immunodeficiency syndrome, AIDS**) and, while HIV is not known to be involved in schizophrenia, this discovery has added weight to the theory that a virus may be involved in the cause (see environmental factors). Perhaps other antipsychotic drugs, or their metabolites, work by a similar viral blocking action in the long term.

Clozapine has a wide range of receptor activity, particularly D_4 and 5-HT2A (Table 10.5).

Drug therapy has become the main mechanism in the management of patients' symptoms. However, one problem with drug therapy in schizophrenia is that of poor patient compliance, particularly within the community. Failure to take the drugs regularly results in the repeated return of some patients to hospital. To improve patient compliance, some drugs are available as **depot** injections, i.e. oil-based slow-releasing intramuscular medication that can be given by the nurse on anything from a weekly to a twelve-weekly basis. This is one of several ways in which nurses can improve patient compliance with their medication regime (Coffey 1999).

The dosage of antipsychotics used in acute psychotic patients is sometimes quite high. It is thought that as many as 25 per cent of inpatients with schizophrenia are prescribed high doses by psychiatrists. A high dose is defined as that which exceeds the maximum dose identified by the British National Formulary (BNF). The problem has been highlighted because a number of patients on high-dose antipsychotics have died suddenly, and ECG (electrocardiogram) changes (notably QT prolongation) have been seen in patients on a high dose. The link between high-dose antipsychotics and sudden death is not accepted by everyone, but it would be a precautionary measure to maintain as many patients as possible on dose ranges identified in the BNF, and to carefully assess every patient for risk of cardiac disorder before a high dosage is prescribed.

Neuroleptic malignant syndrome (**NMS**) is a rare but potentially dangerous reaction to antipsychotic drugs, both typical and atypical. The syndrome is thought to be due to inadequate dopamine activity in the brain, probably caused by excessive D_2 receptor antipsychotic blockade. The symptoms include fever, unstable blood pressure, muscle rigidity, sympathetic dysfunction, changes in cognitive abilities, agitation, delirium and coma. Treatment includes withdrawal of the antipsychotic drugs.

Pharmacokinetics of the antipsychotics

Oral antipsychotics are well tolerated by mouth and absorbed quickly from the digestive tract. There is extensive first pass metabolism and this may be linked to the variable blood plasma concentration seen between patients on the same dosage of

Table 10.5 Receptor affinity for the major antipsychotic drugs (approximated from available data) (Labbate et al. 2010).

Antipsychotic	High receptor affinity	Intermediate receptor affinity	Low receptor affinity
Chlorpromazine	D2, α1, M, H1	D1	
Haloperidol	D2, D3, D4	5-HT2A, α1	D1, H1, 5-HT2C,
Olanzapine	5-HT2A, D2, H1, 5-HT2C, α1	Other 5-HT	D3, D4, D1, M,
Risperidone	5-HT2A, D2, D3, D4, α1, H1	5-HT7	α2, D1
Clozapine	D4, 5-HT2A, H1, 5-HT2C, α1	Other 5-HT, D2, D1, M1,	D3, α2
Quetiapine	α1, H1	5-HT2A, 5-HT6, 5-HT7	D1, D2, 5-HT2C, α2, D3, D4

the same drug. The oral bioavailability is different between the various drugs (e.g. low for chlorpromazine at 10–33 per cent, high for pimozide at up to 80 per cent). The half-lives vary from some drugs with short half-lives (e.g. quetiapine = 6 hours), to those with long half-lives (e.g. pimozide = 55 hours), and this will have an influence on the frequency with which drugs are administered. As a general rule, drugs with short half-lives tend to be administered more frequently than those with long half-lives. These drugs are metabolised in the liver and excreted from the kidneys.

Key points

- Schizophrenia is a polygenetic neurodevelopmental disorder.
- The symptoms of schizophrenia fall into two categories, positive (Type I) and negative (Type II).

Genetics

- The risk of developing schizophrenia is about 1 per cent for the population as a whole.
- Multiple genes linked to schizophrenia have been found, and some environmental factors are implicated.

Brain pathology

- Some abnormalities have been reported in the brain. These include enlarged ventricles, a reduction in brain weight of about 5 per cent and a shortening of the length of the brain.
- The entorhinal cortex and the anterior hippocampus both show neuron losses of about 20 per cent, and a change in the cytoarchitecture.
- Preschizophrenia, the pre-symptom childhood stage, causes the child to have poor abilities to mix and socialise with friends, with attention and language problems causing them to underachieve at school.
- The mesolimbic system is thought to be the pathway most involved in positive symptoms.

Brain biochemistry

- Increased dopamine activity in the brain is thought to be the main cause of the positive symptoms of psychosis.

Environmental factors

- Two factors stand out as significant environmental contributors to the cause of schizophrenia: a history of birth trauma and maternal influenza during pregnancy.

The antipsychotic drugs

- The antipsychotic drugs fall into two main groups: the typical and atypical forms.

- These drugs are dopamine antagonists, i.e. they block dopamine receptors and reduce dopamine activity in the brain.
- The most important pathway in which to block dopamine is thought to be the *mesolimbic* tract, but phenothiazines also block dopamine receptors in other tracts, resulting in side-effects.
- Extrapyramidal side-effects are caused by blockade of dopamine receptors in the nigrostriatal pathway.
- Atypical drugs have a range of receptor blockade, but especially D_2 and 5-HT2A.
- This, and their different 'hit and run' profile, results in fewer side-effects.
- The problem of non-compliance in drug administration may be overcome by the use of depot injections.

References

Blows W. (2000) Neurotransmitters of the brain: serotonin, noradrenaline (norepinephrine), and dopamine. *Journal of Neuroscience Nursing*, **32** (4): 234–238.

Carlson N. R. (2010) *Physiology of Behavior* (10th edition). Allyn and Bacon, Boston.

Coffey M. (1999) Psychosis and medication: strategies for improving adherence. *British Journal of Nursing*, **8** (4): 225–230.

David A. S. and Busatto G. (1999) The hallucination: a disorder of brain and mind, in Ron M. A. and David A. S. (eds), *Disorders of Brain and Mind*. Cambridge University Press, Cambridge.

Fletcher P. (1998) The missing link: a failure of fronto-hippocampal integration in schizophrenia. *Nature Neuroscience*, **1** (4): 266–267.

Furlow B. (2001) The making of a mind. *New Scientist*, **171** (2300): 38–41.

Holland M., Baguley I. and Davies T. (1999) Psychological methods of treating hallucinations and delusions: 1. *British Journal of Nursing*, **8** (15): 998–1002.

Iyer S. N., Boekestyn L., Cassidy C. M., King S., Joober R. and Malla A. K. (2008) Signs and symptoms in the pre-psychotic phase: description and implications for diagnostic trajectories. *Psychological Medicine*, **38** (8): 1147–1156.

Labbate A. L., Fava M., Rosenbaum J. F. and Arana G. W. (2010) *Handbook of Psychiatric Drug Therapy* (6th edition). Wolters Kluwer, Lippincott Williams and Wilkins, Philadelphia.

Maier M. (1999) Magnetic resonance spectroscopy in neuropsychiatry, in Ron M. A. and David A. S. (eds), *Disorders of Brain and Mind*. Cambridge University Press, Cambridge.

Nolen-Hoeksema S. (2007) *Abnormal Psychology* (4th edition). McGraw-Hill, Boston.

Ross C. A. and Margolis R. L. (2009) Schizophrenia: a point of disruption. *Nature*, **458**, 976–977.

Stahl S. M. (2003) Describing an atypical antipsychotic: receptor binding and its role in pathophysiology. *Primary Care Companion Journal of Clinical Psychiatry*, **5** (suppl 3): 9–13.

Stefansson H., et al. (2009) Common variants conferring risk of schizophrenia. *Nature*, **460** (7256): 744–747

Taylor E. (1999) Early disorders and later schizophrenia, in Ron M. A. and David A. S. (eds), *Disorders of Brain and Mind*. Cambridge University Press, Cambridge.

Thompson P. M., Vidal C., Giedd J. N., Gochman P., Blumenthal J., Nicolson R., Toga A. W. and Rapoport J. L. (2001) Mapping adolescent brain change reveals dynamic wave of accelerated gray matter loss in very early-onset schizophrenia. *Proceedings of the National Academy of Sciences of the USA*, **98** (20): 11650–11655.

11 Depression

- Introduction
- Factors in the aetiology of depression
- Brain pathology
- Biochemistry and immunity in depression
- Depression in young people
- Post-partum depression (PPD) and seasonal affective disorder (SAD)
- The antidepressant drugs
- Mood-stabilising drugs
- Key points

Introduction

It is not unnatural to be unhappy as a result of certain life events, such as loss of a close family member, and this kind of reaction is expected. It is also expected that the depressive state will resolve itself after a reasonable period of time, allowing the individual concerned to return to their usual state of mind and to function normally. Depressive illness (also called **affective disorder**; **affect** = mood) occurs either when the depressed state has no apparent cause or reason or when the period of depression is prolonged beyond what is considered normal, with no signs of recovery. The depth of depression is important also. A depressive illness dominates the person's life, committing them to an existence in misery with no end in sight. Suicide becomes an attractive way out of this despair and many depressive patients succeed in killing themselves to end their suffering. Such patients need help to recover the purpose of living and, with treatment, many are returned successfully to a happier existence. Such an outcome is more likely now than it has ever been as a result of better understanding of what is happening in the brains of depressed patients and of the introduction of improved drug treatment. Depression has long been associated with other serious and long-term debilitating disorders, e.g. cancer, coronary artery disease and chronic infections, and is often linked with the elderly (Hestad et al. 2009).

Depression is possibly the commonest mental health disorder. The World Health Organisation (WHO) estimate a worldwide incidence of depression at more than 150 million people, approximately 4 per cent of the world's adult population, but this may be an underestimate due to problems related to reporting and diagnosing cases in some regions of the world (Westly 2010).

Various attempts have been made to classify different depressed states and some of these classifications have been adopted and used more commonly than others (Table 11.1). The current view is that there are two main types of depressive illness, **unipolar depression** (having symptoms of depression only) and **bipolar depression** (having symptoms of depression coupled with alternating periods of **mania,** an acute borderline psychotic state involving symptoms of euphoria; see Table 11.2). This classification is supported by growing evidence concerning the

Table 11.1 Previous and current classifications of depression.

Previous classifications	Explanation
1. Primary	Not associated with any other disorder
Secondary	As a result of some other disorder
2. Neurotic	Mild depression, associated with symptoms of a nervous nature, like anxiety
Psychotic	More severe depression, associated with psychotic symptoms akin to schizophrenia
3. Reactive	Caused by a sad or unfortunate life event, and continued from there
Endogenous	From within, i.e. no identifiable life event is recognised as the cause
Current classification	
Unipolar	Depressive symptoms only
Bipolar	Depressive symptoms plus bouts of mania

Table 11.2 The symptoms of depression.

Symptom	Further explanation
Low level of mood (flattening of affect)	Misery which does not improve; patient looks very unhappy.
Pessimistic thoughts	Feelings of hopelessness, unworthiness, no self-confidence.
Low energy	
Psychomotor retardation	Slow body movements, delayed responses to stimuli.
Sleep disturbance and tiredness	Early morning waking, difficulty in returning to sleep.
Poor appetite and weight loss	
Slow speech and thought	Protracted conversations.
Loss of libido	
Sometimes anxiety, agitation or restlessness	
Severe depression is sometimes associated with loss of reality and pessimistic delusions	These symptoms are akin to those of schizophrenia. Delusions are of doom and gloom.
Sometimes mania (in bipolar depression)	Mania is the sudden outburst of overactivity, rapid speech and thinking, expanded optimistic ideas, increased appetite and libido, possibly aggression and psychotic symptoms like hallucinations. Manic events occur between depressive periods but are rare compared to the depressive phases.
	Bipolar I (BP I) indicates these manic states are severe. Bipolar II (BP II) indicates states of mild or very mild mania (hypomania) which may not impede everyday function.

underlying biology of depression (Carlson 2010). Depressed patients demonstrate the symptoms we now associate with disturbed receptor and neurotransmitter levels in the brain (Table 11.2).

Gender differences in the symptoms are becoming better recognised. There are approximately twice as many women with depression as men. Women's symptoms are typical of depression, i.e. various degrees of sadness, crying and despair. Men, however, show symptoms of anger, irritation and recklessness. These differences are thought to be due to social pressures on men not to succumb to what may be considered to be weak emotions (such as crying), rather than any biological differences (Westly 2010).

Another disorder, in which depressive symptoms appear to be chronic and directed *outwards* towards the world in the form of anger or irritability, is called **dysthymic disorder**. *See page 223*

Factors in the aetiology of depression

The cause of depression is basically unknown. Genes have been implicated for many years because some forms of depression appear to be familial, particularly the more severe manic-depressive bipolar disorder. For the population as a whole, the risk of any one person developing unipolar depression is 6 per cent, and for bipolar depression the risk is 1 per cent (the same as for schizophrenia). Mild forms of depression carry a general population risk of approximately 10 per cent. The first-degree relatives of a patient with bipolar depression have a concordance rate of 19 per cent – i.e. a 19 per cent chance of developing the disease – while for unipolar depression the concordance rate is 10 per cent. The concordance rate for bipolar depression in monozygotic (identical) twins is about 65 per cent, and in dizygotic (fraternal) twins the concordance rate is about 14 per cent. Affected twins are most likely to have the same disorder, i.e. if one has the bipolar form then the other will have the bipolar form, although occasional crossing over has been seen. All these figures are much greater than for the population as a whole, suggesting a powerful genetic influence in the causation of this disorder.

A number of important genes are now known to be linked to bipolar disorder (**MAFD** = Major Affective Disorder):

- **MAFD1** (18p); **MAFD2** (Xq28); **MAFD3** (21q22.3); **MAFD4** (16p12); **MAFD5** (2q22–24); **MAFD6** (6q23–24); **MAFD7** (22q12); **MAFD8** (10q21); **MAFD9** (12p13).

Additional genes have also been linked to depression (**MDD** = Major Depressive Disorder):

- **MDD1** (12q22–23.2) is linked to unipolar depression.
- **P2X7** (or **P2RX7**) (12q24) is an ATP (adenosine triphosphate) ionotropic cell-surface receptor, mutations of which are linked to bipolar depression.
- **MTHFR** (1p36) codes for an enzyme involved in **folate (folic acid)** metabolism and linked to depression.
- **CREB1** (2q34) is linked to unipolar major affective disorder (MAFD).
- **FKBP5** (6p21) is involved in regulation of the HPA axis (see page 223)

and linked to the response to antidepressants and recurrence of episodes of depression.

- **DYT1** (9q34) is linked to early age (before 30) recurrent major depression.
- **DRD4** (11p15) dopamine D4 receptor gene is linked to unipolar depression.
- **TPH1** (11p15) is a tryptophan hydroxylase gene.
- **TPH2** (12q21) is another tryptophan hydroxylase gene which may be involved in some cases of unipolar depression.
- **SLC6A4** (17q) is a serotonin transporter gene linked to unipolar depression.
- **BRC** (21q11) is linked to major depression.

The difference between unipolar and bipolar disorder is emphasised by the fact that the incidence for the unipolar form in females is double that seen in males, while in bipolar disorder there is no difference between the sexes. Bipolar disorder has shown a tendency to develop more often in those persons born in the winter months (not unlike schizophrenia), leading to a suspect viral origin. One proposed virus is **Borna virus**, which is known to infect animals, notably horses, and humans. It is responsible for a significant number of horse deaths from neurological disease. There is no *direct* evidence of Borna virus disease in humans, but it is known to be a virus that infects the nervous system, especially the limbic system, and some studies have demonstrated the presence of **anti–Borna virus antibodies** in several groups of patients with psychiatric disorder (Fukuda et al. 2001; Miranda et al. 2006). Viruses fall mainly into two types, the **DNA (deoxyribosenucleic acid)** form, and the **RNA (ribosenucleic acid)** form. Borna virus is a single-stranded RNA virus that has apparently found its way from animals to man. The evidence for the presence of Borna virus in depressed patients is growing (Bode and Ludwig 2003), but this is just one of several suggested environmental factors that are possibly involved in the cause of depression. Other factors include maternal deprivation, unstable parental relationships and disturbance in the home life, all factors resulting in an unhappy childhood. These factors will have led to various *losses*, i.e. loss of a loved one, loss of a job or a home. Sudden loss events, such as a bereavement or parental separation, may trigger the first bouts of depression in a vulnerable individual. Environmental factors appear to play a much bigger role in the aetiology of unipolar depression, while genetic factors are more important in bipolar disorder.

Suicide is a phenomenon that is often triggered by environmental factors such as poor social conditions or very difficult personal circumstances, all of which cause chronic stress. Somewhere in the world, one person dies from suicide every forty seconds. The highest suicide rates in the world occur in northern and eastern European countries, Russia, Australia and in Asian countries (notably China) (Figure 11.1). The Indian rate of suicide may be five times higher than recorded because suicide there is a crime and families do not want this stigma recorded as the cause of death. Therefore many suicides are recorded as other causes of death. China has 22 per cent of the world population but 40 per cent of the world's suicides. Here there are more women killing themselves than men (suicide in China accounts for one in four female deaths between the ages of 15 and 44), although everywhere else the male suicide rate is greater than the female rate (approximately four males die from suicide for every female suicide death). The high female rate in China may have something to do with the fact that Asian societies are male

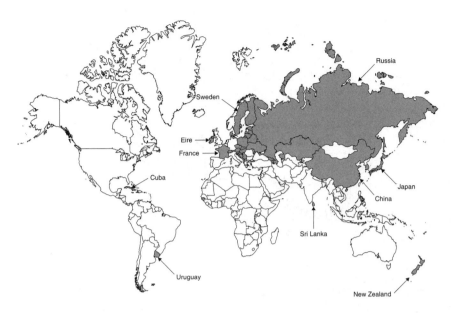

Figure 11.1 The high suicide rate areas of the world.

dominated and that women are given less value in society. Despite the high rate of suicide in these areas it is generally considered that mental illness, and in particular depression, probably accounts for only a low percentage of these deaths. In China, only about 50 per cent of the suicidal deaths are caused by mental illness, the others are caused by social conditions. While links between brain chemistry and suicide can be established in many cases (see serotonin), it is clear that environmental factors are extremely important. The UK, when compared with these high-rate countries, shows a significantly lower rate of suicide.

Brain pathology

The evidence of physical changes identified in the brain during depression is limited. In many cases, the brains of depressed and normal persons, previously examined at post mortem, but more recently seen on brain scans, are virtually identical. Changes are sometimes observed which are akin to those found in schizophrenia; for example, between 10 per cent and 30 per cent of depressed patients have some degree of ventricular enlargement and some patients show a reduction in the size of the temporal lobe. The frontal and temporal lobes also suffer some cell losses in *elderly* depressed patients, but the extensive loss of cells from the cerebral cortex seen in a significant number of schizophrenic patients has not been found in bipolar depression (Ron 1999). Lesions are sometimes found in the periventricular white matter, i.e. the axons surrounding the ventricles. Studies of cerebral blood flow indicate various changes in the left anterior and right posterior areas of the cerebrum in a number of patients, including reduced blood flow to the left anterior cingulate gyrus and the left dorsolateral prefrontal cortex (Figure 11.2). Ron (1999) suggests that symptoms of mood disorder are most likely to arise in the case

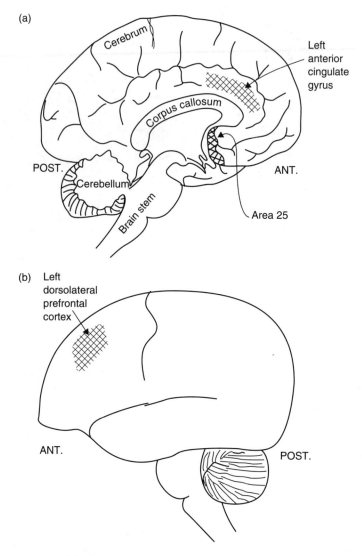

Figure 11.2 Areas of the brain involved in depression. Reduced blood flow is sometimes found in (a) the left anterior cinglulate gyrus (seen here in midline section of the brain). Also shown is Area 25, called the subgenual cingulate, which is overactive in depression. Blood flow is also often reduced in (b) the left dorsolateral prefrontal cortex (seen here in left lateral view).

of dysfunction of the temporal and frontal lobe cortex (or subcortex), combined with either the temporal lobe associated limbic areas, or the pathway from the basal ganglia to the cortex via the thalamus.

Part of the **cingulate region** of the brain, called the **subgenual cingulate** (also called Brodmann area 25), is a narrow band of frontal cortex folded beneath the corpus callosum (Figure 11.2). Functional Magnetic Resonance Imaging (fMRI) studies have demonstrated that this area is in a state of hyperactivity in major depression (Dobbs 2006). Normally area 25 has large amounts of serotonin transporter which moves serotonin from the synaptic cleft back into the presynaptic bulb, i.e. *re-uptake* of serotonin. This has the effect of concentrating serotonin in the synapses of this area. Overall, area 25 is thought to have a powerful influence over many brain areas involved in memory, the sleep-wake cycle, mood, thought and self-esteem. Many of these functions are disrupted in depression. Overactivity of area 25 was coupled with reduced frontal and limbic activity is most patients. Relief of depression using antidepressant therapy corrected these abnormal activity levels in area 25 and the frontal cortex. However, a number of patients who responded well to **cognitive behaviour therapy** (**CBT**) showed a significant reduction in area 25, to levels seen in non-depressed persons, plus they also had a *lowering* of frontal lobe activity. This is possibly because the group responding well to CBT had excessively high frontal activity which settled down with therapy. It may be possible to distinguish between those patients who will recover best with drugs and those who will recover best with CBT on the basis of their frontal lobe activity levels. **Deep brain stimulation** is a surgical procedure in which electrodes are placed within the brain in white matter adjacent to area 25, and are connected to an electrical source that gives stimulation to the area. This appears to switch off area 25 activity, and gives good results in lifting depression.

Biochemistry and immunity in depression

The main changes seen in the brains of depressed patients begin at the molecular level. Overall, this is a disease of brain chemistry disturbance, an imbalance between several neurotransmitters and their receptors. The following text should be read in conjunction with Chapter 4.

Serotonin (5-hydroxytryptamine, or 5-HT)

Serotonin is a major neurotransmitter in one of the two **diffuse modulatory systems**. The serotonergic system extends from the **raphe nuclei** of the brain stem to many other brain areas (Figure 11.3a) (Blows 2000a). Serotonin levels have been identified as a factor in depression. The neurotransmitter's metabolites (waste products for excretion), derived from degraded serotonin and measured in the cerebrospinal fluid (CSF), are significantly *reduced* in depression, indicating a lower than average turnover of the transmitter at the synapses. Low levels of serotonin will also occur if the dietary intake of the amino acid **tryptophan** is low. Tryptophan is required for the production of serotonin (Figure 4.8). Male brains appear to suffer less than female brains from this loss. Very low levels of serotonin have been linked to increased violent behaviour, both against the self, as in suicide, or against others, as in violent crime including murder (see also aggression). In addition, increases in the numbers of serotonin receptors have been identified in some patients, and this greater receptor density is to be expected if the neurotransmitter is low. The additional receptors are often of the subtype 2 (i.e. 5-HT2), and this is regarded as a compensatory *up-regulation* of the receptor to maximise the binding of what serotonin there is present. The subtype 2 receptor is thought to be the most important of all the receptor subtypes involved in mood regulation. There is some evidence indicating that the effects of low serotonin are further aggravated by a reduction in serotonin receptor activity (i.e. receptors function less well even when the neurotransmitter binds) and by a loss in the number of neurons within the serotonin pathways, leading to reduced serotonin synthesis.

Serotonin has some effect on the production of noradrenaline in the second diffuse modulatory system of the brain. As with the serotonergic system, this secondary system starts in the brain stem and passes out to many parts of the brain (see noradrenaline below). Lower than normal serotonin levels reduce the noradrenergic neurons' ability to produce noradrenaline. Thus a low serotonin level has a *knock-on* effect in causing a lower noradrenaline level in the brain.

Serotonin is also taken up by **platelets** (**thrombocytes**), which are blood cells important for the prevention of bleeding by the formation of a **thrombus** (a blood clot). Serotonin released from platelets has a local effect on blood vessels which may have a bearing on migraine. The role of serotonin directly on platelets is to enhance their ability to become active as part of the thrombus formation process. In depression, the platelets show less ability to take up serotonin and thus are less able to be activated.

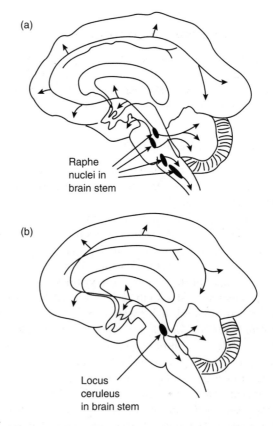

Figure 11.3 The diffuse modulatory systems. (a) The serotonin pathways from the raphe nuclei in the brain stem extend to many areas of the brain. (b) A similar pattern of noradrenaline pathways extends out from the locus ceruleus of the brain stem.

Noradrenaline

Noradrenaline pathways form the second of the two diffuse modulatory systems in the brain, noradrenaline being centred on the **locus coeruleus** in the brain stem, with pathways to many diverse parts of the cerebral cortex and limbic system (Figure 11.3b) (Blows 2000a). Some evidence indicates disturbance in the numbers and density of noradrenaline receptors in depression. Of the two major noradrenaline receptors that are known, alpha-adrenergic and beta-adrenergic, the increased density appears to be of the beta-adrenergic type. As noted, some serotonin pathways from the raphe nucleus extend to areas that involve noradrenaline secretion, and it seems likely that noradrenaline levels are disturbed because there is a loss of serotonin regulation of noradrenaline secretion.

Noradrenaline is the neurotransmitter of arousal, i.e. it causes increased levels of brain activity, and it is therefore most active during the day (Blows 2000a).

Dopamine and others

Dopamine is not the major player in the aetiology of depressive symptoms that it is in schizophrenia. Not only is serotonin a regulator of noradrenaline secretion, it also regulates the secretion of dopamine, so disturbances of the serotonin levels seen in depression are likely to have a knock-on effect on dopamine production. It is possible that severe bipolar depressive states that show psychotic symptoms such as hallucinations have some disturbance to the dopaminergic systems, although direct involvement of dopamine in depression has not been demonstrated (Carlson 2010).

The inhibitory role of gamma-aminobutyric acid (GABA) may also be impaired, and disturbance of glutamate is found in states of **mania**.

Mania

The biology of mania is now becoming clearer at the cellular level (Figure 11.4). **Protein kinase C (PKC)** is an enzyme involved in the activation and deactivation of many other proteins, some of which are part of the cell signalling mechanism (one method by which cells signal to each other) in many tissue types. Overactivity of the PKC cell signalling system, especially within the prefrontal cortex, is now strongly implicated in causing the symptoms of mania. PKC is itself activated by the second messenger **diacylglycerol** and serotonin in brain cells. PKC activation is reduced by an enzyme which, if coded by a mutant gene, would fail to regulate PKC. Excessive PKC activity causes reduced prefrontal lobe function and ultimately loss of some prefrontal mass. This loss of prefrontal cortex function appears to be a key factor in the production of manic symptoms. Regulation of the PKC system is achieved by the drugs **lithium**, **valproate** and **tomoxifen** given in therapeutic doses. Tomoxifen is used in breast cancer treatment as an anti-oestrogen, and its possible future use in bipolar disorder comes as a surprise. In addition, the omega-3 unsaturated fatty acids **DHA (docosahexaenoic acid)** and **EPA (eicosapentaenoic acid)** have an inhibitory effect on PKC, whilst mild stress and lead poisoning increase PKC activity (Figure 11.4a). *See page 38*

PKC activity in **platelets** is also increased in depression, causing an increase in intracellular calcium. PKC inhibitors used in platelets from depressed patients cause

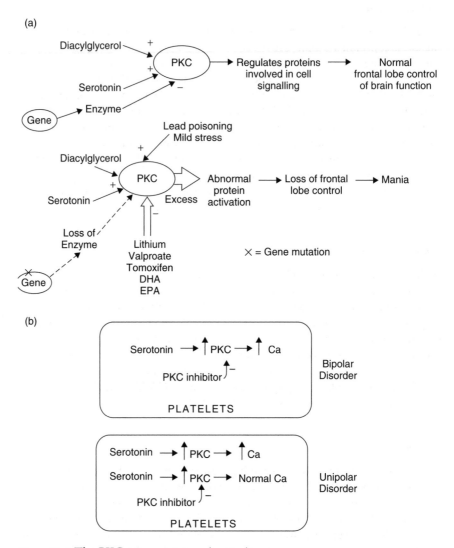

Figure 11.4 The PKC enzyme system in mania.

a reduction of calcium in unipolar depression but not in bipolar disorder, supporting the notion that these are distinct disorders with different pathologies (Figure 11.4b).

Hormones

Hormonal abnormalities are also well recognised in depression. Depressed patients often show reduced levels of secretion of several pituitary hormones, especially growth hormone and thyroid hormone. Depression is frequently associated with hypothyroidism and thyroid hormone is given to a number of depressed patients along with their antidepressant medication. This combination is considered by many to improve the results from the antidepressant. Chronic stress, with persistently high levels of cortisol, and in particular prolonged elevated levels of

corticotrophin-releasing factor (**CRF**), can also lead to depression. In this case the **hypothalamus–pituitary–adrenal axis** (**HPA axis**) (Figure 11.5) goes into prolonged hyperactivity, resulting in enlargement of both the adrenal and pituitary glands. This hyperactivity is probably due to malfunction of the CRF-producing neurons in the hypothalamus and can happen either as a result of external chronic stress or as a result of a direct problem with the neurons. CRF produced in elevated quantities does more than just cause the release of ACTH, it also suppresses sleep (causing insomnia), reduces appetite (causing anorexia), inhibits reproductive behaviour and causes withdrawal in unfamiliar environments – all symptoms that are seen in depression. Some of these are disturbances of the body 'clocks'. They are often called **circadian rhythms** because some, such as the sleep-wake cycle, take about a day to cycle (circadian means 'about a day'). Circadian rhythm disturbance is involved in causing many of the symptoms of depression, especially in children (see childhood depression). CRF levels are found to be high in the cerebrospinal fluid (CSF) of depressed patients but return to normal with treatment. The increased activity of the HPA axis results in persistently high levels of circulating cortisol, the protective hormone released in stress. Normally, a high level of cortisol in the blood is short-lived, as a result of the hormone binding to receptors in the brain; the brain responds to this by signalling the reduction of cortisol production and release through the HPA axis (Figures 11.5 and 11.6). In depression, these cortisol receptors are not functioning adequately; the brain's ability to suppress cortisol production is reduced and cortisol levels remain high.

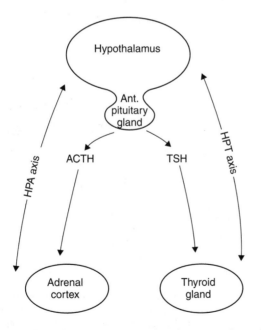

Figure 11.5 The HPA (hypothalamo–pituitary–adrenal axis) involves adrenocorticotropic hormone (ACTH). The HPT (hypothalamo–pituitary–thyroid axis) involves thyroid-stimulating hormone (TSH). Depression often involves a prolonged hyperactivity of the HPA, whilst dysthymic disorder involves a dysfunction of the HPT.

In **dysthymic disorder**, there is less evidence for the involvement of the HPA, but there are indications of dysfunction of the **hypothalamus–pituitary–thyroid axis (HPT)** (Figure 11.5) causing thyroid hormones abnormalities in many cases.

Immunity

The relatively new science of **psychoimmunology** is pointing the way towards a better understanding of how the mind (or the brain) affects the immune system and vice versa. Stress and depression are said to be the major players in this field, with significant changes occurring in the immune system in both these disorders (Hestad et al. 2009). However, the problem of 'cause or effect' comes into play, and much detail has to be worked out to determine whether the changes seen cause depression or whether they are the result of depression. Different researchers have

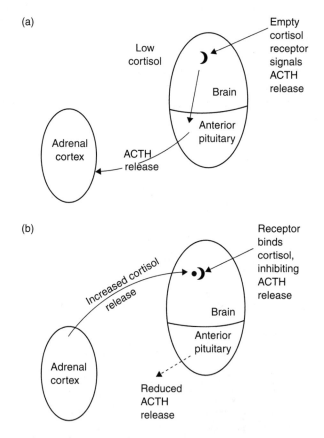

Figure 11.6 Low levels of cortisol in the blood cause a release of adrenocorticotropic hormone (ACTH), which stimulates cortisol release from the adrenal cortex (a). This is because cortisol receptors in the brain remain empty and signal the anterior pituitary where ACTH is produced. Increased cortisol in the blood (b) binds with the brain receptors, and this deactivates the signal to the anterior pituitary, which reduces ACTH release. In depression, the receptors are possibly malfunctioning, and ACTH release is not turned off even when cortisol levels are high.

Table 11.3 The psychoimmunological changes reported in depression.

Psychoimmunological change	Possible effects on the patient
Lower circulating active monocytes	?Affects immune response to infection
Lower circulating active NK cells	?May disturb sleep and cause psychomotor retardation
Lower lymphocyte proliferation	?Affects immune response to infection
Increased circulating cytokines, especially PGE$_2$, TNF-α and IF-γ.	?May be involved in the cause of depression, see text.
Raised acute-phase proteins (APP)	?Part of an acute immune response
Raised anti-serotonin antibodies	?Antibodies lower serotonin in blood + CNS
Raised anti-ganglioside antibodies	?Antibodies lower gangliosides (part of serotonin receptors) in CNS
Raised circulating T-cells	Unknown if any
Disturbed blood lipid levels, especially high density lipoproteins (HDL)	Unknown if any
Lower circulating beta-endorphin	Associated with lower NK cells
Raised leukocytes, e.g. neutrophils	Unknown if any

reported a wide range of immune changes in depression (Brown 2001), but the main changes are as listed in Table 11.3.

Monocytes are phagocytic white cells; that is, they engulf **antigens** (foreign particles) as part of the fight against infection. **NK (natural killer) cells** are white blood cells that are normally active against virally infected and some malignant cells. **Lymphocytes** are white cells which provide the main defence against invading antigens. There are two types of lymphocytes: **B-cells**, which produce proteins called **antibodies** that attack antigens (B-cell defence is called **humoral immunity**), and **T-cells**, which attack and destroy specific antigens (T-cell defence is called **cell-mediated immunity**). Lymphocyte studies in depression appear conflicting, with overall numbers down but T-cells levels raised. This is possibly because different subgroups of depressive patients show different lymphocyte results, with overall disturbance affecting cell-mediated immunity more than humoral immunity. Humoral antibody production sometimes involves anti-serotonin antibodies, the presence of which is associated with a poor response to treatment. Understanding these variations is a goal for further research. **Gangliosides** (Table 11.3) are **glycolipids** (i.e. lipids with sugars attached) found in the brain and nervous system. **High-density lipoproteins** (HDL) are blood lipid particles containing **cholesterol**.

See page 84

Cytokines are chemicals involved in 'cell signalling' during an immune response. Those raised in depression are reported as **interleukin-1beta (IL-1β)**, **interleukin-6 (IL-6), tumour necrosing factor-α, gamma-interferon (γ-IF; IFNγ)** and **prostaglandin E$_2$ (PGE$_2$)**. Cytokines are naturally produced during infections by activated immune cells, i.e. leukocytes such as monocytes and lymphocytes, but they are also given as drugs for various conditions, such as cancer therapy. Observations of people with active immune systems during infections, or during cancer treatment with cytokine therapy, show them often to be sad, not eating or sleeping well, with poor concentration, constant tiredness with fatigue and complaining of multiple aches and pains. These are symptoms akin to those of depression, and this is sometimes called **'sickness behaviour'** or **'sickness syndrome'**. It may be that antidepressants could have an anti-inflammatory effect and therefore have a role to play in treating people with sickness syndrome, and there is growing evidence that some antidepressant drugs could act as a *prophylaxis*, i.e. have a preventive effect, if given before or during cytokine therapy.

In depression, PGE_2 and Il-6 appear to enhance each other in a loop which is suppressed by antidepressants. IL-1β and II-6 appear to be involved in the disturbance of the HPA axis and in the disorder of serotonin metabolism. Brown (2001) reported that patients taking either one of two drugs to boost their immune systems to fight infection or cancer were becoming depressed, and even suicidal. These drugs are **alpha-interferon (α-IF)** and **interleukin-2 (IL-2)**, and it is this kind of observation that provides further weight in support of the 'immune theory' of depression. The mechanism is still not fully sorted out, but it would appear that cytokines reduce the level of **tryptophan**, the precursor of serotonin, possibly leading to a serotonin shortage. Tryptophan is degraded by the enzyme **idoleamine 2,3 dioxygenase (IDO)** which converts tryptophan into a metabolite in the brain. In depression, raised levels of tumour necrosing factor-α and gamma-interferon caused raised levels of IDO. This creates more tryptophan metabolite than expected, and it is this increased metabolite level that appears to induce the depressive symptoms seen in sickness syndrome. Drugs which block the action of IDO may become a valuable mechanism of treatment for the future.

The large circulatory cytokine molecules, such as interleukin, are not generally able to cross the blood–brain barrier, so their role is copied by smaller molecules such as **prostaglandins** and **nitric oxide** *inside* the brain. These smaller molecules stimulate glial cells in the brain to produce further inflammatory cytokines, which then bind to receptors on neurons of the cerebellum, the hippocampus and the hypothalamus, areas where mood and behaviour are moderated.

As noted, cortisol levels are high in depression, and this has implications for the immune system. Apart from the glial cells of the brain, the immune cells in the blood also have cortisol receptors and can therefore bind cortisol. As well as the HPA axis, inflammatory cytokines also trigger cortisol release, but the rise in cortisol causes the inflammatory cells to reduce cytokine production in a double feedback mechanism (Figure 11.7). If brain cortisol receptors are not working well, inflammatory cell receptors may not be functioning properly either, and the high cortisol levels fail to reduce the cytokine level. A vicious circle is created in which the cytokines continue to stimulate further cortisol release, which is then unable to turn the cytokines off.

Some of these findings may also be useful as **markers** of depression since their blood measurement is fairly consistent and they could be used as part of the diagnostic procedure to identify depression. The markers include raised **leucocyte** (white cell) numbers, especially the **neutrophils** (phagocytic cells, of the **granulocyte** white cell group), and the **HDL (high density lipoproteins)** findings.

Whether these immune changes are triggered by a viral infection, as suspected by some, remains to be confirmed. Perhaps depression is of viral origin, or perhaps the effect of depression is to degrade the immune system and to allow viral infections to gain entry.

Depression in young people

Compared to adult depression the incidence in children is lower: about 2.5 per cent of children, 8.3 per cent of adolescents and 16 per cent of adults suffer the disorder.

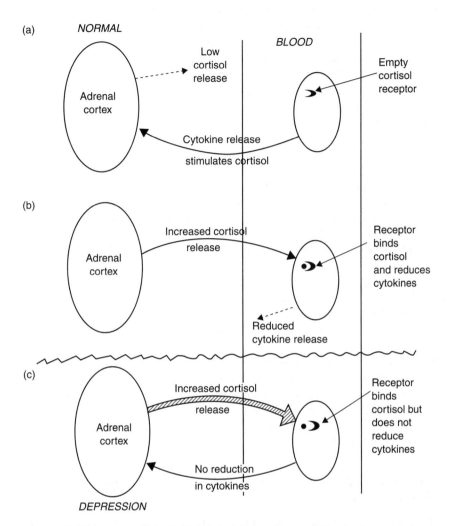

Figure 11.7 (a) Immune cells in the blood produce cytokines, which stimulate cortisol production when this is low. (b) As cortisol levels rise, cortisol binds to cortisol
receptors in the immune cells and this reduces cytokine production. (c) In depression, the receptors do not function so well, resulting in continued cytokine
production when cortisol level is high.

As identified in this chapter, there is growing evidence that bipolar depression is
linked to disturbance of the body's biological rhythms (i.e. circadian rhythms), such
as the sleep–wake cycle, eating habits, body temperature and hormonal balance. *See page 72*

The bipolar cycles from depression to manic states and back to depression again
occur more quickly in children than in adults. The changes in the circadian rhythms
are in some way linked to these rapid mood swings, but the molecular mechanism
remains unclear. Disturbances of the circadian rhythms are dominant among the
symptoms of this disorder in children. It now appears that in children with bipolar
disorder the disturbance to these biological rhythms may be due to as many as four

mutations of the **RORB** (**RAR-related orphan receptor B**) gene at 9q22. The full function of the protein coded for by this gene is unknown but it possibly has some importance in expression of other genes. It is involved in the regulation of the circadian cycles which go wrong in depression. One example is sleep loss, which is a major, and possibly early symptom in childhood bipolar depression.

The long-term detrimental effects (i.e. the psychological 'scars') of a period of depression in childhood (to a greater extent) and in adolescence (to a lesser extent) are as follows:

* Impairment of social skills, in particular interpersonal skills. The childhood dependence on adults comes under considerable strain during depression, and the effects of this strain can be long-lasting.
* Developmental skills, especially the learning skills developed at school, are likely to suffer as a result of a depressive phase, with gaps in knowledge occurring which are difficult to make up at a later date.
* The development of the concept of 'self' is a feature of childhood (mostly) and adolescence. Depression at an early age may distort the perception of 'self' for years after.
* Extended periods of negative thinking may be reinforced by a depressive episode during childhood, causing low self-esteem, fatigue, poorer social skills, difficulty with concentration and learning.

From about 13 years of age onwards, depressive states become more common amongst girls than boys. The reasons are not entirely clear, but may be partly due to hormonal changes that result in different ways boys and girls view the physical effects created by the hormones. Social pressures to conform to certain stereotypes, often led by celebrities or advertising, have a greater impact on girls than on boys (Nolen-Hoeksema 2007).

Post-partum depression (PPD) and seasonal affective disorder (SAD)

Depression can occur during pregnancy, with a peak of incidence between weeks 18 to 32 of gestation, but most cases of depression happen soon after delivery of the baby. **Post-partum depression** occurs in some women at any time from 3 days to 6 weeks after giving birth. The cause is unclear, but a hormonal or immune imbalance, stress or a genetic predisposition to mood disorders have all been suggested as contributing factors. Protein deficiency has also been suggested as a potential cause, or a contributing factor to PPD, given that the mother's protein intake over the period of gestation was required to accommodate for both the growing child and her own protein needs. This is easily corrected by providing an increase in the protein content of the mother's diet, and it may be a safe and valuable method of reducing the risk of PPD in women who could be vulnerable.

During pregnancy, the uterine contents, notably the fetus, are *immunologically privileged* in the sense that the fetus is foreign, or alien tissue (i.e. it is potentially an **antigen**) that has to be tolerated by the mother's immune system. Very soon after birth, the mother's immune system changes significantly. There is an increase in those factors that promote inflammation, i.e. activation of type 1 T-helper cells

(Th1 cells), increased levels of **interferon gamma (INFγ)** and **tumour necrosing factor alpha (TNFα)**, and these factors are associated with post-partum depression. About a third of all sufferers have a previous history of a psychiatric disorder and about a quarter will have more than one episode.

Some women may show signs *before* giving birth which suggest that a depressive illness could follow labour; such signs include lack of preparation for the baby, denying the pregnancy or expressing future plans that clearly do not involve the baby. The range of severity is wide, from a mild form (often called *baby blues*) to an intense suicidal psychotic depression.

- *Post-partum blues (baby blues)*, a mild depression that lasts 1 to 14 days after the birth, often peaking on the fifth day, in which the new mother feels low and cries easily. She may show hostility towards the baby or even the father. It affects between 20 and 75 per cent of mothers, the figure varying between different studies.
- *Post-partum depression*, a more severe syndrome occurring at any time up to six months after the birth and which lasts for most of the first year. These mothers show loss of emotion, anxiety, reduced appetite, sleep disturbance and guilty feelings. Most of the women have no intentions of harming themselves or the baby. It affects between 10 and 15 per cent of mothers.
- *Post-partum psychosis*, the most severe form, in which the mother loses contact with reality and show signs of psychosis (hallucinations, delusions and disorientation). The depression takes the form of unipolar or bipolar depression, with harmful tendencies towards the baby (who may be seen as the cause of their problem) or themselves. It affects about 0.2 per cent of mothers.

Seasonal affective disorder (SAD) is a depressive state that occurs during the winter months when shorter days are accompanied by less sun, i.e. when light levels are lower. Exposure to natural daylight is therefore at a minimum. Daylight is an important external cue for several biological rhythms which the brain goes through, each rhythm taking about a day (approximately 24 hours) to complete. These rhythms are known as **circadian rhythms** (circa = about, diem = day), such as the **sleep–wake cycle**. But sunlight is also involved in mood regulation.

Serotonin is used by the **pineal gland** (found immediately behind the hypothalamus, Figure 11.8) to make a hormone called **melatonin. Pinealocytes** (cells of the pineal gland) concentrate serotonin, which is then converted first to **N-acetylserotonin**, then to melatonin. Melatonin can cross membranes better than serotonin and it binds to receptors to form complexes that interact with cellular activity. The pineal gland is sensitive to light levels on the retina (part of the retinal output to the brain goes to the pineal gland via the hypothalamus, the **retinohypothalamic tract**). During periods of darkness, noradrenaline levels rise and this acts on the pineal gland to create melatonin from serotonin. Melatonin may be the true trigger of sleep, as it is involved in the normal sleep–wake cycle. Melatonin levels are very low during the day, when noradrenaline levels are lower. The winter months of long nights and lower daytime light levels can maintain a higher than expected melatonin level and this may trigger a persistent depressive mood throughout winter. SAD can sometimes be treated with artificial light (called **phototherapy**) (Birtwistle and Martin 1999).

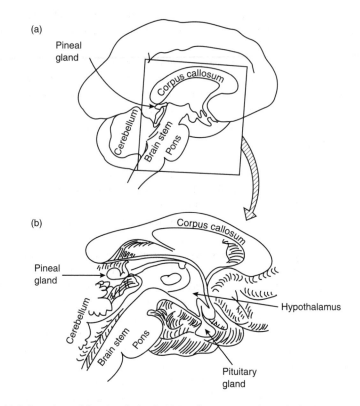

Figure 11.8 Location of the pineal gland. (a) Midline section through the brain, view from the right. (b) Close-up of the upper brain stem, hypothalamus and corpus callosum, showing the pineal gland.

The antidepressant drugs

The main neurotransmitters involved in depression are the *monoamines* serotonin and noradrenaline (Blows 2000a, b). The **monoamine hypothesis** of depression came from two important observations made in the 1950s:

- Some patients treated for hypertension with a drug called **reserpine** were becoming depressed.
- Some patients treated for tuberculosis with a drug which is no longer in use for this purpose, called **para-amino salicylic acid (PAS)**, were becoming happier.

Reserpine was later found to deplete the synapses of both serotonin and noradrenaline, thus inducing a depressive state. PAS, however, was noted to block the enzyme that breaks down the neurotransmitter, thus allowing the neurotransmitter to increase in the synapse and therefore relieving depression. The enzyme concerned is **monoamine oxidase**, which is found in association with the mitochondria of the presynaptic bulb. After use in the synaptic cleft, many neurotransmitters are returned to the presynaptic bulb (*re-uptake*) for conversion to a **metabolite** before removal from the brain. This creates two possible mechanisms for increasing the amounts of neurotransmitter in the synaptic cleft:

- Blocking the re-uptake so that the chemical stays in the cleft. This is the principal mode of action of the **tricyclic antidepressants** and *some* **atypical antidepressants**.
- Blocking of the breakdown by inhibiting the enzyme so that the chemical stays in the synapse. This is the principal mode of action of the **monoamine oxidase inhibitors (MAOI)**.

Tricyclic antidepressants

These drugs are named after the three-ringed (*tri-cyclic*) nature of the their chemistry, known as the **dibenzazepine** structure (Figure 11.9a). They work by blocking the re-uptake of the neurotransmitters serotonin and noradrenaline into the presynaptic bulb, with the result that these transmitters accumulate in the synaptic cleft. Two of the drugs in early use were **imipramine** (the first antidepressant, which came into clinical practice in the late 1950s) which is more selective in blocking noradrenaline, and **amitriptyline** (Figure 11.9a), which has approximately equal activity in blocking both neurotransmitters. Other typical tricyclic antidepressant drugs are **doxepin, clomipramine, dosulepin, lofepramine, nortriptyline** and **trimipramine**.

This drug group had the problem that symptoms of depression were not relieved until up to six weeks into treatment (known as a **therapeutic delay** or **latency period**). This was difficult to understand; after all, the very first dose of the drug

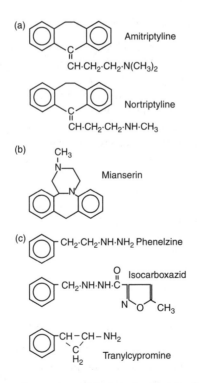

Figure 11.9 Structure of some important antidepressants: (a) tricyclic drugs; (b) atypical drugs; (c) monoamine oxidase inhibitor (MAOI) drugs.

given was active in raising the neurotransmitter levels at the synapse, so why was mood taking so long to return to normal? It is now thought that the delay is due to the time it takes to down-regulate receptors (see Figure 11.10) or to improve receptor sensitivity. This therapeutic delay can increase the risk of suicide because during this time the patient acquires more energy and severely depressed patients with more energy are greater suicide risks. There had to be another way round this delay. One step forward was the development of drugs which were more selective for blocking the re-uptake of either serotonin (the **selective serotonin re-uptake inhibitors**, or **SSRI**) or noradrenaline (Table 11.4). These drugs are said to have a shorter therapeutic delay than the tricyclic drugs.

The side-effects of the tricyclic antidepressants are drowsiness, dry mouth, blurred vision, urinary retention and constipation, all of which are **antimuscarinic** effects. Muscarinic receptors bind the neurotransmitter acetylcholine. Muscarine is a plant alkaloid that binds to this receptor, thus giving its name to the receptor. As muscarinic antagonists, the tricyclic antidepressants prevent acetylcholine from binding to muscarinic receptors, and in this way cause the side-effects. Other side-effects include **hyponatraemia** (low blood sodium levels) in the elderly and occasionally **cardiac arrhythmias** (abnormal rhythms of heart activity) such as **heart block** (failure of electrical conduction through the heart). The most likely tricyclic drug interactions are with the MAOI drug group. The switching of treatment from tricyclic to MAOI, or from MAOI to tricyclic medication, should only be done after a time gap of two weeks or more.

Selective serotonin reuptake inhibitors (SSRI)

These drugs selectively inhibit the reuptake of serotonin, therefore increasing the serotonin levels in the cleft. **Fluoxetine** was one of the first SSRIs to be introduced into clinical practice in the late 1980s. It is perhaps still the best known and most often prescribed antidepressant. Others SSRI drugs include **citalopram, escitalopram, paroxetine, sertraline** and **fluvoxamine**.

SSRIs are said to have fewer side-effects and are safer than tricyclic drugs if taken as an overdose because they have less powerful cardiac effects. The SSRI drugs also have fewer antimuscarinic side-effects, but they do sometimes cause varying degrees of nausea and vomiting, dizziness, fatigue and headache. Some of these unwanted effects become less troublesome as patients begin to tolerate the drug. These drugs are thought to have a short-term and a long-term effect, both of which are explained in Figure 11.10.

Fluoxetine has been found to increase neurogenesis in the brain. The drug causes a 50 per cent increase in the activation of **progenitor** cells, i.e. those cells from which new neurons are produced. It is still unclear if this has any influence with regard to resolving depression, or if other drugs have a similar effect.

Serotonin and noradrenaline re-uptake inhibitors (SNRIs)

Venlafaxine and **Duloxetine** are SNRI drugs which, similar to the tricyclic drugs, block the reuptake of both serotonin and noradrenaline, but as with the SSRIs they have much fewer side-effects and shorter therapeutic delay that the tricyclic drugs. Venlafaxine has variable effects at different dosages. At low dose it

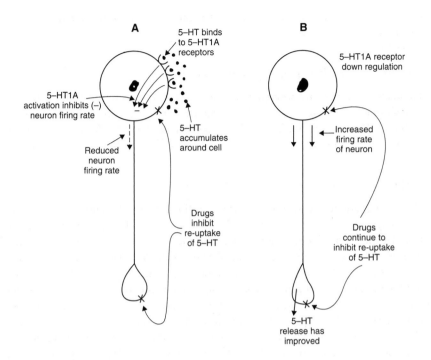

Figure 11.10 The short-term and long-term effects of SSRI drugs on the serotonin neurons. A. In the short term, the blockage of re-uptake at the synapse and cell body causes serotonin to accumulate around the neuron. This raised serotonin level actively stimulates the 5-HT1A autoreceptor on the cell body, which in turn decreases neuronal firing. B. In the longer-term, this causes the cell to down-regulate the 5-HT1A autoreceptor so the neuron can restore the impulse firing rate. This increases serotonin release at the synapse, which is prevented from re-uptake, and therefore will accumulate.

Table 11.4 Selective serotonin and noradrenaline inhibitors.

Serotonin-selective re-uptake inhibitors	*Noradrenaline-selective re-uptake inhibitors*
Fluoxetine Sertraline Paroxetine Citalopram Fluvoxamine `Escitalopram	Nortryptiline
	Reboxetine

Table 11.5 Some atypical antidepressants.

Atypical antidepressant	*Notes*
Mirtazapine	Blocks presynaptic α_2-adrenoceptors, which causes an increase in noradrenaline release
Mianserin (Figure 11.9b)	Reduces sensitivity of postsynaptic β-adrenoceptors (which alters the balance of postsynaptic adrenoceptor activity); it also blocks presynaptic α_2-adrenoceptors, which causes an increase in noradrenaline release
	Agomelatine A melatonin receptor agonist and selective serotonin receptor antagonist.
Flupentixol	An antipsychotic which can be used as an antidepressant in low dose.

inhibits the re-uptake of serotonin, but at higher doses it inhibits the re-uptake of serotonin, noradrenaline and dopamine.

Selective noradrenaline re-uptake inhibitors (NRIs)

Reboxetine inhibits the reuptake of noradrenaline only, and the resulting increase in noradrenaline is thought to enhance the neurotransmission of the serotonergic pathways. Reboxetine has fewer side-effects than the tricyclic drugs, including less serious cardiac effects.

Atypical antidepressants

These drugs are newer than the other groups (Figure 11.9b). While some do block the re-uptake of neurotransmitter at the synapse, others do not (Table 11.5). The fact that some relieve depression without interfering with the re-uptake of neuro-transmitter adds weight to the notion that blocking re-uptake is not the primary mechanism for relieving depression. These drugs, either exclusively or partially, modify the function of serotonin or noradrenaline receptor sites (Table 11.5) and this gives a clue as to the mechanism by which all antidepressant drugs ultimately work. Drugs of this atypical group appear to relieve symptoms faster than the tricy-clic drugs and they are known to be active in the limbic areas of the brain. Because some do not block transmitter re-uptake, they tend to cause fewer side-effects than the tricyclic group.

Monoamine oxidase inhibitors (MAOI)

The introduction of MAOI drugs (Figure 11.9c) that block the enzyme monoam-ine oxidase was one of the earliest treatments available for depression. Monoamine oxidase is an enzyme located on the outer membrane of mitochondria in the presy-naptic bulb, particularly in the dopaminergic, adrenergic and serotonergic path-ways. The enzyme inactivates the neurotransmitter after it has done its work in the synaptic cleft and has been taken back into the bulb. When the enzyme is blocked with the inhibitor drug, the neurotransmitter cannot be reduced to its metabolites for excretion and remains in the synapse. The transmitter levels then rise in the bulb and cleft. This action is more pronounced in noradrenergic and serotonergic synapses than in dopaminergic synapses.

Two forms of MAO exist, MAO-A and MAO-B, but the human brain has mostly MAO-B. Both forms of the enzyme degrade all three neurotransmitters (dopamine, noradrenaline and serotonin) when these transmitters are in high con-centration, but when they are in lower concentrations the enzymes become more specific. Both forms of the enzyme also exist in many tissues outside the brain, in particular the gut wall and the liver. The purpose of having the enzyme in these digestion-related sites is to facilitate the degradation of monoamines found in the diet, mostly **tyromine**. If tyromine enters the blood unmodified by MAO it can cause a hypertensive crisis. A throbbing headache is an early sign of this potentially dangerous condition. This is what happened to some patients given MAOI drugs for depression before it was realised that dietary monoamines were the cause of their crisis. To allow continuation of the treatment with the MAOI drugs it became necessary to remove monoamines from the diet. Patients were then issued with a list of foods to avoid, particularly those that contain the monoamine tyromine: foods such as cheese, pickled herring, red wine, and yeast or meat extracts to name a few. On the surface, it does seem paradoxical to issue potentially suicidal patients with tablets and a list of foods that may, in combination, kill them! In reality, of course, it was more selective and controlled than this picture would suggest, with potentially suicidal patients admitted for observation. However, occasional fatalities did occur and it became apparent that this was not the ideal way to cope with the problem.

All the original MAOI drugs worked by the *irreversible* blocking of the enzyme MAO, which meant that the enzyme had to be degraded, removed and replaced by a new enzyme. The problem of potentially dangerous hypertensive crisis led to the development of the newer *reversible* MAOI (RIMA) drugs. These work by locking on to and inhibiting the enzyme when the monoamine levels are low, thus allowing the levels to accumulate and rise. Should there be a sudden rise in monoamines – for example, in the digestive tract and the liver following the eating of a cheese sandwich – the drug will unlock from the enzyme, which then becomes free to act on the monoamines in the diet. Meanwhile, the same drug will remain active in the brain where the monoamine levels are low, thus exerting its antidepressant qualities. The action of the drug is therefore dependent on the amine levels in the area where it is found. As a result, the presence of monoamines in the diet has become a less important issue, although patients should still avoid consuming large amounts of these foods. The only RIMA drug currently available in clinical practice in the UK is listed in Table 11.6, but others are available outside the UK.

MAOI drugs can cause side-effects such as **postural hypotension** (low blood pressure on standing up from a sitting or lying position, a particular problem for elderly patients on these drugs) and dizziness. Other noted side-effects include dry mouth, drowsiness, insomnia, headache, fatigue, gastrointestinal disturbances, difficulty with **micturition** (passing urine) and many more, some potentially serious. For all these reasons, MAOI drugs are usually a second-line choice of treatment, used when the SSRI or atypical drugs have failed.

If, as has been seen, the relief of depression is not (at least not entirely) dependent on the increase in neurotransmitter levels in the brain, how do antidepressants really work? The full answer remains unknown. The current thinking is that all the antidepressant drugs work to relieve depression by two possible mechanisms:

- re-adjustment of the sensitivity of the receptors for serotonin and noradrenaline;
- modification of the transport of these neurotransmitters across the presynaptic membrane.

Table 11.6 MAOI antidepressants (Figure 11.8c).

Irreversible MAOI drugs	Reversible MAOI drug (RIMA)
Phenelzine	Moclobemide (MAO-A specific)
Isocarboxazid	
Tranylcypromine	

It seems likely that depression is the combination of defective neurotransmitter transporter, poor receptor activity and low neurotransmitter at the synapse. The antidepressants work to correct these defects and in so doing readjust the HPA axis to normal at the same time. They may also go some way in correcting the immune system abnormalities.

Pharmacokinetics and pharmacotherapeutics of the antidepressants

All these drugs are well absorbed from the gut so oral administration is not normally a problem. The tricyclic drugs have variable first pass metabolism and this means the dose does not always correlate with the therapeutic response. They are highly protein bound in circulation and tend to have long half-lives. The SSRI drugs also have long half-lives running into several days, and good bioavailability following first pass metabolism. The SNRI venlafaxine has limited first pass metabolism resulting in a high bioavailability (more than 90 per cent). The half-life of five hours for this drug is extended by the fact that the major metabolite is the primary active agent, with a half-life of eleven hours. Reboxetine (the NRI drug) has 100 per cent bioavailability, i.e. no first pass metabolism, and a fifteen-hour half-life. MAOI drugs tend to have short half-lives (typically one to three hours) and so may need to be given more frequently.

Since antidepressants are not addictive in the classical sense of the word, withdrawal of antidepressants should not be a problem provided it is done slowly. Sudden withdrawal after long-term use may induce unwanted effects, such as stomach upset, flu-like symptoms, sweating, insomnia, anxiety, dizziness, tremor, confusion, vivid nightmares, sexual dysfunction and sensations similar to small electric shocks (described as 'brain zaps', 'brain shocks' or 'head shocks'). These unwanted effects are often referred to as '**SSRI discontinuation syndrome**' (sometimes called '**SSRI withdrawal syndrome**' or '**SSRI cessation syndrome**').

There is no clinical justification for administering two different antidepressants for the same patient at the same time. This is likely to cause dangerous drug interactions. The MAOI drugs must never be administered immediately before or after the tricyclic drugs. At least a two-week gap should be allowed before commencing one of these groups after stopping the other. The potential for causing a hazardous interaction between these drug groups is very high. RIMA drugs are particularly dangerous if prescribed with other antidepressants due to the prospect of hazardous drug interactions.

Serotonin syndrome

Sometimes called '**serotonin toxicity**', '**serotonin storm**' or '**hyperserotonaemia**', this is a potentially life-threatening adverse drug reaction where excessive serotonin is produced in the brain and leaks into the blood. The result is overactivity of serotonergic receptors in both the brain and the body. The cause may be very high antidepressant dosage, or sometimes even normal dosage of one antidepressant drug; or a reaction between two antidepressant drugs (which should never happen; see the preceding paragraph) or the use of some illicit drugs. The symptoms occur rapidly, and they include confusion, mania, agitation, hallucinations, headache, shivering, sweating, low blood pressure, nausea, muscle twitching and tremor, raised body temperature, fast pulse rate, diarrhoea and dilated pupils. These symptoms can range from quite mild to very severe, even fatal. Discontinuation of any antidepressant drugs must be the first line of treatment, followed in severe cases by the administration of a serotonin antagonist. Benzodiazepine sedation may also be useful.

Mood-stabilising drugs

The drugs described under this heading are those used to prevent the swings in mood associated with bipolar depression, in which long periods of deep depression are interrupted by occasional bouts of mania. **Lithium carbonate** is very effective in this role by controlling the manic state when used in a prophylactic manner, i.e. over a lengthy time period. It has no role to play in the management of unipolar depression or acute manic states.

Lithium is given orally and is rapidly absorbed from the gut, peak levels being reached in the blood within 24 hours of commencement. The mechanism by which lithium balances mood is now becoming better understood. The drug shows several biochemical effects occurring together, and until recently, deciding which of these resulted in the desired effect was difficult.

Lithium is a **cation** (a positively charged particle) and can act as a substitute for other cations such as sodium (Na^+), potassium (K^+), magnesium (Mg^{2+}) or calcium (Ca^{2+}). Lithium can penetrate the neuronal cell body membrane and accumulate within the cytoplasm. This increases the intracellular cation population, repelling some K^+, which is forced out of the cell. This results in a partial *depolarisation* of that neuron, and in turn slows the *repolarisation* phase, thus reducing the excitation of the neuron. However, the main action of lithium in prevention of mania appears to be its role in inhibiting the PKC enzyme, which becomes excessively active and cannot be shut down in mania. Lithium inhibits this enzyme, thus preventing the PKC cause of mania.

Lithium has several other effects:

- It inhibits **ATPase** (the enzyme that produces **ATP, adenosine triphosphate,** the cell's high-energy molecule), causing a reduction in the level of ATP in the cell.
- It has a similar inhibitory effect on **cAMP (cyclic adenosine monophosphate)** and **inositol**. *See page 59*
- It slows down the uptake of choline into the neurons that synthesise acetylcholine and this neurotransmitter is therefore reduced.
- It causes reduced release of serotonin and reduced serotonin receptor density in the hippocampus.
- It prevents dopamine receptors in the corpus striatum from becoming supersensitive to dopamine, a possibility that can occur after long-term use of the **neuroleptic** drugs. This particular action of lithium is probably quite an important mechanism leading to the desired antimanic effect.
- It has significant antiviral effects, especially against the **herpes virus**.
- It has modulatory effects on cell-mediated and humoral immunity. This suggests a possible role for viral infections in depression.

Toxic levels of lithium are achieved rapidly if the dose is not carefully controlled. Blood levels of the drug are monitored. The toxic effects of lithium, which may be worsened by a low blood sodium level, include tremor, **ataxia** (unsteady walking), nausea, dizziness, convulsions and coma. Lithium can also cause a wide range of other side-effects, such as endocrine disturbance, notably **thyroid disorders**, by inhibiting iodine uptake into the thyroid gland and reducing thyroid hormone production. Alterations of the thyroid receptor concentration in the hypothalamus as a result of lithium treatment may have some bearing on its mood-stabilising role, given the importance of the thyroid for brain activity. Lithium can also cause **polyurea** (a large urine output) with **polydipsia** (excessive thirst), weight gain, oedema and gastrointestinal disturbances. Changes in the electrical rhythm of the heart may be noticed on the **electrocardiogram** (**ECG**). Clearly, the decision to use lithium is not taken lightly, and usually involves specialist advice.

Carbamazepine is also available for the prophylaxis of mania, especially in those patients who are unresponsive to lithium. It is particularly useful in patients who have a rapid cycle of manic and depressive episodes (i.e. four or more such episodes per year). This drug is an important anti-epileptic and as such is discussed in Chapter 12.

Key points

Depressive illness

- Depressive illness occurs when the depressed state has no apparent cause or when the period of depression is prolonged beyond what is considered normal.
- Two main types of illnesses occur, unipolar depression (depression only) and bipolar depression (symptoms of depression with periods of mania).

Risk

- For the population as a whole, the risk of developing unipolar depression is 6 per cent, and for bipolar depression the risk is 1 per cent.
- First-degree relatives of a bipolar depressed patient have a concordance rate of 19 per cent, while for unipolar depression the concordance rate is 10 per cent.
- The concordance rate for bipolar depression in monozygotic twins is about 65 per cent; in dizygotic twins the concordance rate is about 14 per cent. This indicates that bipolar depression is a genetically based disease.

Cause

- Some twenty genes are implicated in the causation of major affective disorder.
- Environmental factors, e.g. the Borna virus, may play a role in the aetiology of unipolar and bipolar depression.

Brain pathology

- There are some limited physical changes in the brains of depressed patients; some have ventricular enlargement and a reduction in the size of the temporal lobe.

- Brodmann area 25, part of the cingulate region of the brain, appears to be hyperactive in depression, and deep brain stimulation can treat depression by reducing this activity.

Biochemistry and immunity

- Serotonin and noradrenaline are reduced and a low turnover of these transmitters occurs at the synapse of the diffuse modulatory systems.
- Very low levels of serotonin have been linked to increased violent behaviour, such as suicide.
- The serotonin subtype-2 receptor (5-HT2) is thought to be the most important receptor involved in mood regulation.
- A prolonged hyperactivity of the hypathalomo–pituitary–adrenal (HPA) axis occurs, causing chronic CRF (corticotropin-releasing factor) and cortisol release.
- There are significant immune system changes in depression.

Post-partum depression

- Post-partum depression, in which women become depressed after birth, is an umbrella term for three conditions: post-partum blues (a mild depression), post-partum depression (a more severe syndrome) and post-partum psychosis (the most severe form).

SAD

- Seasonal affective disorder (SAD) is a depressive state occurring during the winter months when there are shorter days and low light levels.

Tricyclic antidepressants

- Tricyclic antidepressants work by blocking the re-uptake of serotonin and noradrenaline into the presynaptic bulb, so these transmitters accumulate in the synaptic cleft.
- Some tricyclic antidepressants are more selective for noradrenaline.

SSRI antidepressants

- Selective serotonin re-uptake inhibitors (SSRIs) are more selective for blocking the reuptake of serotonin.

Atypical antidepressants

- Atypical antidepressants reduce the side-effects seen with other drugs and shorten the therapeutic delay.

MAOI antidepressants

- Monoamine oxidase inhibitors (MAOI) block the enzyme monoamine oxidase, which normally breaks down neurotransmitters.

- Antidepressant drugs relieve depression mainly by increasing neurotransmitter levels, by readjusting the sensitivity of the receptors for serotonin and noradrenaline and by modifying the transport of these neurotransmitters across the presynaptic membrane.
- MAOI drugs require restriction of oral intake of the monoamine tyromine to prevent hypertensive crisis.
- Different antidepressant drugs should not be prescribed without at least a two-week gap between them to prevent drug interactions.

Lithium

- Lithium is a prophylactic mood-stabilising drug used to control the manic phases of bipolar depression.
- Lithium works mainly by inhibiting the PKC enzyme system within the neuron.
- Lithium can reach toxic levels quickly and must be carefully monitored.

References

Birtwistle J. and Martin N. (1999) Seasonal affective disorder: its recognition and treatment. *British Journal of Nursing*, **8** (15): 1004–1009.

Blows W. T. (2000a) Neurotransmitters of the brain: serotonin, noradrenaline (norepinephrine), and dopamine. *Journal of Neuroscience Nursing*, **32** (4): 234–238.

Blows W. T. (2000b) The neurobiology of antidepressants. *Journal of Neuroscience Nursing*, **32** (3): 177–180.

Bode L. and Ludwig H. (2003) Borna disease virus infection, a human mental health risk. *Clinical Microbiology Reviews*, **16** (3): 534–545.

Brown P. (2001) A mind under siege. *New Scientist*, **170** (2295; 16 June): 34–37.

Carlson N. R. (2010) *Physiology of Behavior* (10th edition). Allyn and Bacon, Boston.

Dobbs D. (2006) Turning off depression. *Scientific American Mind*, **17** (4): 26–31.

Fukuda K., Takahashi K., Iwata Y., Mori N., Gonda K., Ogawa T., Osonoe K., Sato M., Ogata S., Horimoto T., Sawada T., Tashiro M., Yamaguchi K., Niwa S. and Shigeta S. (2001) Immunological and PCR analyses for Borna disease virus in psychiatric patients and blood donors in Japan. *Journal of Clinical Microbiology*, **39** (2): 419–429.

Hestad K., Aukrust P., Tønseth S. and Reitan S. (2009) Depression has a strong relationship to alterations in the immune, endocrine and neural system. *Current Psychiatry Reviews*, **5**: 287–297.

Miranda H., Nunes S., Calvo E., Suzart S., Itano E. and Watanabe M. (2006) Detection of Borna disease virus p24 RNA in peripheral blood cells from Brazilian mood and psychotic disorder patients. *Journal of Affective Disorder*, **90** (1): 43–47.

Nolen-Hoeksema S. (2007) *Abnormal Psychology*. McGraw-Hill, Boston.

Ron M. A. (1999) Psychiatric manifestations of demonstrable brain disease, in Ron M. A. and David A. S. (eds), *Disorders of Brain and Mind*. Cambridge University Press, Cambridge.

Westly E. (2010) Different shades of blue. *Scientific American Mind*, **21** (2): 30–37.

12 Epilepsy

- Seizures: types and causes
- The electroencephalogram (EEG) in epilepsy
- Factors involved in the cause of epilepsy
- The epileptogenic focus
- Tonic–clonic (grand mal) seizures
- The hippocampal involvement in seizures
- Temporal lobe seizures (psychomotor epilepsy)
- Jacksonian seizures
- Infantile spasms and febrile convulsions
- The anticonvulsant drugs
- Key points

Seizures: types and causes

Epilepsy is a term used to cover a very wide range of complex disorders, all character-ised by the presence of seizures or fits and sometimes convulsions. **Seizures**, or **fits**, are brief periods of high frequency, high voltage electrical discharges from the brain. They are associated with altered consciousness and accompanied by changes in sen-sory and motor function, causing momentarily abnormal behavioural patterns. The altered state of consciousness may mean a short period of either total or partial loss of consciousness, or simply a state of unawareness. **Convulsions** are powerful, often violent, rhythmic muscular contractions of the trunk and limbs occurring during a seizure. The word **ictal** is used to indicate a fit, with **interictal** meaning the period between two successive fits. Seizures occur in a variety of major or minor types, and are basically the result of **cerebral irritation**, meaning anything that directly disturbs the function of neurons in the brain (see Table 12.1 on page 246). The majority of these *one-off* fits are caused by temporary self-correcting or curable problems.

Idiopathic, or **primary epilepsy** (indicated as **1°**) is of unknown cause; that is, the existing pathology cannot be explained, and may be due to a developmen-tal malformation of the brain structure. **Symptomatic**, or **secondary epilepsy** (indicated as **2°**) is caused by distinct and explainable brain pathology, either in structure or function. There are also various syndromes involving fits and special forms of epilepsy (see Table 12.2 on page 247; see also text for temporal lobe and Jacksonian epilepsy).

It is estimated that the total number of people in the United Kingdom who have ever had a fit is about 5 per cent (including febrile convulsions). The occurrence of one fit does not mean the sufferer has epilepsy and of this 5 per cent group only about 0.5 per cent will go on to develop true epilepsy after their first fit.

Generalised seizures

Generalised seizures are characterised by changes in consciousness due to spread of an electrical discharge to many areas of the brain, and they are often associated with convulsions. They account for about 30 per cent of all epilepsies. *Generalised epilepsies* can be classified into four types: **absences**, **generalised tonic–clonic**, **myoclonic** and **atonic**. Of these four types, the first two are the most common.

Absence (formally the **petit mal** or **minor fit**) describes a transient loss of awareness during which the person will stop what they are doing, then stare vacantly into space for about 30 seconds or so, perhaps fumble with objects around them, then return to normal. There is no perceptive or cognitive function for the duration of the fit and afterwards there is no memory of the event. The person does not fall to the ground because normal **muscle tone** is maintained. Occasionally **automatism** (mechanical-like automatic movements) is seen, particularly if the duration of the fit is longer than 30 seconds. Petit mal usually starts at around the age of 5–7 years and stops at puberty, but can go on into adulthood. **Atypical absences** show a similar clinical picture, but the person may also show muscle twitching or some other abnormal movement.

Generalised tonic–clonic fits (the **grand mal** or **major fit**), are those in which the person loses consciousness, falls to the ground and convulses. They are discussed in the section 'Tonic–clonic (grand mal) seizures'. This form of epilepsy is the type most people think of as a fit in the full sense of the word. Such fits occur in three ways: as *primary generalised epilepsy*, where there is no other neurological abnormality; as a *partial seizure* which becomes generalised; and as a symptom associated with *diffuse brain dysfunction*.

Myoclonic fits (**myo** = muscle, **clonus** = rapid; alternating contractions and relaxations of skeletal muscle) are those in which muscle jerks occur in the arms or legs for a short period of about 1–5 seconds.

Atonic (a = without, tonic = tone, also called **drop attacks**) fits are those in which there is a sudden loss of muscle tone, resulting in collapse of the person. They last only a few seconds.

Partial (or focal) seizures

Focal seizures are centred around one particular part of the brain with some spread of the impulses, but spread is more limited than in generalised seizures. This is the most common type of seizure. The neurons involved fire rapid bursts of action potentials which are then synchronised in other neuron groups as the wave of impulses spreads.

Consciousness is often preserved (**simple partial**), but sometimes lost (**complex partial**) depending on the cause of the seizure, the location of the initial site and the spread of the electrical impulse. Behavioural changes are often a feature. The areas of the brain usually involved are:

- *Frontal lobe.* Seizures originating here cause predominantly motor symptoms, especially of the legs and the head. These seizures last for just a few seconds and occur several times a day.
- *Parietal lobe.* Seizures originating here can cause sensory and motor symptoms as in **Jacksonian epilepsy**.
- *Temporal lobe.* Seizures originating here cause personality symptoms, as typified in **temporal lobe epilepsy**.
- *Occipital lobe.* Seizures originating here cause disturbance of the visual cortex, resulting in the patient seeing visual phenomena such as flashing lights or sparks. *See page 6*

There is some evidence to suggest that at least one form of partial seizure, called **Rasmussen's encephalitis** (**RE**), may be **autoimmune** in origin (Acharya 2002). Autoimmune means that the immune system reacts to a normal part of the body as though it is a harmful agent introduced from the environment. Research in this area is currently limited, but changes in the body's immune response are part of the pathology of this disease.

The electroencephalogram (EEG) in epilepsy

The EEG is a very useful tool in the investigation of epileptic syndromes but it cannot be used alone to diagnose epilepsy. It does have a value in helping to distinguish between the different categories of epilepsy. Basically, the EEG is a recording of the overall pattern of electrical signals generated by millions of active neurons across the brain surface. A characteristic epileptic feature on the EEG is the *spike*, a pointed feature in the wave pattern not seen on the normal tracing, as shown in Figure 12.1. During seizures the wave patterns and spikes show increased frequencies and abnormal irregularities as the seizure spreads. The following patterns are usually seen.

- Absences show a 3-per-second spike and wave activity (Figure 12.2).
- Simple partial seizures show localised slow but sharp wave activity (Figure 12.3).
- Complex partial seizures show a medium-voltage spike activity centred on one brain area, increasing in intensity as it spreads (Figure 12.4).
- Generalised tonic–clonic seizures show rhythmic high-voltage activity leading to the clinical appearance of convulsions, with bilateral multispiked wave patterns during convulsions (Figure 12.5).

Factors involved in the cause of epilepsy

Fits are either of known or unknown aetiology. The designation unknown probably means that the underlying pathology remains undetected. Examples of those caused by known pathology are listed in Table 12.1.

Other factors include:

Age. The incidence of fits increases with age; 12 per 100,000 people between 40 and 59 years of age are affected and this figure rises to 80 per 100,000 in the population over 60 years. A quarter of the epileptic population is over 60 years old.

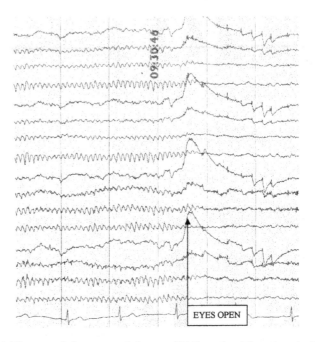

Figure 12.1 The normal electroencephalogram (EEG) tracing. There is no 'spike' feature, as is often seen in epilepsy.

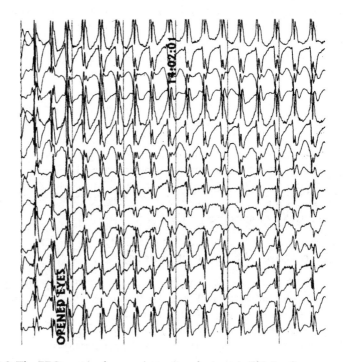

Figure 12.2 The EEG seen in absences (or petit mal seizures). This is a 3-per-second wave pattern.

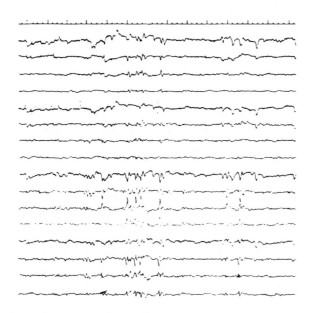

Figure 12.3 The EEG seen in simple partial seizures.

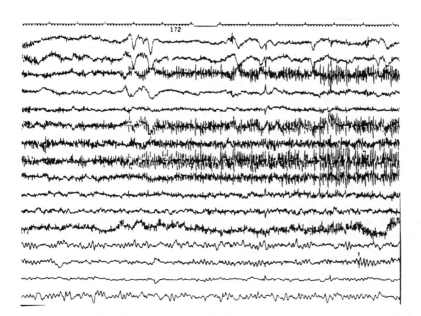

Figure 12.4 The EEG seen in complex partial seizures.

Genetics. Epilepsy can be familial, but the picture is often complicated by the effects of several genes involved acting together (polygenic), or by varying amounts of genetic penetrance. There are over 250 genetic causes of epilepsy; many are disorders that carry an increased risk of epilepsy as a common feature. Some are

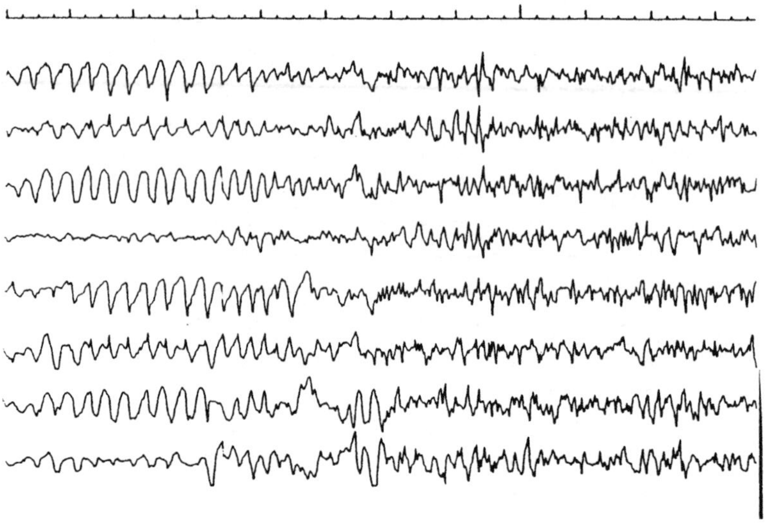

Figure 12.5 The EEG seen in general tonic–clonic (or grand mal) seizures.

Table 12.1 The known causes of seizures.

Cause of seizures	Notes
Congenital defects	Caused by disruption to neuronal function
Head injury (accidental or birth)	From brain damage or raised intracranial pressure (RICP)
Brain tumours and CNS disorders	Caused by pressure and disruption to neuronal function
Intracranial infections	Caused by irritation of the brain surface
Febrile convulsions	Caused by high temperature in children under seven
Drugs and alcohol withdrawal	Caused by removal of depressive effect on neuronal function
Metabolic	Caused by disturbance of neuronal biochemistry
Psychological	Invented by the patient for a specific purpose

See page 43 **autosomal recessive** whilst others are **autosomal dominant, X-linked** or even **mitochondrial DNA** (see Table 12.2).

Not all the genes responsible for epilepsy are found in the karyotype. DNA, the molecular basis of genes, is also found in **mitochondria**, the cellular organelles charged with the task of energy production. Mitochondria need their own genes to code for the proteins involved in the energy cycle. One mitochondrial gene mutation that can cause seizures is **MERRF (myoclonic epilepsy and ragged red fibres)** (Figure 12.6, Table 12.2). The 'ragged red fibres' are the accumulations of mitochondria seen on biopsy below the cell membrane of skeletal muscle. A change from the DNA base adenine to guanine in the normal gene causes a mutation that reduces mRNA production and thus protein synthesis. Skeletal muscle then deteriorates and the person becomes deaf and demented before the seizures, myoclonus and ataxia begin (Mancuso et al. 2004).

Table 12.2 Some genetic epileptic disorders.

Genetic epilepsy	Notes
West syndrome (generalised); at Xp22	About 17 per cent of West syndrome is caused by genetic factors. Involves infant developmental delay, muscle spasms and long-term intellectual handicap.
Lennox–Gastaut syndrome (generalised); at 4q21.3	Multiple tonic or atonic seizures per day, sometimes absences, drop-attacks or myoclonus. Slow mental development or even intellectual regression with learning difficulties.
Myoclonic epilepsy and ragged red fibres (MERRF) Mitochondrial gene	Seizures with myopathy (muscle deterioration) (see text).
Lafora disease (or **Lafora progressive myoclonic epilepsy**) 2 genes at 6q & 6p22	Neurons and other tissue cells have Lafora bodies (intracellular inclusions). Starts in adolescence with myoclonus, seizures and drop attacks associated with gradual dementia. Usually fatal around mid-twenties.
Progressive epilepsy with mental retardation; at 8q	Generalised tonic–clonic seizures begin at five to ten years of age, increasing until puberty, and then declining in frequency to thirty-five years, when the person remains seizure-free. Mental deterioration begins about five years after seizures begin and requires nursing care.
Benign familial neonatal convulsions (BFNC); at 20q	Seizures from second or third day after birth cease at about six months of age. Development after that is normal.

A number of epileptic fits are caused by an **epileptogenic focus** (Hickey 2008; McCance et al. 2010). This is a lesion at any specific site in the brain where, as a result of damage or changes in their biochemistry, the neurons are in continuous state of partial depolarisation and are therefore hyperexcitable. The surrounding

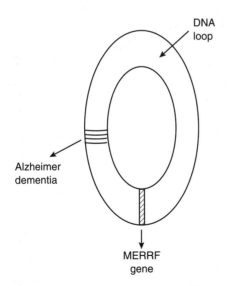

Figure 12.6 The mitochondrial DNA loop. Two genes on this loop are important for mental health, one associated with Alzheimer's dementia, and the myoclonic epilepsy and ragged red fibres (MERRF) gene, which causes a syndrome that includes epilepsy.

GABA neurons inhibit the excessive activity of the focus, but on occasions the focal activity exceeds the inhibitory neurons and a seizure results. The abnormal discharges spread to other parts of the brain, e.g. the cerebral cortex (affecting consciousness) and subcortical parts, and this spread causes a generalised fit. It is useful to think of a fit as an electric *storm* in the brain spreading from one particular point. Where the epileptogenic focus is known and has been studied, several interesting characteristics have been found (Figure 12.7):

- The neurons of the focus may suffer some degree of **deafferentation**, i.e. a loss of **dendritic spines**, the afferent component of the neuron. This means there is a reduction in synaptic density because dendrites, and the branches from dendrites (dendritic spines), are the location of many synaptic connections. The reason for this loss is not fully understood, but it causes a chronic state of depolarisation and excitability in the neurons.
- The normal passage of an action potential is from the cell to the synapse, and this is described as an **orthodromic** impulse. There is some evidence to suggest that the epileptogenic focus can sometimes generate **antidromic** impulses, which return abnormally from the synapse back up the axon. This is possibly one reason for a rapid depolarisation in the axon of the focal neurons. The antidromic impulses may also generate other orthodromic impulses, creating a cycle.
- There are neurotransmitter differences at the focus. Focal neurons have reduced GABA activity; i.e. less inhibition from the GABA neurons that occur in the vicinity of the focus. This creates an imbalance between excitation and inhibition, with excitation overwhelming the inhibitory activity. The process

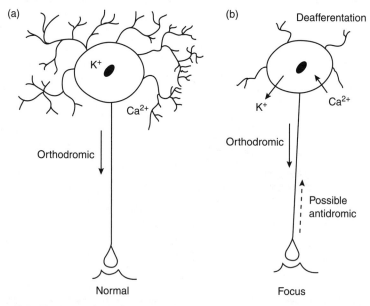

Figure 12.7 Changes at the epileptogenic focus neuron. Deafferentation, calcium entry, and possible antidromic impulses are some of the features that cause greater electrical activity at the focus.

is made worse by increased excitatory glutamate activity at the NMDA gluta-mate receptors. The focus is also more sensitive to acetylcholine (ACh) which binds to ACh receptors for longer than it does on normal neurons.

- The cells of the focus and other neurons have increased permeability to ions. This is due to an increase in the numbers of ion channels within the cell membrane, a process called **up-regulation**. Chief amongst these chan-nels involved in epilepsy are calcium and potassium channels. Calcium (Ca^{2+}) is normally in greater concentrations outside the neuronal cell body, with potassium (K^+) inside. There are several types of calcium channels in the cell membrane, and the channels involved in epilepsy are known as **T-type chan-nels**. Changes in the genetic expression of these channels result in an increase in T-type channels in the membrane. This kind of gene disorder which affects ion channels is sometimes called **channelopathies**. T-type calcium and potas-sium channelopathies are the best studied in relation to epilepsy. During a sei-zure, focal neurons leak calcium *into* the cell through the T-type channels, and this displaces potassium *out of* the cell. These ionic changes cause increased depolarisation of the membrane and further hyperexcitability of the neuron (McCance et al. 2010). Some drugs are now in clinical use which block T-type calcium channels to reduce cellular hyperexcitability and therefore help to prevent fits. *See page 255*
- Occasionally, a **primary (1°)** epileptogenic focus (the real focus) can induce changes in normal brain cells nearby so that they act as a **secondary (2°, or false focus)** during a seizure. This induction process is known as **kindling**. In some cases, the primary focus is present in one hemisphere of the brain (either cortical or subcortical), whilst a secondary focus (also called a **mirror focus**) can be traced in the opposite hemisphere (Figure 12.8) (Hickey 2008). The primary focus communicates with the false secondary focus through the corpus callosum. The secondary focus is essentially normal brain tissue act-ing along with the true focus to cause the seizure. However, given enough time, the secondary focus will be converted to epileptogenic tissue which can

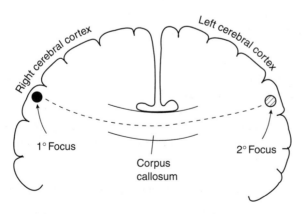

Figure 12.8 The primary focus (1°) sometimes causes a secondary focus (2°) to form at the mirror image position on the other side of the brain. They link through the corpus callosum. Removal of the primary focus causes the secondary focus to disappear.

function independently. This means that early surgical removal of the primary focus is important, as is possible in some patients, before this permanent conversion of the secondary focus occurs. This surgery, if done early enough, will result in the restoration of normal structure and function of the secondary focus (Acharya 2002).

The net effect of all these changes at the epileptogenic focus is to produce a small area of neurons which are hyperactive with a low threshold for firing impulses. They are likely to discharge action potentials easily and rapidly, up to 1,000 impulses per second during a fit, sparking off a wave of high-voltage abnormal electrical activity across the brain.

During a fit the brain increases its use of ATP (adenosine triphosphate) as an energy source by 250 per cent. This huge energy requirement must be met by an increase in the blood supply, which also increases by 250 per cent. The oxygen consumption of the neurons increases by 60 per cent, but still this massive supply becomes depleted. The brain moves into anaerobic metabolism, with the result that lactic acid production, acidosis and cellular exhaustion occur (McCance et al. 2010). Fits rarely last for more than one or two minutes. The question of what causes the fit to stop has been controversial. Previously it was considered to be due to either the neurotransmitters becoming depleted or because of the rapid accumulation of waste products which cannot be removed fast enough from the cell body. A more modern view suggests that since the fit was the result of excessive excitatory activity, the cessation of the fit may be due to restoration of inhibitory activity to restore the balance (see next section on tonic–clonic seizures). In either case, any further abnormal neuronal activity would be prevented.

Tonic–clonic (grand mal) seizures

Generalised tonic–clonic fits may be due to an epileptogenic focus or caused by a more widespread irritation of brain cells. Some factors that lead to this form of grand mal seizure are listed in Table 12.1, and this list illustrates why those having an epileptic-type fit for the first time must undergo extensive investigations to identify the presence or absence of a focus and, in the case of the latter, to determine what may have been the cause.

The fit occurs in four stages, as shown in Table 12.3. The **tonic stage** involves muscle rigidity due to a strong increase in muscle tone. This is caused by the spread of abnormal impulses to the subcortical regions, notably the thalamus, brain stem and spinal cord. The **clonic stage** is the convulsive stage, and involves inhibitory responses from the thalamus, basal ganglia and cortex which interrupt the tonic phase to allow brief moments of muscle relaxation followed by restoration of rigidity. These bursts of inhibitory impulses become more dominant and gradually gain control of the fit, causing the fit to stop.

Table 12.4 indicates the nurse's role at each stage of the fit.

Two important myths are associated with the management of fits are discussed further here:

- **Do not put anything in the mouth**. The placing of a hard object between the teeth to stop the person from biting their tongue is usually done *too late* and therefore becomes a dangerous procedure. By the start of the tonic phase the

Table 12.3 Stages of a tonic–clonic fit.

Stage of the fit	Notes
1. **Aura**, or warning	Occurs in the form of confusion, aggression, or hallucinations such as flashing lights or strange smells. Many patients do not have an aura, and some who have an aura do not recognise it as such.
2. **Tonic**	Fall to the ground followed by increased muscle tone which causes stiffness and arching of the body on the ground. Lasts about 15–30 seconds, during which breathing stops and the patient becomes somewhat cyanosed.
3. **Clonic**	The convulsive stage. The patient thrashes about with rapid, powerful muscle contractions. They may be incontinent. Breathing is spasmodic and excessive salivation causes frothing at the mouth. Lasts for about 30–60 seconds.
4. **Recovery**	Starts when the patient stops moving. Breathing gradually settles down. Patient goes from unconsciousness into sleep, and then wakens. They may be a little confused or disorientated, but should recover from this quickly. There is no memory of the event. Lasts about 5–10 minutes or so.

Table 12.4 Nurse's skill at each stage of the fit.

Stage of the fit	Nurse's (or first-aider's) role at each stage
1. **Aura**	Assist the patient to the ground in a clear area to avoid injury when falling or convulsing. Loosen tight clothing around neck, chest and waist. Note the time.
2. **Tonic**	Work from the head end away from the body. Do not restrain the patient. Keep other people away from the patient's body. Keep the airway as clear as possible. Do not try to put anything between the teeth as this will cause oral damage and bleeding into the mouth. Clear the area around the patient.
3. **Clonic**	Continue to work from the head end away from the body. Do not restrain the patient. Observe and facilitate breathing by clearing the airway of any obstruction. Check the pulse (carotid is best) and skin colour for cyanosis.
4. **Recovery**	Turn into the recovery position when convulsion stops. Stay at head end to maintain clear airway and check breathing, pulse and skin colour. On the patient's awakening, get them into a resting position gradually. Note the time again.

jaw will already be clenched tightly shut, and to open the jaw would require a considerable force, causing injury to the patient's mouth. Bleeding into the mouth and dental damage would cause a further risk of airway obstruction and distress when the patient wakes up. If the person is going to bite their tongue, this will have happened by the start of the tonic phase. Any such damage to the tongue is not common and can be treated. The aura, therefore, is the only stage at which it is possible to take preventative action. Since an aura does not always occur, and if it does it is over very quickly, it is best to relegate this procedure to the history books.

- **Do not restrain the patient**. The restraining of the body during the convulsion is another very dangerous practice. Anyone attempting this is putting themselves and the patient at considerable risk of injury, and it is unnecessary. The patient's limb movements are powerful, and they may kick, punch or throw off anyone holding them. In addition, it has been shown that restraint causes more limb injuries to the patient than allowing them to be free. Emptying the space around the patient's body to give them room is a useful thing to do, to prevent them hitting against hard objects. Everyone should keep clear of the patient's body, while the nurse stays at the head end.

The **recovery stage** is an important time for nursing care. The patient should be placed in the *recovery position* as soon as the clonic phase ends. The nurse should remain with the patient at all times, unless there is no choice but to leave to get help. If going to get help is the only choice, leave the patient in the *recovery position* or wait until they are awake. The patient may go into a second fit, so the nurse should, whenever possible, remain to assist should this happen. Staying at the head end, the nurse should *maintain a clear airway* and *observe for breathing, carotid pulse and cyanosis* (cyanosis = blue colour of the skin, indicating a lack of oxygen). Check the patient's *level of consciousness* every few minutes by talking to them (Blows 2001). On return to consciousness, allow the patient time to rest, reassure them, and help them orientate themselves to time, place and what happened. The patient can sit up *slowly*, when ready to do so. The nurse should make a note of the time at each stage of the fit, but especially the time taken for recovery. A prolonged recovery phase, i.e. longer than 30 minutes, may be a sign of complications. Be aware of the possibilities of complications and seek help if required. Some of the possible complications are:

- The patient may go into another fit. If this happens then they must receive urgent medical care to prevent further fitting. **Status epilepticus** means the occurrence of multiple fits lasting 30 minutes or more without regaining consciousness between fits, and this is a very serious complication. **Impending status epilepticus** (multiple fits lasting 5 minutes or more without regaining consciousness between fits) often precedes status epilepticus and acts as a warning that the patient may be deteriorating. Status epilepticus is dangerous because patients can die from exhaustion or heart failure and prolonged convulsions create a shortage of oxygen to the brain, causing brain damage.
- **Postepileptic (interictal) twilight state** is a prolonged period of confusion and disorientation following a fit. Restless wandering and abnormal behaviour can accompany a twilight state. Patients do not know what they are doing and may unknowingly carry out bizarre, dangerous and even criminal acts. Again, urgent medical help is needed to safeguard the patient and others around him.

The hippocampal involvement in seizures

Some seizures are triggered by abnormal activity from the hippocampus. The hippocampus is described in Chapter 1 and also in Chapter 10 in relation to schizophrenia.

The cells most prone to epilepsy within the hippocampus are those of the **CA3** cell collection because they have strong excitatory connections. The least prone to epilepsy are the **granulate cells** because they have strong inhibitory connections. Normally, granulate cells provide inhibitory impulses that resist any onset of epileptogenesis within the hippocampus. Variation in the synaptic circuitry may change granulate cells to epileptogenic status which may then initiate a fit. The exact changes that cause granulate cells to trigger a fit are still under examination, but they centre on the formation of abnormal synaptic connections and the local reduction of inhibition (Acharya 2002).

Temporal lobe seizures (psychomotor epilepsy)

Epilepsy caused by temporal lobe lesions has a specific set of characteristics. The main occurrence is an abrupt change in personality and restless automatic behaviour patterns, with or without a concluding loss of consciousness. Hallucinations of an **olfactory** (smell) or **gustatory** (taste) nature sometimes occur and the patient may experience **déjà vu**, i.e. the sense of events repeating themselves, or **jamais vu**, the sense of being a stranger in familiar company or environments. Psychotic symptoms can present with aggressive overtones and emotional or mood swings. This sudden change in the behaviour and personality can be very frightening to the witness, who is often a member of the patient's family, and the nurse's support is needed to allay their fears. The sudden onset of the symptoms and the quick return to normal are strong indications that the cause is a seizure, even in the absence of convulsions.

The temporal lobe lesion responsible is often **medial temporal sclerosis**, a hardening of the temporal brain tissue, which occurs often in the hippocampus, notably that part called **Ammon's horn** (see the anatomy of the hippocampus). This lesion is associated with cerebral anoxia, especially as a fetus, or can result from febrile convulsions early in childhood, particularly if they were complicated or prolonged. The child grows up free from seizures for many years, but then develops temporal lobe epilepsy in early adulthood.

One part of the temporal lobe is the *limbic portion* (i.e. the area that connects and works with the limbic system), and epilepsy caused by a lesion here is referred to as **medial temporal epilepsy syndrome** (or simply **limbic epilepsy**). Again, the characteristics of this syndrome involve behavioural difficulties and psychotic, schizophrenia-like symptoms. There is also an **interictal syndrome** (i.e. symptoms occurring between fits), identified by reduced sexual behaviour, increased religious convictions (e.g. compulsive church attendance) and **hypergraphia** (excessive compulsive writing). The presence of psychosis as part of an epileptic illness is confusing, since without the fits these patients may well be diagnosed as schizophrenic. Often this raises the question: *Does the epilepsy cause this psychosis, or is this a schizophrenic illness with the patient having fits as well?* One suggested distinction between the 'psychosis of epilepsy' and the 'psychosis of schizophrenia' is that the former is a milder psychosis with fewer negative symptoms, no thought disorder, full preservation of affect and a distinct increase in religious delusions (Trimble 1999).

Jacksonian seizures

Jacksonian fits begin with a unilateral twitching of muscles in one part of the body – for example, the small finger of the *left* hand – and from there the convulsion spreads to all other parts of the same side of the body, and then onto the other side. The patient becomes unconscious and has a full convulsion. The muscles involved at the start indicate which part of the cerebral primary motor cortex was generating the fit, i.e. the focus of the lesion. In the example given here, the lesion would be in the *right* motor cortex (Brodmann 4), the area that controls the little finger. Notice that the *right* motor cortex controls the *left* side because the motor fibres cross to the other side, most crossing in the brain stem. The lesion in the motor cortex could be a tumour, inflammation or scar tissue. The disease manifestations are extremely varied, and other symptoms include sudden head and eye movements, tingling, numbness and smacking of the lips. Keen observation by the nurse can pinpoint the muscles involved at the start of the twitching and thereby assist the doctor in the diagnosis and location of the lesion.

Infantile spasms and febrile convulsions

Infantile spasms are attacks of head nodding and flexing of the body that begin in the early months of life. They cause a type of EEG trace known as **hypsar-rhythmia**, which is a very disorganised and chaotic brainwave recording with no recognizable patterns. Gross abnormalities of the brain are one cause of this form of epilepsy, and in this case it can lead to progressive mental retardation. However, another cause is a deficiency of **vitamin B6 (pyridoxine)** in the diet and treatment simply involves replacing the vitamin.

Infantile (or febrile) convulsions are not true epilepsy and very few cases go on to develop epilepsy later in life. The cause is a high temperature in children below the age of seven when the temperature control centre in the hypothalamus is still immature. Prevention of the convulsion can sometimes be achieved by the administration of **paracetamol** in syrup form when the child is conscious and able to swallow, during the early stages of a raised temperature. Paracetamol is thought to help reduce body temperature, although scientific evidence for this is lacking. Nursing measures are aimed at body temperature reduction, and include reducing the clothing, cooling the *room* (not the child directly) with a fan, and tepid sponging. If consciousness is lost and convulsions commence, do not attempt to give anything further by mouth. Maintain a clear airway, continue cooling the child and seek medical assistance as quickly as possible (Blows 2001). Drug treatment, usually with **diazepam** administered by injection or rectally by a doctor, may be required to stop the fitting, as prolonged fits can cause brain damage.

The anticonvulsant drugs

There are several classes of drugs used in the treatment of epilepsy (Table 12.5). They act in two main ways: on the epileptogenic focus and other cells to prevent the abnormal electrical discharge from happening; or on the brain as a whole to prevent spread of the discharge.

There are a number of different ways of preventing spread of the seizure (see Figure 12.9 on page 256).

- *Sodium channel blockers* act by blocking the channels through which sodium influxes through the axonal membrane during an action potential. This prevents the action potential from travelling any further down the axon and the discharge is blocked from spreading. In this way these drugs stabilise the axonal

Table 12.5 The classification of the antiepileptic drugs.

GROUP	DRUGS
Aldehydes	Paraldehyde
Barbiturates	Phenobarbital
Benzodiazepines	Clobazam Clonazepam Diazepam Midazolam Lorazepam
Carboxamides	Carbamazepine Oxcarbazepine Eslicarbazepine
Fatty acids	Sodium valproate Vigabatrin Tiagabine
Fructose derivatives	Topiramate
GABA analogues	Pregabalin Gabapentin
Hydantoins	Phenytoin Fosphenytoin
Pyrimidinediones	Primidone
Pyrrolidines	Levetiracetam
Succinimides	Ethosuximide
Sulfonamides	Zonisamide
Triazines	Lamotrigine
Others	Rufinamide Lacosamide

Rufinamide has an unknown mechanism of action, possibly it prolongs closure of sodium channels. It is used in Lennox-Gastaut syndrome (Table 12.2).
Lacosamide acts on sodium channels at sites that have long-term depolarisation, such as the epileptogenic focus, and is used for partial onset seizures.
Vigabatrin and progabide are also analogues of GABA.

membrane. The drugs in this group are **phenytoin, carbamazepine** and **sodium valproate**.

- Other drugs *promote GABA activity* by binding to the $GABA_A$ receptor complex (Figures 4.13 and 12.9). This enhances the action of GABA, which opens the chloride channels and causes inhibition of any further action potentials, preventing spread of the discharges across the brain. The drugs in this group are the **benzodiazepines** (e.g. **diazepam, clonazepam** and **lorazepam**, which are used in several types of epilepsy) (Table 12.6) and the **barbiturates** (**phenobarbital** is the drug of this group used in epilepsy).

- Increasing the amount of GABA available in the brain is another way of improving inhibition of action potentials, and the drug **sodium valproate** achieves this by preventing the breakdown metabolism of GABA after use, so that the neurotransmitter builds up in quantity at the synapse.

- Phenobarbital also *suppresses glutamate activity*, glutamate being the excitatory neurotransmitter of the cerebrum. Suppressing the excitatory action of glutamate, particularly on the NMDA receptors, will reduce the ability of the abnormal discharge to spread across the cerebrum. This drug is especially useful in having a dual role in combating the spread of seizures (see also the $GABA_A$ receptor).

- *Calcium channel blockers* have been tried as anticonvulsant therapy, with some success in clinical trials. They prevent the influx of calcium into the neuron cell body and this reduces the ability of the epileptogenic focus to discharge action potentials. The drug ethosuximide, currently regarded as the best treatment for infantile absences, has long been considered to be a T-type calcium channel blocker, but this hypothesis has been challenged. Now the evidence is giving greater support to this mechanism of action. Other drugs are undergoing trials and may be released for clinical use in the future.

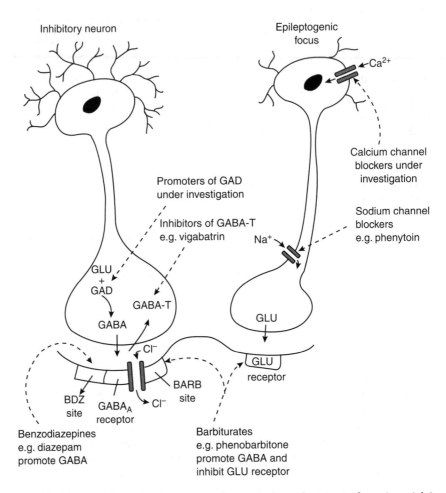

Figure 12.9   The action of anticonvulsant drugs. At the epileptogenic focus (top right) calcium enters abnormally and excites the cell. Calcium channel blockers may be useful to prevent cell excitation. The abnormal action potentials (impulses) from the focus pass down the axon where sodium influxes. Blocking the sodium channels would halt the progress of the impulses. At the synapse, glutamate is released. Blocking the glutamate receptor will halt the impulses at that point. The inhibitory neuron (top left) produces gamma-aminobutyric acid (GABA), which blocks impulses. Promoting glutamic acid decarboxylase (GAD) or inhibiting GABA-transaminase (GABA-T) will increase the level of GABA at the synapse. Drugs that increase GABA activity at the $GABA_A$ receptor will help to inhibit abnormal impulses.

Particular drugs are used to treat specific epileptic categories, as indicated in Table 12.6.

The pharmacokinetics of the antiepileptic drugs

The antiepileptic drugs are well tolerated by mouth, making oral administration easy. Oral administration involves first-pass metabolism (see Chapter 7) . Binding

Table 12.6 Drugs used in specific epileptic categories.

Epileptic category	Drugs used in the treatment
Partial seizures	
Simple	Carbamazepine, lamotrigine, sodium valproate, oxcarbazepine
Complex	Carbamazepine, lamotrigine, sodium valproate, oxcarbazepine
Generalised seizures	
Absences	Ethosuximide, sodium valproate,
Tonic–clonic	Carbamazepine, lamotrigine, sodium valproate
Myoclonic	1st: Sodium valproate, 2nd: clonazepam, levetiracetam
Status epilepticus	Diazepam, clonazepam, lorazepam, paraldehyde, phenytoin phenobarbital (preventive)
Infantile spasms	Clonazepam, also effectively treated with ACTH
Infantile (febrile) convulsions	Diazepam

to protein (mostly albumin) in plasma varies between 80–90 per cent (phenytoin) to 50 per cent (phenobarbital). Induction of liver enzymes occurs, particularly with phenobarbital and phenytoin, and this may cause drug interactions if given with other medication. Some drugs have short half-lives (e.g. oxcarbazepine at 1 to 2.5 hours) whilst others have intermediate half-lives (e.g. phenytoin at 7–60 hours) or much longer half-lives (e.g. phenobarbital at 50–150 hours). Long half-life drugs may be administered less often or in lower dosage than those with shorter half-lives. Most drugs are metabolised in the liver and excreted through the kidneys.

The side-effects of the anticonvulsant drugs

These are quite extensive and relate to the specific drugs listed in Table 12.5. Sedation is a problem with some drugs, notably the benzodiazepines and phenobarbital, and this may cause difficulties with some activities. Phenytoin side-effects are numerous, including dizziness, nausea, skin rashes, insomnia and gastrointestinal disturbance, **nystagmus** (rapid, involuntary flicking of the eyes), **ataxia** (unsteady walking) and **diplopia** (double vision). However, it still has a valuable contribution to make to anticonvulsive therapy. Carbamazepine and ethosuximide both have similar lists of extensive side-effects, including headache, dizziness, drowsiness, ataxia and gastrointestinal problems. More serious side-effects, such as **agranulocytosis** (reduced white blood cell counts), **aplastic anaemia** (low red blood cell counts due to reduced bone marrow activity) and even mental depression are less often reported. Sodium valproate can cause nausea, ataxia, gastric irritation, tremor, increased appetite and weight gain, transient hair loss and occasional blood disorders. This drug can also be toxic to the liver and can disturb the blood clotting mechanism, so careful patient selection and persistent monitoring of blood clotting and liver function are important.

Anticonvulsant drug interactions and withdrawal

Drug interactions are also a problem and this is a good reason for patients to be given **monotherapy**, i.e. treatment with one drug only. The patient is unlikely to benefit from several drugs at once and toxic effects can occur quickly, with an unpredictable outcome. Care must be taken to ensure that the anticonvulsant drug prescribed is compatible with any other form of medication the patient may be taking. It is important to check with the drug interaction information in the prescription handbooks. Withdrawal of any anticonvulsant drug must be done slowly, with staged reductions in dosage. This particularly applies to the benzodiazepines and barbiturates. Abrupt withdrawal of the drug, or sudden change of one drug to another, may cause *rebound seizures* to occur.

Key points

Types of seizures

- Generalised fits are characterised by unconsciousness; partial (or focal) seizures are centred on one particular part of the brain with limited spread.
- Generalised fits include absences and generalised tonic–clonic, myotonic and atonic seizures.
- Partial fits may be simple (no loss of consciousness) or complex (loss of consciousness), and may become generalised.
- The generalised tonic–clonic fit (the grand mal, or major fit) causes the patient to lose consciousness, fall to the ground and convulse.

Electroencephalogram

- EEGs have value in helping to distinguish between the different categories of epilepsy.

Factors involved in the cause of epilepsy

- The incidence of fits increases with age.
- Some epilepsies are genetic and run in families.

The epileptogenic focus

- Many epileptic fits are caused by an epileptogenic focus, a lesion at a specific site in the brain that can trigger a fit.
- The neurons of the focus appear to suffer some degree of deafferentation, abnormal glucose and protein metabolism, changes in ion permeability, reduced GABA activity and possibly the production of an orthodromic–antidromic loop.
- The primary focus is sometimes linked to a secondary focus.

Tonic–clonic (grand mal) seizures

- The four phases of a grand mal fit are aura (if present), tonic, clonic and recovery.
- Nurses should not force anything between the patient's teeth during a fit.
- Nurses should never restrain a convulsing patient.
- Work from the head end during a fit to clear the airway and maintain observations.

- Place the patient in the recovery position when the recovery stage begins.
- Get help if complications arise, such as in status epilepticus or post-epileptic twilight state.

The hippocampal involvement in seizures

- The **CA3** cells are most prone to epilepsy within the hippocampus.
- Reduced GABA inhibition and abnormal synaptic connections may be responsible for hippocampal induced seizures.

Temporal lobe seizures (psychomotor epilepsy)

- Temporal lobe epilepsy (or psychomotor epilepsy) is characterised by an abrupt change in personality and restless automatic behaviour patterns, with or without a concluding loss of consciousness.
- The lesion is medial temporal sclerosis, a hardening of the temporal lobe brain tissue, often in the hippocampus.
- Interictal syndrome (symptoms occurring between fits), involves reduced sexual behaviour, increased religious convictions and hypergraphia.

Jacksonian seizures

- Jacksonian fits begin with a unilateral twitching of muscles in one part of the body, and it spreads from there to all other parts of the body.

Infantile spasms and febrile convulsions

- Infantile spasms involve head nodding and flexing of the body that begin early in life.
- Infantile (or febrile) convulsions are not true epilepsy.
- The cause is a high temperature in children below the age of seven, due to the hypothalamic temperature control centre being immature.

Anticonvulsant drugs

- Benzodiazepine and barbiturates act by binding to the $GABA_A$ receptor and promote the opening of the GABA-mediated chloride channels to inhibit any action potentials.
- Phenytoin, sodium valproate and carbamazepine are sodium channel blockers, blocking the entry of sodium into the axon during an action potential.
- Monotherapy is preferred to prevent drug interactions and toxicity.
- Withdrawal of anticonvulsants should be gradual.

References

Acharya J. N. (2002) Recent advances in epileptogenesis. *Current Science*, **82** (6): 679–688.
Blows W. T. (2001) *The Biological Basis of Nursing: Clinical Observations*. Routledge, London.

Hickey J. V. (2008) *The Clinical Practice of Neurological and Neurosurgical Nursing* (6th edition). Wolters Kluwer/Lippincott Williams & Wilkins, Philadelphia, PA.

Mancuso M, Filosto M, Mootha VK, et al. (2004) A novel mitochondrial tRNAPhe mutation causes MERRF syndrome. *Neurology* **62** (11): 2119–2121.

McCance K. L., Huether S. E., Brashers V. L. and Rote N. S. (2010) *Pathophysiology, The Biological Basis of Disease in Adults and Children* (6th edition). Elsevier-Mosby, London and Oxford.

Russell A. and Hanscomb A. (1997) Epilepsy: the most common serious neurological condition. *Nursing Times* **93** (21): 52–55.

Trimble M. R. (1999) A neurobiological perspective of the behaviour disorder of epilepsy, in Ron M. A. and David A. S. (eds) *Disorders of Brain and Mind*. Cambridge University Press, Cambridge.

Wallace D. C. (1997) Mitochondrial DNA in aging and disease. *Scientific American* Aug.: 22–29.

13 Subcortical degenerative diseases of the brain

- Introduction: the basal ganglia
- Parkinson's disease
- The anti-Parkinson's drugs
- Huntington's disease
- Wilson's disease and Harvey's disease
- Key points

Introduction: the basal ganglia

The subcortical degenerative diseases, often called the **subcortical dementias**, are included here because, like the cortical dementias (Chapter 14) they sometimes fall into the care of the psychiatric nurse. The reason is that they are often associated with depression and psychoses (Kaplan and Sadock 1996). These disorders are essentially caused by degeneration of the basal ganglia, those parts of the brain below the conscious cortex that have a powerful influence over body movements and muscle tone (Aird 2000). The basal ganglia form part of a loop that regulates motor function. This loop starts with the **frontal cortex**, which projects fibres to the **corpus striatum**. The striatum has connections with both the **globus pallidus** and the **substantia nigra pars reticulum**, which then connect to various nuclei of the **thalamus**. Finally, the thalamus connects back to the frontal lobe, completing the loop (Figure 13.1). Degeneration of any part of this loop can cause both motor symptoms (basal ganglia) and psychotic symptoms (frontal lobe). Central to the production of symptoms in these disorders is the disturbance to dopamine metabolism. Dopamine depletion in the basal ganglia causes motor deficits, while dopamine problems in the frontal lobes generate cognitive and psychotic symptoms.

The basal ganglia are five separate nuclei of neuronal cell bodies (see Figure 1.7). The main pathways between the nuclei and their connections with other brain areas are shown in Figure 13.2. The **caudate nucleus** and the **putamen** (together called the **corpus striatum**) have an input from the cerebral cortex (the *higher centres* of the brain) that involves the neurotransmitter **glutamate**. Two outputs from the caudate nucleus to the **globus pallidus** use GABA as the neurotransmitter; one is an inhibitory pathway to the **medial globus pallidus** (**GP$_m$**), the other is an inhibitory pathway to the **lateral globus pallidus** (**GP$_l$**). The putamen has an output to part of the **substantia nigra** called the **pars reticulata** (abbreviated

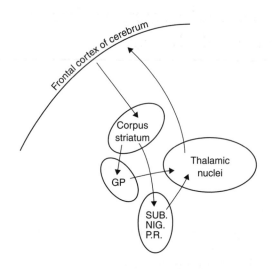

Figure 13.1 The motor loop, from frontal cortex to the corpus striatum, then to both the globus pallidus and the substantia nigra pars reticulum (SUB. NIG. P.R). From here the connection is with the thalamus, then back to the cortex.

to **SN$_r$**). The other part of the substantia nigra, the **pars compacta (SN$_c$)**, has dopaminergic feedback loops to both components of the corpus striatum, i.e. an excitatory loop back to the putamen, an excitatory loop back to the GP$_m$ caudate nucleus output, and an inhibitory loop back to the GP$_l$ caudate nucleus output. The output from GP$_l$ to the **subthalamic nucleus (STN)** utilises GABA, while the outputs from the STN to both the SN$_r$ and the GP$_m$ are facilitated via glutamate. Both the SN$_r$ and the GP$_m$ have GABA-mediated outputs to the **thalamus** (Bear et al. 1996). All these pathways can be visualised using Figure 13.2.

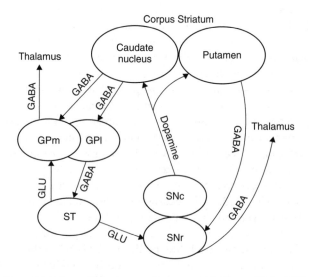

Figure 13.2 Normal basal ganglia pathways. Compare with Figure 13.3. GLU = glutamate; GABA = gamma-aminobutyric acid; SN = substantia nigra; ST = subthalamus.

From Chapter 1 we recognise that *the substantia nigra is responsible for lowering muscle tone and it does this through its dopaminergic pathways to the corpus striatum*. This statement is fundamental to our understanding of Parkinson's disease.

See page 13

Parkinson's disease (PD)

James Parkinson (1755–1824) was an apothecary surgeon working in Hoxton, an area of Shoreditch, East London. During his regular walks through East London he noticed six people who had a stiffness to their gait and shaking limbs. In 1817 he wrote a description of these people, and this was published as *An Essay on the Shaking Palsy* (a disease he called **paralysis agitans**, which means *agitated paralysis*). It became known as Parkinson's disease (PD) some 60 years later.

PD affects about 2 people per 1,000 in the UK population. Muscle stiffness (or **rigidity**) and shaking of the limbs (or **tremor**) have become the classic signs of the disease. The major features of Parkinson's disease are therefore as follows:

- Progressive muscle rigidity due to increasing muscle tone. The body and limbs become stiff and movement is very limited (i.e. an **akinesia** = a muscular paralysis, or a **bradykinesia** or **hypokinesis** = slow voluntary movements) (Borrell 2000) causing difficulty in initiating movement, which is sometimes known as **freezing**. These are often relieved during sleep.
- Shaking of the limbs, both *coarse* tremors of the whole limb and *fine* tremors of the hand and fingers. These are reduced during intentional movement of the limb, but become very marked at rest. Fine tremors of the hand are sometimes called *pill rolling*, because they resemble the hand movements used to roll handmade pills before the days of quality control.
- People with PD adopt a forward stance, i.e. leaning slightly forwards, and walk with a shuffling gait. When walking, the top half of the body tends to move forwards faster than the feet, and there is a risk of falling forwards onto the face. In one study, 59 per cent of people with PD had falls, and of these falls 49 per cent resulted in injuries (Gray and Hildebrand 2000). Factors that increase the risk of falling were identified as the severity of the symptoms of the disease, the effectiveness of the medication, the activities and the location of the person at the time of the fall and the degree of fatigue they were suffering at the time (Gray and Hildebrand 2000).
- The arms are held in a bent fashion, in a position similar to that seen in the insect called a praying mantis.
- The facial muscles are paralysed by the excessive muscle tone and this results in the inability to adopt a facial expression, known as the **Parkinsonian mask**.
- Speech becomes difficult and is reduced to a low, mumbled and hurried voice that is almost impossible to understand.
- The mouth tends to hang open and produce excessive saliva (called **sialorrhoea**). This results in patients dribbling saliva down their front. Having one's mouth open all the time is embarrassing, so patients often try to solve both these problems by putting a handkerchief in their mouth. The handkerchief soaks up the excess saliva and blocks the open mouth.
- Swallowing becomes difficult as the disease progresses and towards the latter stages other methods of feeding are required, e.g. nasogastric tube feeding.

- The patient's handwriting becomes impossible to read and communication with the patient becomes very difficult.
- **Oculogyric crisis** is a phenomenon that occurs perhaps several times a day. The eyes rotate upwards so that the iris is hidden under the upper lid and they are held there for a minute or so before returning to normal. This muscular spasm of the eye muscles is said to be very painful.
- Other associated symptoms include constipation, sexual dysfunction, **orthostatic** or **postural hypotension** (low blood pressure on standing), and bladder dysfunction, all due to disturbance of the **autonomic nervous system** (i.e. the component of the nervous system that maintains automatic organ functions) (Herndon et al. 2000). Observations by the nurse during their day-to-day management of the patient may identify specific autonomic problems which will need to be addressed.
- Sleep disturbances occur often in PD and the nurse is in the best position to be able to assist the patient and to advise the family concerning interventions that promote adequate rest (Crabb 2001).
- Psychiatric symptoms can occur, such as **depression** (up to 16.5 per cent of PD patients) and **hallucinations** (up to 37 per cent of PD patients) and these require specific management (Herndon et al. 2000). Nurses need to be alert to this and report any symptoms of depression (e.g. sleep disturbance) or **psychosis** that they observe.
- **Dementia** has been identified in as many as 25 per cent of patients with PD (Herndon et al. 2000), further complicating both the clinical appearance of the disease and its management.

What is happening in this disorder is that, for reasons that remain unclear, the substantia nigra is gradually degenerating, neurons of this nucleus are dying and are not being replaced. Since the function of the substantia nigra is to lower muscle tone (and the function of the cerebellum is to increase muscle tone), there is normally a balance between the two. The gradual loss of the substantia nigra upsets that balance in favour of the cerebellum (which remains normal). Muscle tone therefore increases unopposed, but the symptoms only become apparent quite late in the disorder because the deterioration of the substantia nigra is very slow and because the neurons are able to compensate to some extent for the losses. Symptoms do not usually appear until the substantia nigra has lost 60 per cent of its cells (Roberts et al. 1993), so that patients diagnosed with Parkinson's disease have had the disorder for many years without symptoms. This is one reason why the disease usually affects those over 60 years of age, although occasionally it is seen in some patients earlier in life. The substantia nigra (which means *black substance*) is so called because its neurons contain a large quantity of **neuromelanin**, a pigment that gives the cells a dark coloration. As these cells die in Parkinson's disease, the neuromelanin is released, and antibodies in the blood that are specific to neuromelanin are increased. This increase *may* prove to be useful as a test in the early detection of the disease long before symptoms arise (Nowak 2000).

Prior to the cells losses, affected cells also develop **Lewy bodies**. These are intracellular collections of neurofilamentous material (i.e. made of neurofilaments) surrounding a central core of α-**synuclein**, a protein. The cause of these bodies and their effect on the cells are still not clear, although it seems that affected cells are likely to degenerate and die. In Parkinson's disease, the substantia nigra is the main site of Lewy body formation, although they can sometimes be identified in other parts of the brain, for example in the cortex when dementia or psychoses also occur. Lewy bodies are also seen in a variety of other neurological disorders, notably in dementia.

As part of their role, the neurons of the substantia nigra pars compacta (SN_c) produce dopamine, but the loss of cells in Parkinson's disease means that the SN_c becomes unable to produce dopamine. Within the pathway that extends from the substantia nigra to the corpus striatum, i.e. the **nigrostriatal pathway**, dopamine levels drop very low. The symptoms of the disease are related to this effect (Figure 13.3), but there is a threshold of 80 per cent loss of dopamine in this pathway before symptoms occur. Clearly a loss of 80 per cent dopamine takes a very long time to achieve.

The gradual loss of the doperminergic nigrostriatal pathway has a knock-on effect on the remaining basal ganglia (follow these steps by comparing Figure 13.2 with Figure 13.3):

- Low dopamine excitation from the SN_c to the putamen results in lower GABA activity from the putamen to the SN_r. This reduced GABA inhibition of SN_r allows an increased GABA inhibition of the thalamus.
- Low dopamine inhibition from the SN_c to the caudate nucleus allows an increase in the GABA inhibitory effect from the caudate nucleus on GP_l. GP_l inhibition is increased, causing lower GABA inhibition of the subthalamus (STN).
- The loss of the inhibitory effects of GABA from the GP_l on the STN allows the STN to increase the excitatory glutamate pathways to both the GP_m and the SN_r, and thus cause increased GABA inhibition of the thalamus.

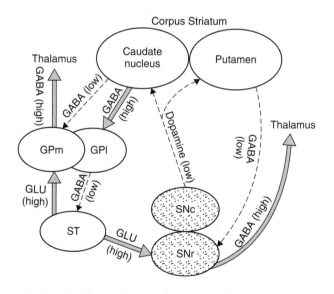

Figure 13.3 In Parkinson's disease, the lack of dopaminergic pathways from the dying substantia nigra (shown dark) to the corpus striatum causes increased GABA activity in the other pathways shown. The result is excess motor disturbance to the thalamus. (Abbreviations as in Figure 13.2.)

- Low dopamine excitation from the SN_c of the caudate nucleus reduces the caudate nucleus GABA activity to GP_m. This results in a low caudate nucleus GABA inhibition of the GP_m. The GP_m is now free to increase its own GABA inhibition of the thalamus.

- The thalamus is now receiving increased GABA inhibition from both the GP_m and the SN_r, causing inhibition of the thalamus is its vital motor role.

The cause of the disease is unknown, although a number of factors are emerging as candidates:

- *Genetics.* Mutations in the *LRRK2, PARK2, PARK7, PINK1* and *SNCA* genes are known to cause Parkinson's disease (Table 13.1). Mutations of the *GBA, SNCAIP* and *UCHL1* genes increase the risk of developing Parkinson's disease. Most cases are sporadic, but these appear to be the result of complex interactions between genes and environmental factors. Unfortunately, the genetic involvement of the majority of sporadic cases of PD remains unclear. A smaller number of patients are found in family groups and those presenting with symptoms at less than 50 years of age, and these are likely to be the result of inherited genetic factors. Mutations of the α-synuclein (**SNCA**) gene (Table 13.1), which is found in some PD families, code for α-synuclein protein, which is found within Lewy bodies. Evidence is accumulating that a metabolite of dopamine, called **DOPAL (3,4-dihydroxyphenylacetaldehyde)**,

Table 13.1 The genetic involvement in Parkinson's Disease.

Gene	Locus	Notes
LRRK2	12q12	Codes for the poorly understood kinase enzyme called **dardarin**, or **Leucine-rich repeat kinase 2**. Mutations are a cause of PD.
PARK2	6q25.2-q27	Codes for the protein **parkin** which has a part in destruction of unwanted or damaged proteins. Mutations are a cause of PD.
PARK7	1p36	Codes for the protein **DJ-7** which appears to have multiple but poorly understood functions in the cell. Mutations are a cause of PD.
PINK1	1p36	Codes for **PTEN-induced putative kinase 1**, a poorly understood enzyme related to mitochondrial function. Mutations are a cause of PD.
SNCA	4q21	Codes for the protein α-**synuclein** which has a poorly understood role in synaptic function (see text). Mutations are a cause of PD.
GBA	1q21	Codes for the lysosomal enzyme **beta-glucocerebrosidase** which breaks down unwanted cellular products. Mutations increase the risk of PD.
SNCAIP	5q23	Codes for two proteins: **synphilin-1** and **synphilin-1A** which have poorly understood roles in synaptic function. Mutations increase the risk of PD.
UCHL1	4p14	Codes for the protein **ubiquitin carboxyl-terminal hydrolase L1** which is involved in the degradation of unwanted proteins. Mutations increase the risk of PD. It is interesting that a single gene locus, 1p36, contains two gene mutations capable of causing PD.

is toxic to neurons, and contributes to neuronal losses in PD. DOPAL is 1,000 times more toxic to neurons than dopamine itself. This appears to be due to DOPAL's ability to generate intracellular **free radicals**, chemicals which react and damage cellular components. Free radicals appear to causes α-synuclein to aggregate, with resulting loss of function. DOPAL may be a target for future anti-Parkinson's therapy.

- *Environment.* A neurotoxin has been identified that induces the disease in animals and also in those humans who have accidentally made contact with it. The neurotoxin is called **N-methyl-4-phenyl-1,2,3, 6-tetrahydropyridine** (or **MPTP**). Some drug addicts in America injected this substance into themselves by mistake, since it is a by-product of 'homemade' cocaine, and they soon developed advanced, irreversible Parkinson's disease. MPTP probably works by being changed first to **1-methyl-4-phenylpyridinium** (**MPP**) by the action of the enzyme MAO-B. By interfering with the energy cycle within the mitochondrion, and by inducing the formation of damaging chemical agents called **superoxide radicals**, MPP is more neurotoxic than its precursor MPTP. As such, the presence of MPP results in depleted energy levels, neural damage and cellular losses (Figure 13.4). The discovery of MPTP has opened the way to new research that may lead to a better understanding of this disease. Questions still need to be answered, such as, *How do ordinary people who have never taken illegal drugs, or their related chemicals, get exposure to MPTP?* The answer is probably, *They dont!* Some other possible neurotoxins acting against the basal ganglia are suspected, mostly in form of pesticides used in the agricultural industry. Increasing evidence is pointing at an association between organophosphate pesticides and between farming or agricultural work and Parkinson's disease. There was seven times as great a risk of developing Parkinson's disease in people exposed to these pesticides.

There may be alternative mechanisms that can account for the energy losses in these neurons. Deletions of some mitochondrial DNA, i.e. the genes that code for enzymes of the energy chain within the mitochondria, have been found in some Parkinson's disease patients. Loss of these genes would result in the failure of energy production within the neuron, leading to cell death (Figure 13.4). Mitochondrial DNA mutations are known to be a factor in the cause of **Alzheimer's disease** (a form of dementia, see Chapter 14) and **Leigh syndrome** (a progressive loss of movement and speech due to basal ganglia degeneration in children).

The anti-Parkinson's drugs

It might sound reasonable to treat Parkinson's disease by simply replacing the missing neurotransmitter, dopamine, with dopamine in drug form, thus restoring the muscle tone balance between the substantia nigra and the cerebellum. There are two main problems with this scenario:

- Dopamine does not cross the blood–brain barrier and, moreover, dopamine outside the brain (in general circulation) causes unpleasant side-effects, particularly concerning cardiac function.

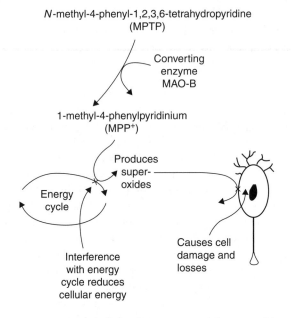

Figure 13.4 The pathway in which MPTP causes neuronal damage and losses.

- Simply replacing dopamine does not stop the relentless deterioration of the substantia nigra, the main cause of the symptoms, so this can never be a cure.

Nevertheless, this notion of replacing dopamine in order to improve quality of life has become the mainstay of treatment. Since dopamine cannot be given directly, the precursor called **levodopa** (**l-dopa**), which does cross the blood–brain barrier, is used. Conversion from levodopa to dopamine is made in the neurons of the basal ganglia. Remember, however, that the dopaminergic neurons of the substantia nigra are slowly dying, so their ability to convert levodopa to dopamine is in gradual decline. In the 1960s, the use of levodopa was shown to have dramatic effects in relieving symptoms. Some decades on, it has become clear that levodopa has some serious long-term problems:

- The amount of conversion of levodopa to dopamine in the brain is somewhat unpredictable. While the dose of levodopa administered can be controlled, what happens after that cannot be controlled. The same levodopa dose can have different results on different days. A way around this problem is to give the minimum dose in combination with other drugs.
- The amount of conversion of levodopa to dopamine declines with time. After five years of treatment with levodopa, the patient needs higher dosages to achieve a reasonable result. Higher dosages mean more side-effects. One cause of this is that dopamine receptors are losing their sensitivity and more neurotransmitter is needed to stimulate them. A way around this is to give the patient a **drug holiday**. This means removing them from all their medication (except antibiotics if they happen to be on them) for about two to four

days. During this drug-free time the patient suffers the full symptoms, but the dopamine receptors are resensitised and on reinstatement of levodopa the patient will become symptom-free on a lower levodopa dosage. However, this problem is minimised in modern treatment by using low-dose levodopa in combination with other drugs.

- The enzyme that converts levodopa to dopamine, called **dopa decarboxylase**, is found also in other tissues outside the brain, so part of the levodopa dose is converted to dopamine in the body. Of course, once converted to dopamine it cannot cross the blood–brain barrier. So the dopamine levels in circulation build up, causing side-effects. To prevent this, another drug, called a **dopa-decarboxylase inhibitor**, is given to block the enzyme *outside* the brain (but *not inside* the brain since the inhibitor cannot cross the blood–brain barrier) so that more of the levodopa enters the brain and is converted there. These inhibitor drugs are **benserazide** and **carbidopa**. In modern Parkinson's disease therapy, the inhibitor drug is given built into the levodopa; for example, benserazide with levodopa is called **co-beneldopa**, and carbidopa with levodopa is called **co-careldopa**.

- Some patients suffer the **on–off phenomenon**, which means the sudden switching from a near symptom-free state to severe symptoms, and back again, several times throughout the day. This gets worse as the length of the treatment period increases. The sudden nature and severity of this switching is distressing, but can be reduced by splitting the dose from once per day to several times throughout the day, or by giving **modified-release** (i.e. slow release levodopa) medication. This gives a better regulation of blood levels of levodopa, and improves the control of symptoms.

- **End-of-dose deterioration** means that the period of symptom-free benefit after each dose becomes progressively shorter. Again, a change to modified-release preparations can help to overcome this problem. The drug **selegiline**, a **monoamine oxidase B** inhibitor, can help to reduce this problem when used with levodopa. Monoamine oxidase B is an enzyme that breaks down neurotransmitters, including dopamine, and inhibiting this enzyme allows dopamine to increase in the brain.

The side-effects of levodopa are anorexia, nausea, dizziness, **tachycardia** (fast pulse rate), **arrhythmias** (abnormal changes in heart rhythm), insomnia and **postural hypotension** (low blood pressure when standing upright).

Other drugs

Antimuscarinic drugs are antagonists (or blockers) of acetylcholine muscarinic (M) receptors. These drugs work by reducing the effects of acetylcholine on the receptors. Acetylecholine is a neurotransmitter of the parasympathetic nervous system and activates muscarinic receptors. Excessive acetylcholine, and therefore excess parasympathetic activity, has occurred as a result of low dopamine in PD, and these drugs help to restore the normal balance between the two systems. The drugs are **trihexyphenidyl**, **orphenadrine** and **procyclidine**. They are less effective than levodopa in controlling symptoms, but are useful in reducing some symptoms, notably the sialorrhoea (excess of saliva). They also facilitate some decrease in rigidity and tremor. However, their main use is in the early stages of the disease as they become less effective as the symptoms worsen.

Dopamine agonists are drugs that act like dopamine in the brain and stimulate dopamine receptors. However, since they are not dopamine they have no problems crossing the blood–brain barrier and require no enzyme conversion. The drugs in this group include **bromocriptine, carbergoline** and **pergolide**. They can be used to augment the role of levodopa and are being used as part of first-line treatment. They can help to prevent the *on–off phenomenon*.

See page 269

They can cause some side-effects, such as nausea, vomiting, headaches, dizziness, hypotension, drowsiness and confusion. **Ropinirole** and **bromocriptine** are D_2 receptor agonists and **pramipexole** is an agonist for both the D_2 and D_3 receptors. **Apomorphine** is a potent D_1 and D_2 receptor agonist which is useful in the management of the *on–off phenomenon*, but it is a powerful **emetogenic**, i.e. it causes vomiting, which may contribute to poor patient compliance.

Monoamine oxidase B inhibitors (**rasagiline** and **selegiline**) are drugs which, at low dosage, selectively blocks the enzyme **monoamine oxidase (MAO) B**. MAO breaks down neurotransmitters after re-uptake from the cleft has taken place. Two types of MAO occur in the brain, MAO-B is found in the corpus striatum, whilst MAO-A is widely found in the CNS and elsewhere. Selegiline prolongs the action of levodopa and is used with levodopa to relieve the end-of-dose deterioration. It also reduces the required dose of levodopa by about a third, reducing levodopa side-effects.

Amantadine is a weak dopamine agonist, but it is thought to improve dopamine release from the presynaptic bulb and block dopamine re-uptake from the cleft. It has only a short-lived effect on Parkinson's disease because the patient develops tolerance.

Catechol-O-methyl transferase (COMT) inhibitors (e.g. **entacapone** and **tolcapone**) are, as the name indicates, drugs that inhibit the COMT enzyme which breaks down between 10 and 30 per cent of levodopa inside and outside the brain. When combined with a dopamine decarboxylase inhibitor, this drug doubles the half-life of levodopa and creates a 50 per cent increase in motor activity per dose of levodopa. Entacapone is therefore useful in the prevention of the end-of-dose deterioration.

Modern treatment of Parkinson's disease is tailor-made to suit the patient, because so many factors are involved, such as the patient's age, the stage of the disease and drug reactions. Many patients are treated with a combination therapy of some levodopa together with an enzyme-inhibiting drug, and perhaps another additional drug given as an adjunct therapy to overcome the problems of levodopa.

Huntington's disease (HD)

George Huntington (1850–1916) was an American doctor in general practice. He was the son and grandson of doctors and all three of these men had noticed the strange symptoms, known as **chorea**, that this disease produced in several American families. In 1872, at the age of just 21, George Huntington published a paper in which these patients were briefly described. The affected families, ultimately involving about 1,000 patients over 12 generations, were centred on the east end of Long Island, New York. They could trace their ancestry back to two brothers in

Sussex, England, indicating the strong genetic basis of this disorder. The origins of the gene mutation are not clear, but it may have first occurred centuries ago in East Anglia, England, and is now widely disseminated across the world.

Huntington's disease (HD) is a neurodegenerative disorder of the GABA neurons within the basal ganglia, notably the caudate nucleus first, followed by the putamen (i.e. the corpus striatum), with concurrent enlargement of the lateral ventricles (Figure 13.5) (Carlson 2010). The disorder starts to produce symptoms between the ages of 30 and 45, in other words usually after the affected person has had their family and has passed the affected gene to their offspring. Up to ten years prior to the onset of movement disorder, a number of patients show mild psychotic and behavioural symptoms, possibly due to the stress of living in a family with a genetic problem. A reduced cognitive ability, including learning and memory deficits in pre-symptomatic gene carriers may be present compared to their non-carrier relatives.

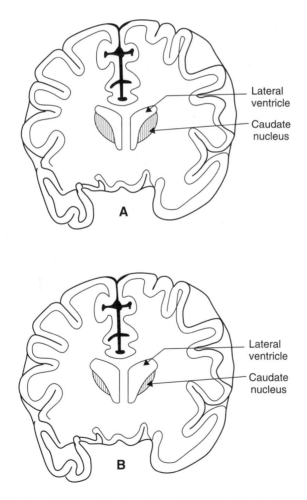

Figure 13.5 Huntington's disease. Sections through the brain showing (A) the size of the normal lateral ventricles and (B) the increased ventricle size in Huntington's disease due to destruction of the caudate nucleus (cross hatched area).

Huntington's disease is a progressive disorder for which there is no cure, so the survival rate is anything from 10 to 20 years from the onset of movement symptoms. The symptoms of Huntington's disease involve involuntary, uncontrollable, jerking movements of the limbs, head and trunk. These movements are called **chorea** ('chorea' means *dance*) and they disrupt the patient's normal daily existence and dominate their every purposeful movement. These patients also suffer an ataxia, an eventual loss of speech (a **dysarthria** = imperfect articulation of speech), and behavioural changes, including depression, apathy and irritability (Hofmann 1999). There is often an intellectual decline associated with the disorder. Some develop a degree of dementia and others have schizophrenic-like psychoses, with excitable outbursts, to complicate the picture. The psychotic symptoms are suspected to be caused by the degeneration of the dorsal part of the caudate nucleus (Hofmann 1999).

The overriding cause of this disorder is undoubtedly a genetic error that has been mapped to **chromosome 4**, specifically **4p16.3** (Figure 13.6). This is an autosomal dominant gene and an affected parent has a 50 per cent chance of passing the mutated gene to any of their offspring. The normal gene codes for a protein named **huntingtin** (**Htt**) and patients with Huntington's disease produce both the normal and abnormal forms of the protein.

The gene mutation is called a **trinucleotide repeat**, where the repeated bases are **CAG** (**cytosine–adenine–guanine**). The normal gene changes by duplicating this CAG trinucleotide base many times; the number of repeats present determines the onset or not of symptoms. Those without the disorder have fewer than

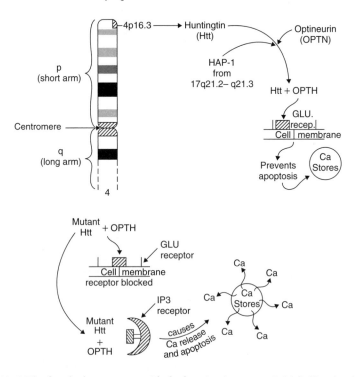

Figure 13.6 The fourth chromosome with the huntingtin gene at 4p16.3. Huntingtin binds with huntingtin-associated protein-1 (HAP-1) from chromosome 17.

36 repeats (most people have fewer than 34 repeats), but the presence of more than 38 repeats causes symptoms of the disease. Juvenile HD (early-age onset) is caused by more than 70 repeats (see also **anticipation**).

See page 102

Early-age onset HD is characterised by slow speech, awkward gait, difficulty in starting a movement coupled with slow movements (**bradykinesia**), abnormal eye movements, abnormal muscle spasms (**dystonia**), occasional fits and muscle rigidity. It is the later-age onset (40 years old or more) which is usually characterised by chorea (uncontrollable jerky movements).

If the gene is passed to the offspring from the mother, the number of repeats tends to be copied faithfully: given a mother with, say, 43 repeats, the offspring will receive 43 repeats. But if the mutant gene is passed to the offspring from the father (which is more common), variation can occur in the number of repeats the offspring receives.

CAG codes for the amino acid **glutamine** and multiple repeats of CAG result in a huntingtin protein (Htt) with a long glutamine 'tail' (mutant Htt). Much research has cast light on how the mutant form of this protein can cause the disease (Figure 13.7).

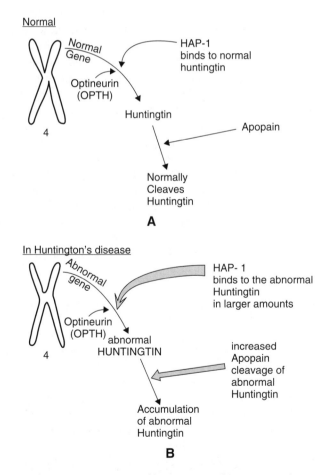

Figure 13.7 Huntingtin protein in normal brain tissue and Huntington disease.

Normal huntingtin. It is known that the normal huntingtin protein (Htt) is expressed widely in the brain and is essential for normal brain development, but importantly, it protects the cell against **apoptosis (programmed cell death)**. Htt binds to two other proteins: **huntingtin–associated protein-1 (HAP-1)** and **optineurin (OPTN)**. There is now evidence to suggest that normal huntingtin, after binding to optineurin, acts by further binding to specific glutamate receptors which have a cellular protective role, i.e. they prevent neuronal cell death (apoptosis). Apoptosis would be achieved by releasing the stored calcium in the cell. The presence of normal huntingtin (Htt), bound to specific glutamate receptors, would prevent the loss of neurons by blocking this natural destruction of cells.

Mutant Htt. The mutant form of huntingtin (mutant Htt), bound to OPTN, also binds to the specific glutamate receptors but has the effect of antagonising (blocking) these receptors. This stops the inhibitory function of the receptors which then allows apoptosis to continue. At the same time, mutant Htt binds to excessive quantities of HAP-1. HAP-1 could be an inhibitor of huntingtin, blocking its normal role. The two proteins, Htt and excessive amounts of HAP-1, then bind to IP3 receptors (for IP3 see page 000). In response to this, the IP3 receptors (in the presence of inhibited glutamate receptors) cause Ca^{2+} (calcium) to be released from cellular stores triggering cell apoptosis.

Apopain is a proteolytic enzyme (an enzyme for breaking down proteins), and this enzyme splits the normal huntingtin protein, a process that is increased with the mutant abnormal huntingtin protein. The result is the accumulation of huntingtin fragments, some of which form clumps inside the nucleus. These clumps within the nucleus are called **neuronal intranuclear inclusions (NII)** and they contain mutant huntingtin fragments together with another protein called **ubiquitin**. Ubiquitin is a universal protein found throughout nature (the name comes from *ubiquitous*) and it appears to join with other proteins when those proteins are to be destroyed. It is one of the proteins found in the core of **Lewy bodies**. Experiments have suggested that the mutant huntingtin fragments enter the nucleus and cause damage there. The presence of ubiquitin seems to slow that process down and encourages the formation of NII as a means of tying up the harmful huntingtin fragments to help to prevent the damage (Quarrell 1999). However, this process is probably only a delaying tactic as the damage continues slowly.

This means there are three molecular bases for the possible effects we see in this disease (Figure 13.7):

- increased inhibition of huntingtin by HAP-1, allowing increased apoptosis;
- increased inhibition of specific glutamate receptors which would normally help to block apoptosis;
- increased cleavage of huntingtin by apopain, resulting in damage to the nucleus.

Mitochondrial DNA damage is a feature found in ageing cells and contributes towards age-related neurodegeneration by reducing cellular energy levels. The ageing of mitochondrial DNA leading to damage is caused by **oxidative stress** within the cell (oxidative stress is discussed in relation to Alzheimer's disease, Chapter 14).

See page 290

The formation of highly damaging oxidative species within the mitochondria is due to the nature of the mitochondrial role, i.e. energy production. Manufacturing

adenosine triphosphate (ATP), the high energy molecule needed by all cells for energy purposes, generates oxygen-based radicals which can damage DNA. Normally these radicals are neutralised by **antioxidants**. Raised levels of these oxygen-based radicals have been found in the cells of selective areas of the brain in HD, although the reason is not fully understood. Mutant Htt has also been shown to damage mitochondrial membranes, which causes disturbance to Ca^{2+} levels within the mitochondria, increasing the risk of cell death by calcium-induced **excitotoxicity**. This refers to neuronal cell death caused by activation of excitatory amino acid receptors, such as glutamate receptors. Mitochondrial DNA damage appears also to be implicated in the pathogenesis of not only Huntington's Disease but also in Parkinson's disease and Alzheimer's disease (Yang et al. 2008).

Treatment of Huntington's disease is not really an option at present. There is no cure and there is little in the way of drug treatment to improve quality of life. **Tetrabenazine** can help to control the abnormal movements. This drug reduces dopamine synthesis in doperminergic neurons, but it has caused some patients to develop depression as a side-effect. Sensitive nursing care, both in the patient's home at first and later in hospital, is the mainstay of effective management of this disorder.

Genetic testing has become available for families with Huntington's disease, to see who in the family carries the gene and who does not. However, the implications of this are enormous, given the 100 per cent penetrance of the gene (i.e. if present, the gene will definitely cause the disease). Any individual learning that they carry the gene will know that they will suffer and die from this disease. Worse still, they may have to live with the thought that they may have passed it on to their children. The only advantage would be for those who know they carry the gene and who are without children, as they would then have the ability to make a conscious decision whether or not to have children. It may be worth considering that sometimes not knowing is the better choice to take.

Wilson's disease and Harvey's disease

Dr S. A. Wilson (1878–1937) described a familial lenticular degeneration in 1912. Wilson's disease, as it was later called, is an autosomal recessive disorder of copper metabolism (Figure 13.8). The word *lenticular* refers to the **lentiform nucleus**, a combination of the putamen and globus pallidus. The genetic problem is one of several possible mutations of the gene *ATP7B*, which is localised to 13q14.3–q21.1. The genetic error causes a reduction in the amount of a blood plasma component called **ceruloplasmin**. Ceruloplasmin is normally synthesised in the **Golgi apparatus** of cells, a structure within the cytoplasm that packages, modifies and transports cellular products to a storage site within the cell or out of the cell altogether. Ceruloplasmin is involved in the transportation of copper into the cells, where it becomes integrated into copper-containing enzymes such as **cytochrome oxidase**. Cytochromes are proteins involved in the energy-producing chain found on the inner mitochondrial membrane (Adds et al. 1996). Ceruloplasmin is low in the majority of patients with this disorder. This prevents copper from entering the cell and being used to form enzymes, and that limits the cell's ability to form energy. Cytochrome oxidase is usually found to be in a low state of activity in Wilson's disease. Copper that cannot enter the cells builds up in the body and is deposited in various tissues, notably the liver, the brain and the eyes. The result is both

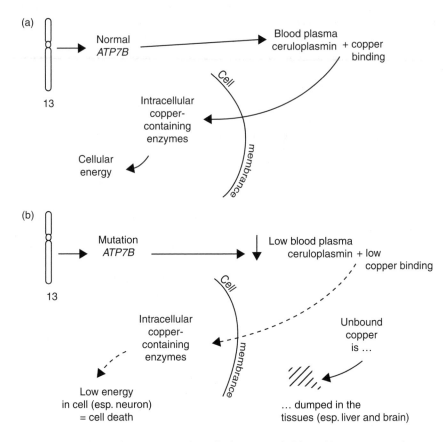

Figure 13.8 Wilson's disease. Normal ceruloplasmin (coded by *ATP7B* gene on chromosome 13) binds copper in the plasma and assists its movement into the cell. Here it is used by the enzymes that generate cellular energy. In Wilson's disease, gene error (mutation) causes low ceruloplasmin, and copper cannot enter the cell. The cell runs low on energy and the spare copper accumulates in the tissues, mostly the liver and the brain.

neurological deficits and liver **cirrhosis** (i.e. hepatic **necrosis**, the death of liver cells). The damage in the brain occurs mostly to the lenticular nuclei and some degree of cerebral dementia can occur. Symptoms include severe involuntary movements at a young age (10–25 years), leading to progressive mental deterioration. Liver failure occurs later in the course of the disease. Unlike brain cells, liver cells are able to regenerate to a certain extent, so the effects of liver involvement are not felt until the disease is more advanced. **Hypercalciuria**, excessive calcium in the urine, is seen in many cases of Wilson's disease and is sometimes found early, before the neurological symptoms occur. It is due to **renal tubular acidosis**, a kidney problem where the proximal tubule fails to control bicarbonate excretion. The excessive renal calcium can cause stones (or **renal calculi**) to form in the kidneys.

Treatment of Wilson's disease is based on the administration of a **chelating agent**, in this case the drug **penicillamine**. Chelating agents form soluble molecular compounds with a metal. In the case of penicillamine, this drug forms a compound with the excess copper, and this promotes the elimination of copper from the body. If it is treated early enough, all further progress of the disease can be halted. The problem remains, however, that the damage already done cannot be repaired.

History: the strange case of Harvey's disease

During training as a psychiatric student nurse between 1965 and 1968 at Bexley Hospital, Kent (now closed, demolished and redeveloped), the author was allocated to a ward called East Hospital. On arrival at this ward, the author was instructed to read a certain set of notes belonging to a patient who was on the ward at that time. The patient was suffering a form of genetically inherited subcortical dementia, which was only present in that one family. The disease had already killed everyone else in his family and our patient was the last family member to die. On his death, the disease would never be seen again as the gene was not passed on to any other generation, nor found in any other family. This was then a very rare example of a genetic disorder becoming extinct.

The symptoms were similar to those of Parkinson's disease or Wilson's disease, but the copper metabolism was normal. He had lost his speech; his mouth was held open and was filled with a handkerchief. He had a very unsteady stiff gait, walking almost on tiptoes, and falling over frequently due to the imbalance caused when the legs could not keep up with the top half of the body.

On the ward his condition was named after him with the family name of Harvey. However, the author has never been able to find any publication concerning this now extinct condition. Surely it must have occurred to a doctor at that time, given the uniqueness of the case, that publication of a paper describing the disease would be useful. Apparently not, and this very brief history, based as it is on the author's memory of the events, may be the only published record of this genetic disease that killed an entire family.

Key points

The basal ganglia

*   The subcortical dementias, essentially degeneration of the basal ganglia, are often associated with depression and psychoses.
*   The basal ganglia form part of a loop that regulates motor function. This loop consists of the frontal cortex, the corpus striatum, the globus pallidus, the substantia nigra pars reticulum, the thalamus, and back to the frontal lobe.

Parkinson's disease

*   Muscle rigidity and tremor of the limbs are the classic signs of Parkinson's disease.
*   The symptoms of Parkinson's disease are caused by a gradual loss of the substantia nigra cells. Muscle tone therefore increases unopposed.
*   The nigrostriatal pathway develops very low dopamine levels, below a threshold of 80 per cent loss of dopamine, before symptoms of the disease occur.

- The low dopamine level causes inhibition of the thalamic role in modifying control of movement by the frontal lobe.
- Both genetic and environmental factors are involved in the cause of this disease.
- Levodopa replaces dopamine in the nigrostriatal pathway and thus improves the quality of life. Long-term problems of levodopa have largely been over-come by multiple drug therapy.
- Nurses must be aware of the constant risk of falls in PD patients due to their instability whilst walking, which is the product of a forward stance with a shuf-fling gait.

Huntington's disease

- Huntington's disease is an autosomal dominant inherited disorder character-ised by a deterioration of the corpus striatum caused by a mutation in a gene on chromosome 4.
- The main signs of Huntington's disease are involuntary jerky movements called chorea, speech loss and intellectual decline.
- The gene mutation is a trinucleotide repeat of the bases CAG (cytosine–adenine–guanine) that causes a glutamine tail repeat sequence on the normal huntingtin protein.
- Accumulations of abnormal huntingtin protein fragments in the neuron nu-cleus and loss of normal huntingtin from the cytoplasm probably cause part of the cellular degeneration.

Wilson's disease

- Wilson's disease is a familial lenticular degeneration caused by an autosomal recessive gene that results in disorder of copper metabolism.
- Mutations of the gene *ATP7B* cause a reduction in the amount of ceruloplas-min in blood, which disturbs copper transport into neurons.
- Energy-producing enzymes that use copper fail to function.
- The result is both neurological deficits, caused by damage to the lenticular nuclei, and liver cirrhosis.
- Treatment of Wilson's disease is with the drug penicillamine, which promotes the elimination of copper from the body.

Harvey's disease

- Harvey's disease may have been a very rare example of a familial genetic basal ganglia degenerative disorder that became extinct in the 1960s when the last affected member of the family died.

References

Adds J., Larkcon E. and Miller R. (1996) *Cell Biology and Genetics*. Nelson, Walton-on-Thames.

Aird T. (2000) Functional anatomy of the basal ganglia. *Journal of Neuroscience Nursing*, **32** (5): 250–253.

Bear M. F., Connors B. W. and Paradiso M. A. (1996) *Neuroscience, Exploring the Brain*. Williams and Wilkins, Baltimore.

Borrell E. (2000) Hypokinetic movement disorders. *Journal of Neuroscience Nursing*, **32** (5): 254–255.

Carlson N. (2001) *Physiology of Behavior*. Allyn and Bacon, Boston.

Crabb L. (2001) Sleep disorders in Parkinson's disease: the nursing role. *British Journal of Nursing*, **10** (1): 42–47.

Gray P. and Hildebrand K. (2000) Fall risk factors in Parkinson's disease. *Journal of Neuroscience Nursing*, **32** (4): 222–228.

Herndon C. M., Young K., Herndon A. D. and Dole E. J. (2000) Parkinson's disease revisited. *Journal of Neuroscience Nursing*, **32** (4): 216–221.

Hofmann N. (1999) Understanding the neuropsychiatric symptoms of Huntington's disease. *Journal of Neuroscience Nursing*, **31** (5): 309–313.

Kaplan H. I. and Sadock B. J. (1996) *Concise Textbook of Clinical Psychiatry*. Williams and Wilkins, Baltimore.

Nowak R. (2000) Early warning for Parkinson's. *New Scientist*, **168** (2266): 14.

Quarrell O. (1999) *Huntington's Disease, The Facts*. Oxford University Press, Oxford.

Yang J-L., Weissman L., Bohr V. and Mattson M. P. (2008) Mitochondrial DNA damage and repair in neurodegenerative disorders. *DNA Repair (Amst.)*, **7** (7): 1110–1120.

14   The ageing brain and dementia

The ageing brain

Like all organs, the brain changes as a result of the ageing process (Figure 14.1), but the functions of the brain can often be retained to extreme late age in many people. This shows the remarkable compensation the brain is able to undergo to make good the deterioration, and demonstrates that dementia is not inevitable.

Age-related neuron losses vary not only between individuals but also between different parts of the brain in the same individual. Naturally occurring neuron loss can begin as early as 23 years of age, but this is very slow at first, increasing after 60 years of age. Rarely, the total losses of neurons could be, in the worst case scenario, as much as 40 per cent – the equivalent of just less than half the brain lost – and yet the brain could retain good cerebral activity. The 40 per cent figure is rare, and the majority of people would sustain far less neuron loss than this. Whatever the losses, the retention of good brain function is the most important point. A very good example of excellent cerebral function in late age is the remarkable English composer Havergal Brian, who wrote *twenty symphonies* between the ages of 80 and 92 years old – an amazing feat of late-age brain activity.

It was thought for many years that neurons were the type of cell that was incapable of replication after birth, so that losses could not be replaced. For the majority of neurons this is still the case. However, humans are now known to be capable of neuronal replication within the dentate gyrus of the hippocampus after birth. Where neuron losses do occur, this is attributed to reduced blood flow to the brain caused by age-related changes in the arteries that supply the head. Neurons

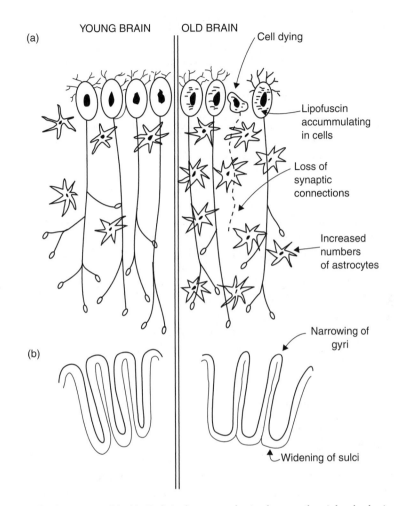

Figure 14.1   The brain gets old. (a). Left is the young brain, but on the right the brain shows cell losses with corresponding synaptic losses, increased astrocytes and lipofuscin deposits in the neurons. (b). Narrowing of the gyri and widening of the sulci is a gross anatomical change in the elderly brain.

are glucose- and oxygen-sensitive and will deteriorate and finally die when faced with a decline in the glucose and oxygen supply. Each neuron can have thousands of synaptic connections, so one neuron lost can account for thousands of lost synapses. Synapses are vital for memory and learning. The neocortex loses glutamate synapses from around the age of 20 onwards, with about 20 per cent lost by the age of 70. Some 40 per cent or so of the glutamate synapses could be lost from the hippocampus with age.

Sustaining good cerebral blood and oxygen flow reduces neuronal losses and improves the brain's ability to compensate for those losses that do occur. Therefore using the brain may be beneficial in preventing neuronal losses, since stimulated areas of the brain use and receive more blood and therefore keep the brain active until a late age.

Neuronal losses are part of the reason for the brain's loss of protein in old age. About 15 per cent of the protein in the brain is lost between the ages of 35 and 70 years and this is partly responsible for the reduction of brain weight with age, from about 1,400 grams in a male aged 20 down to 1,200 grams in the same male aged 80. In contrast, both the volume of extracellular water and the number of astrocytes in the brain *increase* with age, and the ventricles within the brain enlarge. The cerebral cortex shrinks and shows a widening of the **sulci** and a narrowing of the **gyri**, with atrophy of the frontal lobes predominating. **Lipofuscin**, an age-related lipid-based pigment, is deposited inside the ageing cells of the brain and elsewhere. The amount varies in different parts of the brain. Apart from lipids, lipofuscin contains sugars and several metals, including zinc, copper, aluminium, mercury and iron. Several of these metals are known neurotoxic agents, notably mercury. The presence of lipofuscin deposits in tissues is not only age-related but is also linked to Alzheimer's disease and Parkinson's disease. Several neurodegenerative disorders, called **lipofuscinoses**, are also caused by lipofuscin, e.g. **Batten's disease**. This autosomal disorder starts slowly in childhood (between the ages of four and ten) with visual difficulties and fits. Patients develop motor instability, with stumbling and gradual loss of motor skills resulting in immobility. The fits gradually get worse, cognitive abilities decline and speech is slowly lost. Dementia and blindness are usually followed by an early death.

The brain's chemistry also changes with age; noradrenaline and dopamine levels slowly decline in some parts and this has been linked to depression in some elderly people.

The hippocampus and memory

The hippocampus is situated within the hippocampal fissure, close to the parahippocampal gyrus, part of the temporal lobes on both sides (see Chapter 1 and Figures 1.4, 9.1, 10.2, 10.3 and 10.4) (Blows 2000). This area is sometimes called the **hippocampal complex** or **hippocampal formation**, because several structures occur close together and have many interconnections with each other. The components of the complex are:

- **Dentate gyrus**, the innermost cell layer of the hippocampus;
- **Ammon's horn** (see Figure 10.2), another part of the hippocampus, consisting also of a layer of neurons that can be subdivided into four areas, **CA1**, **CA2**, **CA3** and **CA4** (where CA means *cornu Ammonis*, or 'Ammon's horn') (Figure 10.2);
- **Subiculum**, also included in the hippocampus by some authors;
- **Entorhinal cortex**, which lies between the subiculum and the perirhinal cortex (Figure 10.2);
- **Perirhinal cortex**, which lies between the entorhinal cortex and the parahippocampal cortex (Figure 10.2);
- **Parahippocampal cortex**, the outermost component of the complex (Figures 9.1, 10.2).

The connections between these areas and with other parts of the brain are:

- Afferent (incoming) pathways into the entorhinal cortex from the **cingulum**;
- Afferent pathways into the entorhinal cortex from the major sensory association areas of the cortex, e.g. visual, auditory, **somatosensory** (i.e. from the body) and **gustatory** (taste) areas;
- **Perforant pathway**, from the entorhinal cortex to Ammon's horn and the dentate gyrus;
- **Alvear pathway**, from the entorhinal cortex to Ammon's horn;
- **Mossy fibre pathway**, from the dentate gyrus to CA3 of Ammon's horn;
- **Schaffer collateral pathway**, from CA3 to CA1 of Ammon's horn;
- Efferent (outgoing) pathways via the **fornix** (the main axonal pathways leaving the hippocampus) to areas of the frontal cortex, thalamus and the hypothalamus (especially the **mammillary bodies**).

The hippocampus has several important roles. These include maintaining the **short-term memory** (which is closely related to learning) and influencing thinking through connections with the frontal cortex. It also has a part to play in emotions, especially the regulation of **aggression**. It is closely linked to the adrenal hormone cortisol, regulating cortisol release via the hypothalamus and pituitary gland pathway. Cortisol is the hormone that is increased during stress, so the hippocampus is also part of the brain's normal stress response. *See page 84*
See page 167

Memory

There are several ways of classifying memory, one way being the division into **long-term memory** and **short-term memory**, i.e. the difference between remembering events which took place 20 years ago and events that happened 20 minutes ago. Another way is the division into **explicit memory** and **implicit memory**, i.e. the difference between memory that comes with *conscious thought* – for example, trying to remember Aunt Edith's telephone number – and *automatic* or *subconscious* memory such as finding the way from your bedroom to the bathroom at home. These classifications are roughly correlated in that long-term memory is broadly implicit, while short-term memory is more likely to be explicit. The term 'commit to memory' implies a shift of memorised facts or skills from explicit to implicit memory; that is, making the memory automatic or long-term. This is achieved by *rehearsal* of the facts or skill, often many times, in much the same way as an actor memorises the lines of a play, a pianist prepares for a concert or a tennis player practises for a match. There is no substitute for the rehearsal of facts; it is crucial for all implicit (or long-term) memory activities, such as taking examinations. It is the basis of the *learning process*, an essential ingredient of success for all aspiring actors, pianists and tennis stars, as well as those hoping to pass examinations.

At a biochemical level, memory is the result of neurons producing and maintaining a **long-term potentiation** (**LTP**). These involve permanent (or at least semi-permanent) changes in the synapse that allows for enhanced impulse transmission between pre- and post-synaptic neurons both ways across the synaptic cleft. This means the changes appear to allow for **retrograde** impulses to cross back from the post-synaptic to the presynaptic membranes. This occurs in the hippocampus and other parts of the brain as a result of increased levels of activation or repetition by a specific excitatory action potential (or stimulus). The formation of this change, a state of heightened stimulation in the synaptic membrane that occurs each time a specific impulse arrives, requires the function of glutamate acting on AMPA and NMDA receptors, and the presence of calcium. A similar, but depressive (inhibitory), effect on the synapse is called **long-term depression** (**LTD**, not to be confused with the disorder called depression). Between them, LTP and LTD may provide the synaptic mechanism for **declarative memory**, i.e. memory for facts and events. But these changes are temporary (i.e. short-term memory). For these changes to become a long-term memory, further complex molecular manipulation is required, especially with regard to proteins, and including the formation of new synaptic connections.

The brains that are best suited to learning and memory are the brains of children (see Chapter 2). All the anatomy of the brain is in place at birth, but the nervous system is far from mature at that point. The development of the nervous system involves the formation of new synaptic connections, and this continues throughout childhood until puberty, so learning is a major part of this process. The bulk of synaptic formation occurs during the childhood years and this is exactly the time when the brain is best suited to forming the permanent proteins and synapses needed for memory. Adult brains are somewhat more resistant to this kind of change, although of course learning can take place at any age.

The relevance of all this to dementia is that forgetting (and memory loss is a major feature of dementia) can be seen as a loss of the synapses as neurons die. A single neuron can have thousands of synapses, so the loss of key neurons in the brain is likely to interfere with memory significantly. This loss primarily affects short-term memory since long-term memory is better preserved. During the early stages of dementia, patients can remember where they were in the Second World War, but can't remember what they had for breakfast that morning. Eventually, as dementia gets worse, long-term memory is affected. What education in childhood has created, dementia can ultimately destroy.

Memory is not found in one place in the brain; many areas serve to store information which can be retrieved when required, the so-called **working memory**. However, the conscious working memory is primarily the role of the frontal lobes, the prefrontal cortex particularly. Here, memory and thought work together on matters that concern us at any particular moment. The prefrontal cortex is vital for the memory needed for spatial tasks, remembering objects, self-ordered tasks and analytical reasoning (Beardsley 1997). Input into this frontal lobe activity is via the hippocampus. With the retrieval of short-term memory at its disposal, and with the influence it has on thinking and emotions, the hippocampus is a powerful tool in the processing of thought. It is not surprising that problems arising with the hippocampus seriously disrupt not only memory, but also the whole ability to think properly.

Declarative memory is divided into **semantic memory**, i.e. the raw facts and figures, and **episodic memory**, the context in which these facts and figures occur. For example:

- **semantic** = 9 is a number; **episodic** = 9 is the ninth numerate in a set sequence of numerates that start at 1.

- **semantic** = fish have gills; **episodic** = fish have gills which are part of a system by which animal life extracts oxygen from its environments.

Hippocampal memory appears to be the result of LTPs in CA1, and to a lesser extent in CA3, of Ammon's horn. Damage to these cell layers appears to impair episodic memory and cause **anterograde amnesia** (i.e. memory loss occurring after some form of brain injury). To lose *all* declarative memory requires lesions of the brain that involve both the limbic areas of the medial temporal lobe and the hippocampus. In fact, lesions anywhere, from the hippocampus through the fornix to the mammillary bodies and anterior thalamus, can disrupt memory. It would appear that this circuit is critical in the formation and recall of memories (Figure 14.2).

The dementias

Dementia means 'loss of mind' and occurs in various forms depending on both the cause and its effects. Dementia can be caused by brain damage from a head injury; cerebral infections; reduced blood flow to the brain; compression of the brain from a **space-occupying lesion** (**SOL**) or from a biochemical imbalance. Vascular disease, which reduces the arterial blood supply to the brain (i.e. **cerebral ischaemia**) with increasing age and often causes areas of cerebrum to die (i.e. **cerebral infarcts**), accounts for about 15–25 per cent of dementia cases. Starved of blood, the oxygen-sensitive neurons die and may be replaced with scar tissue. Trauma (head injury) accounts for only about 3 per cent of dementias, but is important in relation to sports injuries. **Traumatic brain injury** (TBI) is a growing concern in relation to various sports (in particular, boxing, football and athletics) where the risk of repetitive head injuries is high. TBI can be anything from **mild traumatic brain injury** (**MTBI**, also known as **concussion**) to severe. But it is the repetitive nature of this cause of injury, as the person returns to their sport after recovery from a first injury only to sustain further subsequent injuries, that is most worrying. Multiple repeated minor injuries are known to cause long-term neurological

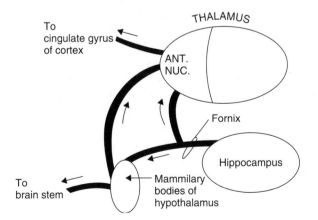

Figure 14.2 Connections of the hippocampus important in memory. Ant. Nuc. is the anterior nucleus.

problems resulting in a higher than expected risk of dementia, depression and death at an early age.

At the molecular level, some of the reasons why brain cells die leading to dementia are becoming evident. The **telomere** is a stretch of deoxyribonucleic acid (DNA) that normally lies beyond the length of the genes at the end of a chromosome. Being outside the gene sequence, the telomere would appear to be of no genetic value. However, it was found that the telomere shortens normally with each cell division, and at a critical point it becomes so short it triggers cell death. It also shortens in response to cellular stress. In patients suffering from non-Alzheimer's dementia, the telomere was shorter than in others of the same age without dementia. Those with long telomeres suffered less cognitive decline than others of their age with shorter telomeres.

As an indication of the variety of dementias occurring, a list of some types is included here:

- **Attentional dementia** with some loss of arousal of the conscious mind;
- **Intentional dementia** with loss of vigilance;
- **Cognitive dementia** with a loss of remote memory;
- **Amnestic dementia** with a loss of recent memory;
- **Multi-infarct dementia**, caused by a number of minor strokes;
- **Binswanger dementia**, due to **hypertension** (high blood pressure), which causes vascular disease in the brain and neuronal white matter destruction;
- **Dementia with cortical Lewy bodies** (**DCLB**) (about 10 per cent of dementias);
- **Pick's disease**, dementia with characteristic cortical Pick bodies;
- **Alzheimer's disease** (**AD**), a form of dementia with characteristic brain changes found at post mortem (about 45 per cent of dementias).

Alzheimer's disease (AD)

Alois Alzheimer (1864–1915) was a German psychiatrist who in 1906 described a dementia with two specific changes found in the brain after death. These changes were the presence of *extracellular* **plaques** and *intracellular* **neurofibrillary tangles** (**NFT**) and these became the hallmarks of this disease, i.e. they were diagnostic for Alzheimer's disease at post mortem.

Two main forms of AD are recognised: an early-age onset (before 65 years) showing a family history of inherited genetic origin (i.e. **familial Alzheimer disease, FAD**) and a late-age onset (after 65 years) of less genetic and more sporadic origin. This disorder has been, and still is, the subject of intensive research for several reasons. First, the pathology of AD is related to other brain-destructive disorders like Parkinson's disease and Huntington's disease. Advances in the understanding of one of these disorders have provided valuable insights into the others (see mitochondrial DNA, Chapter 13). Second, there is a very interesting link between AD and **Down syndrome**. Third, the devastation caused by this disease, both to the patient and to the family, is catastrophic, as it usually occurs at a time of life when an ageing partner is ill-equipped to care for a demented spouse. It reduces formerly highly intelligent people to a pitiful state, with no hope of recovery. The fear that any of us could end our days in this manner drives research forward in an attempt to prevent the tragedy. Estimates put the number of AD sufferers in the UK at around 400,000, with this figure set to rise significantly with the ageing population.

Dementia causes memory losses and erosion of personality; relatives say that the patient is nothing like their former self. Mood changes with emotional blunting occur, with abnormal and inappropriate behaviour, especially restless wandering at any time of the day or night. People with dementia develop a state of self-neglect and need everything done for them. One important form of self-neglect is that these people may suffer from a lack of adequate nutrition. Several factors combine to cause this, including memory losses (e.g. when to eat, how to prepare food), inadequate supervision by family carers or hospital staff, poor oral hygiene and constipation. Nurses can improve the person's overall state of health by effective interventions to maintain a healthy mouth and bowels, and by ensuring that nutritious meals are eaten by the patient daily (Biernacki and Barratt 2001).

Anything from one to four years prior to the diagnosis of AD, the individual goes through a period of *mild cognitive impairment*. This involves a range of problems, from occasional memory lapses to poor decision making. Memory loss and confusion are perhaps the problems for which the more advanced stages of this disorder are best known. **Amnesia** (memory loss) is at first primarily short-term. **Confusion** is not uncommon in the elderly in any case and is often *acute*, i.e. relatively short-lived and caused by a physical problem which may be easily corrected, such as constipation, sleep loss, fever or a drug side-effect. Other, more difficult conditions which can cause confusion, especially in the elderly, are cardiac, renal or liver failure; blood glucose instability in diabetes; other endocrine and metabolic disorders, such as acidosis, epilepsy, vitamin deficiencies, malnutrition or dehydration, post-anaesthetic or other drug withdrawal, head injury, brain tumours, or stress. Confusion which is persistent, after all the physical causes have been eliminated, may be a sign of dementia.

Preserving cognitive and functional abilities in the Alzheimer's disease patient is central to the role of the nurse (Maier-Lorentz 2000b). Nursing interventions can be most valuable in overcoming the problems of failing memory, behavioural difficulties (e.g. wandering), language problems (e.g. errors in the language), impaired **visuospatial function** (e.g. confusion in an unfamiliar environment), sleep disturbance and psychotic episodes (notably depression, delusions and hallucinations) (Maier-Lorentz 2000a, b).

The molecular neurobiology of Alzheimer's disease

Alzheimer's disease is a progressive deterioration of brain function associated with neuronal losses. Before the age of 65 about 1 per cent of the population are sufferers and by the age of 85 the figure is 10 per cent of the population. The devastating effects of the disease on the individual and their family, together with a proportional increase in the elderly population resulting in greater numbers of people suffering from the disease, makes it a major mental health problem. After years of difficulties, much progress has now been achieved in understanding the pathology of Alzheimer's disease and it is expected that research will continue to make strides towards prevention of its worst effects.

The plaques

The plaques described by Alzheimer are made from the central core of an abnormal **amyloid** protein called **Aβ42** (**beta-amyloid 42**, which is 42 amino acids long). Normally Aβ42 exists in very small quantities in the brain, but it accumulates in large amounts in Alzheimer's disease, hence the abnormality.

Amyloid levels in the brain fluctuate according to a circadian rhythm, i.e. a cycle of amyloid production taking about 24 hours to complete, which is controlled by *orexin* (see also eating disorders, Chapter 9) (Kang et al. 2009). The cycle causes higher levels of amyloid to occur when awake and lower levels when asleep, leading to speculation that abnormalities in orexin or its production may lead to insomnia which could increase the risk of AD.

See page 72

A large gene on chromosome 21 called the *APP* gene (Figure 14.3) codes for the normal protein called **APP** (**amyloid β precursor protein**). Normal amyloid precursor protein (APP)'s primary function is in synaptogenesis and synaptic repair after damage. Other functions have been suggested, but supported by only limited evidence. In the cell body, APP is found associated with the **endoplasmic reticulum** (**ER**) of the neuron where it normally undergoes cleavage (i.e. being cut by enzymes) into the **Aβ40** and **Aβ42** forms (Aβ40 is 40 amino acids long, i.e. a shorter chain version than the Aβ42) (Figure 14.4). Cleavage of APP is carried out by two enzymes, **beta-secretase** and **gamma-secretase**. **Presenilin 1** (**PSEN1** or **PS1**) and **presenilin 2** (**PSEN2** or **PS2**) are the APP cleavage components of the enzyme **gamma-secretase**. The genes for coding

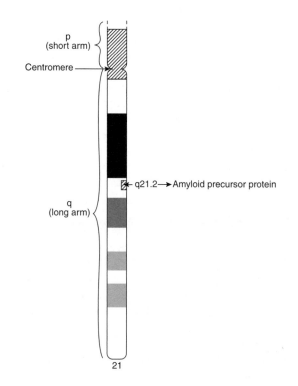

Figure 14.3 Chromosome 21. The amyloid precursor protein (*APP*) gene is at 21q21.2.

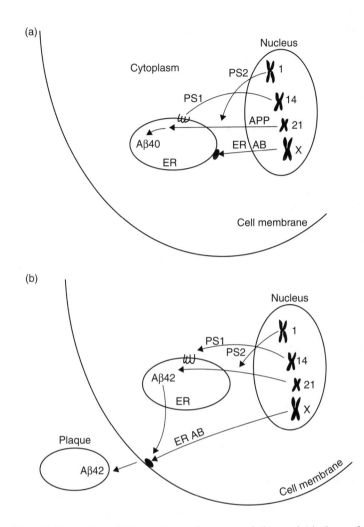

Figure 14.4 (a) Normal amyloid protein production, and (b) amyloid plaque formation outside the cell in Alzheimer disease. ER is the endoplasmic reticulum.

the PS1 and PS2 proteins are on chromosome 14 (PS1) and chromosome 1 (PS2). More is known about PS1 than about PS2. PS1 attaches across the ER membrane, influencing APP cleavage within the ER. PS2 may bind to APP and affect its cleavage by this means.

   One further gene involved is **HSD17B10 (17-beta–hydroxysteroid dehydro-genase X)** (formerly the **ERAB gene**) on chromosome X (Xp11.2). It codes for a mitochondrial **dehydrogenase enzyme** which catalyses (i.e. breaks down) a wide range of fatty acids, alcohol and steroids as part of energy production. This enzyme is overproduced in neurons during AD and interacts with beta-amyloid. In AD, it also relocates to the plasma membrane and is probably involved in the export of amyloid from the cell into the plaques.

   In **Familiar Alzheimer's disease (FAD)**, mutations within the *APP* (chromosome 21), *PSEN1* (chromosome 14), *PSEN2* (chromosome 1) and *HSD17B10* (chromosome X) genes cause errors in the proteins that these genes code for, leading to mistakes in the way these proteins function. Mutations are abnormal changes in the DNA (deoxyribosenucleic acid) code within the chromosome, which create abnormal proteins. In the case of the *APP* gene the mutation results in excessive APP protein, while mutations in the *PSEN1* and *PSEN2* genes cause errors in the cleavage of APP causing excess of the abnormal Aβ42 form. The combination of all three mutations results in a large accumulation of the Aβ42 protein. This Aβ42 must find its way out of the neuron to become extracellular plaques. Mutations of the *HSD17B10* gene may be involved in this process. Once accumulated between the neurons, Aβ42 plaques allows for the development of abnormal glial cell production and accumulation (a **gliosis**, mostly of **astrocytes**), especially around blood vessels (**perivascular gliosis**).

Amyloid imaging involves the use of a radioactive tracer called **Pittsburgh compound B** (**PiB**) injected into a vein. This locks onto amyloid accumulating in the brain, and being mildly radioactive it emits a signal which can be detected by a **positron-emission tomographic** (**PET**) scanner. The brain areas affected by amyloid accumulations create very bright areas on the brain picture obtained, showing exactly where, and by how much, amyloid is replacing brain tissue. Given the battery of new therapies that are under development, including a large number of new and exciting drug treatments awaiting final clinical trials (see section on *the drugs used in dementia*), early detection of plaque accumulation using PiB and PET technology will be very beneficial in allowing very early medical intervention to slow the course of the disease.

The neurofibrillary tangles

The tangles inside the neurons described by Alzheimer are made from an abnormal form of **tau protein**. Normal tau protein is a **microtubule-associated protein**, or **MAP**, which interacts with the protein **tubulin**, the main component of the cell microtubules. Tau is essential for the assembly and stabilisation of the cell cytoskeleton. Microtubules are also vital for functions such as axonal transport and abnormal tau may also be partly responsible for disruption of this process. The abnormal form of tau accumulates as tangles (Figure 14.5).

In AD, the neurons of the temporal and frontal lobes, and also of the hippocampus, lose up to 70 per cent of a particular enzyme called **choline acetyltransferase** (**ChAT**) (not be confused with another enzyme, *acetylcholinesterase*, or *AChE*, which is involved in the drug treatment of AD). The role of ChAT is to combine **choline** (derived from the diet) with **acetyl-CoA** to form the neurotransmitter **acetylcholine** (**ACh**). A loss of ChAT causes a reduction in the choline and ACh content of these cells. The result is an adverse affect on APP cleavage, leading to an increased amount of Aβ protein inside the cell. These higher levels of Aβ protein contribute to a process called **oxidative stress** within the cell, involving an increase in the production of **reactive oxygen species**, highly reactive chemical agents based on oxygen which damage cellular processes. A mechanism for this has been identified whereby Aβ protein binds two metals, iron and copper, and in the process these metals donate electrons to oxygen. The negatively charged oxygen then reacts with hydrogen to form **hydrogen peroxide** (H_2O_2), a highly reactive and damaging compound. In this case, the damage is disruption of the

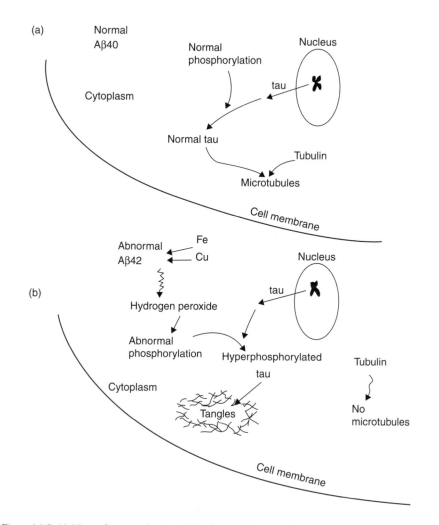

Figure 14.5 (a) Normal tau synthesis and (b) abnormal tau tangles in Alzheimer's disease. Fe and Cu are the chemical symbols for iron and copper, respectively.

normal **phosphorylation–dephosphorylation cycle** of proteins in the cell. The phosphorylation (adding of a phosphate to proteins) and dephosphorylation (removal of a phosphate from proteins) is a mechanism for activating or deactivating proteins. The disruption of this process as a result of oxidative stress causes **hyperphosphorylation** of tau, i.e. tau becomes saturated with phosphate and thus accumulates as tangles (called **tau inclusions**). The absence of normal tau causes tubulin to fail in its role of microtubule formation (Figure 14.5).

Two other proteins are apparently involved in AD. The first is called **ubiq-uitin** which attaches to the abnormal tau at a late stage during tangle formation. Ubiquitin has a range of functions, but its most important role is to attach to, and therefore label, those proteins which are destined for destruction by proteolytic enzymes. This is possibly the function of ubiquitin in tangle formation. The second is a protein called the **AMY antigen** which is produced along with beta-amyloid (an **amyloid-associated antigen**). It coexists with beta-amyloid in plaque lesions found in both sporadic and familial AD and in adult Down syndrome patients.

The genetics of AD

As noted before, the *early-age onset* form of the disease (before 65 years) is more often genetically inherited than the *late-age onset* form (after 65 years). Familial AD studies, especially in the early-age onset group, often show multiple mutations in the three major autosomal dominant genes identified already, namely the *APP* (chromosome 21), *PSEN1* (chromosome 14) and *PSEN2* genes (chromosome 1) (Bentley 1999). In the over-65 age group, the genetic evidence is less compelling, but 20–40 per cent of this group show a genetic error on the ***ApoE*** (**apolipo-protein E**) gene on **chromosome 19**. Three forms of the ApoE gene have been found in studies of the Northern European indigenous population: ***ApoE$_\varepsilon$-2*** (8 per cent of the population), ***ApoE$_\varepsilon$-3*** (77 per cent of the population), and ***ApoE$_\varepsilon$-4*** (15 per cent of the population). Within the human population as a whole, the percentage of allele combinations of *ApoE* are approximated as follows:

$$_\varepsilon\textbf{-2}/_\varepsilon\textbf{-2} = 1\text{-}2\%, \quad _\varepsilon\textbf{-2}/_\varepsilon\textbf{-3} = 15\%, \quad _\varepsilon\textbf{-2}/_\varepsilon\textbf{-4} = 1\text{-}2\%, \quad _\varepsilon\textbf{-3}/_\varepsilon\textbf{-3} = 55\%, \quad _\varepsilon\textbf{-3}/_\varepsilon\textbf{-4} = 25\%, \quad _\varepsilon\textbf{-4}/_\varepsilon\textbf{-4} = 1\text{-}2\%$$

It is the *ApoE$_\varepsilon$-4* version that is the mutation that increases the risk for late-age on-set AD, *ApoE$_\varepsilon$-4* at one allele in the risk of AD starting in the *late* sixties and seventies age group, while the gene present at both alleles doubles the risk of developing the disease and brings the onset age to the *early* sixties. Apolipoprotein E is a protein that binds with fats (lipids) to form lipoproteins. These package cholesterol and other fats for transport through the blood. Apolipoprotein E is an important component of **very low-density lipoproteins** (**VLDLs**). The *ApoE$_\varepsilon$-4* gene adds to the accumulation of Aβ42 in plaque formation, although the mechanism remains unclear. It is possible that apolipoproteins normally breakdown beta-amyloid, but the *ApoE$_\varepsilon$-4* variation is the least efficient of the three alleles at carrying out this process, and therefore allows beta-amyloid to accumulate.

An interesting twist to the story of the *ApoE$_\varepsilon$-4* gene is the fact that *young people* with this gene variation appear to be intellectually brighter than those without the gene variant. They gain higher levels of education and have better attention spans and memory abilities. Some interesting scan results suggest that this increased cognitive ability in youth *may* be partly the reason for early brain deterioration at an older age, i.e. early dementia, but this is still speculative.

Another gene which may have a part to play in the story of AD is the **CETP** (**cholesterol ester transfer protein**) gene. This codes for a protein which controls the size of cholesterol particles. A mutation of this gene, where the amino acid **isoleucine** is replaced by the amino acid **valine**, results in a protein that causes a slower cognitive decline, especially in relation to memory. The mechanism by which this mutation becomes protective to neurons is not fully understood. Lipid levels and functions are becoming important in our understanding of brain activity and decline, partly because the brain houses 25 per cent of the body's cholesterol, and high blood cholesterol is a risk factor for dementia. Drugs which alter *CETP* gene function to replicate this mutation are in development.

Two further genes are under investigation in relation to AD. The **clusterin** protein, coded for by the **CLU** gene at 8p21, is a protein involved in the clearance of cell debris and cellular apoptosis. Mutations have been recently linked to AD. **PICALM (Phosphatidylinositol binding clathrin assembly protein)** is coded for by the **PICALM** gene at 11q14.2. This protein is involved in synaptic function, and gene mutations have recently been associated with late-age onset AD.

Mitochondrial DNA mutations may also have a role to play in some dementias, notably Alzheimer's disease (see Figure 12.6). The relationship between mitochondrial gene errors and AD is not clear, and is controversial. Mitochondrial genes were discussed in Chapter 13 in relation to Parkinson's disease and Huntington's disease, and a similar pathogenesis may apply to AD.

Alzheimer's disease could result from the accumulation of beta-amyloid protein damaging the mitochondrial membrane, which then disrupts membrane permeability. The change in membrane ionic permeability causes oxidation and other forms of damage to the mitochondrial DNA and failure of cellular energy. This would result in neuronal cell death, called apoptosis, if these genes become faulty. Mitochondrial DNA mutations, including point mutations and deletions, may play a more important role in the sporadic (i.e. non-inherited) forms of the disease.

Inflammation in AD

There are a number of risk factors identified for AD (Katzman and Kawas 1998). Observations made on patients with diseases such as arthritis have identified that those patients taking steroids have a low incidence of Alzheimer's disease. The anti-inflammatory effect of the steroids apparently dampens an immune reaction in the brain caused by the protein beta-amyloid and the damage caused by oxidation. This increase in the immune response by immune cells can, itself, cause neuronal cellular damage. The phagocytic cells of the brain, called **microglia**, would normally clear away the debris which occurs in the brain. In AD microglia appear to produce toxic cytokines that can cause neuron destruction. Other mechanisms suggesting an inflammatory component in the cause of cell destruction in AD include:

*   The production of **prostaglandins** which increase levels of glutamate leading to glutamate-induced neuronal apoptosis;
*   The increased release of an inflammatory protein called **tumor necrosis factor** (**TNF**) which induces the vagus nerve to promote an inflammatory response against brain cells which are in a state of chronic inflammation.
*   The release of soluble toxins called **amyloid beta derived diffusible ligands** which may become important in cell destruction.

From this stems the idea that anti-inflammatory drugs may slow the progress of the disease. Not everyone should take steroids, of course, but other **non-steroidal anti-inflammatory drugs** (**NSAIDs**) may benefit the Alzheimer's patient, or could even be given as a preventative measure.

Inflammation is often, but not always, caused by an infectious organism, and some post-mortem brain samples taken from late-age onset Alzheimer's disease patients have revealed the presence of the bacterium *Chlamydia pneumoniae* in some, and the virus *herpesvirus 1* (*HSV1*) in others. The *intracellular* organism

Chlamydia pneumoniae was located in the temporal lobes and hippocampus, the areas affected most by this disease. This does not, of course, prove that the organism is the cause of AD; rather it may increase the risk of developing the disorder. Microglia and astrocytes appear to be the main cells in which this organism survives, and the fact that it also lives *inside* the neuron makes it more difficult to treat. It is suspected that people with the mutant $ApoE_\varepsilon$-*4* gene allele are more susceptible to these infections.

Diet and AD

High levels of the amino acid **homocysteine** have been found in the blood of AD sufferers and very high levels found in non-sufferers appear to increase their risk of developing the disease (Smith et al. 1998). Homocysteine is not obtained from the diet; instead it is regularly produced from the combination of another amino acid called **methionine** (which is derived from protein in the diet) with adenosine from ATP. Part of this combination is used in the metabolism of adrenaline and in the normal function of DNA. What is left is converted to homocysteine, a destructive amino acid which must be rendered harmless. The body does this by turning much of this homocysteine either back into methionine with the help of vitamin B12 (called **cyanocobalamin**) or into **cysteine** with the help of vitamin B6. **Folic acid** (or **folate**) is also involved. If the blood levels of these vitamins are low, homocysteine levels will build up in the blood as its conversion declines. High homocysteine levels appear to be very toxic to nerve cells and blood vessels, increasing the risk of AD. Low levels of vitamin B12 and folate in the circulation suggests that there is a lack of these nutrients in the person's diet. Reducing the levels of homocysteine may be achievable by increasing the dietary intake of these vitamins. However, it is not entirely clear whether the high levels of homocysteine are a cause of AD or whether they are perhaps the effect of early AD before any symptoms occur (i.e. when it is **asymptomatic**). Evidence points more towards the former, but caution is urged before anyone considers taking any vitamin supplements. Excess vitamins can themselves be harmful and a balanced diet would normally provide all the body's needs.

Key risk factors for AD include mid-life obesity, high blood pressure and high serum cholesterol. Any regime that involves increasing physical fitness levels, weight reduction, lowering the blood pressure and lowering blood lipid levels will improve an individual's chance of retaining good cognitive function well into late old age. Chief amongst these protective measures are mild exercise three times per week and the consumption of a healthy diet. These help to stabilise blood glucose in those people with poorly regulated levels, as is often seen in older people. Peaks and troughs in blood glucose levels have been shown to cause damage to the dentate gyrus in the hippocampus, and thus affect memory. Relaxation is also recommended as a means of retaining good cognitive function in older people, since stress-induced cortisol can shrink some brain areas with corresponding loss of function.

See page 105   ### Association of AD with Down syndrome

Down syndrome is a trisomy 21 (three chromosomes 21 instead of two). Chromosome 21 is the site of the *APP* gene, which means that Down syndrome sufferers carry three copies of this gene in every cell. Two interesting correlations have been found to link AD with Down syndrome:

- Down syndrome sufferers develop Alzheimer-like dementia at 30+ years and have been found to have multiple, diffuse plaque formation up to 10 years before dementia symptoms arise.
- Elderly AD sufferers were found on average to have had a higher than expected number of Down syndrome children earlier in their lives.

Those affected with Down syndrome express five times more APP in the brain than normal owing to the 50 per cent extra APP present. The risk of developing AD is proportional to the amount of APP produced by the three copies of the gene present.

Dementia with cortical Lewy bodies (DCLB)

In 1912 Frederick Lewy discovered abnormal intracellular aggregates of protein in cells dying from Parkinson's disease. Lewy bodies, as they became known, are rounded microscopic deposits of the protein alpha-synuclein which are found in deteriorating nerve cells. They can be present in the basal ganglia in Parkinson's disease, and in the cortex of Alzheimer's disease. DCLB, or dementia with cortical Lewy bodies disease, accounts for about 10 per cent of all dementias, but about 20 per cent of Alzheimer's disease patients also have cortical Lewy bodies (i.e. they have a combination of AD with DCLB, and DCLB may be a variation of AD). About 2 per cent of the normal elderly population also have Lewy bodies. The proposed difference between AD, AD with DCLB and DCLB is shown in Table 14.1. The symptoms of DCLB are very similar to those of AD but with greater emphasis on motor symptoms such as extrapyramidal tremors and walking difficulties. Some additional psychiatric symptoms can occur, such as hallucinations and delusions, and a reduction in cognitive ability includes alternating periods of alertness with periods of confusion and unresponsiveness.

Pick's disease

Pick's dementia was described in 1892 by Arnold Pick, earlier than Alzheimer's disease (1906). It is rarer than AD, with few patients showing familial inheritance. This indicates that genes are not a powerful influence in this disease. The cause remains unknown. The onset of symptoms mostly occurs at about 50 to 60 years of age, affecting women more than men. The early symptoms show a predominance of social and personality changes rather than memory and intellectual deterioration (as in AD). This is due to the neuropathology which is characteristic for this disease.

Table 14.1 The distinction between AD and DCLB.

Dementia type	Plaques	Tangles	Lewy bodies
AD	Present	Present	Absent
AD with DCLB	Present	Present	Present
DCLB	Present	Absent	Present

The brain shows a significant atrophy (a loss of superficial neurons) in the anterior *cortical* aspects of the frontal and temporal lobes. The atrophy is rare and less severe in the parietal lobe and extremely rare in the occipital lobe and cerebellum. This is very much a disease of the front half of the brain. Astrocytes proliferate in these areas of atrophy, with gliosis (glial cell proliferation) and fibrous tissue deposited.

Neurons in the affected areas become swollen and oval in shape, with an absence of Nissl bodies. In place of the Nissl bodies, abnormal **Pick bodies** fill the cell cytoplasm, pushing the nucleus to one side. Pick bodies are rounded inclusions of neurofilamentous proteins similar to typical neurofibrillary tangles (but differing in many respects) and, like neurofibrillary tangles, they disrupt the cell's internal cytoskeleton. However, the typical neurofibrillary tangles and the plaques seen in AD are both missing in this disease. **Hirano bodies**, another form of intraneuronal inclusion found mostly in the hippocampus, are present in many cases. These are made from deranged cytoskeletal components. Another feature is the extensive loss of myelination within the white matter coming from the affected cortical areas.

The disease causes changes in the personality and social behaviour patterns in the patient during its early stages. The deterioration of social habits may include inappropriate sexual or criminal activities, the patient showing a loss of normal inhibitions and a lack of insight. Changes in mood may be characterised by either apathy or a state of euphoria. As the disease progresses, the patient suffers speech and language difficulties and in the later stages memory and intellect decline.

Variations of this disease have been noted, such as **Pick's disease type II**, where severe gliosis (predominance of glial cells) occurs within the *subcortical* white matter, nuclei, brain stem and parts of the spinal cord. The cortex is less affected, with shrunken cells (not swollen) and mild gliosis.

The drugs used in dementia

Donepezil, **Galantamine** and **Rivastigmine** are reversible acetylcholinesterase inhibitors, used as a treatment of the symptoms of mild to moderate Alzheimer's disease. They have little effect on patients with advanced disease. These drugs work by blocking the action of acetylcholinesterase, the enzyme that breaks down acetylcholine, thus increasing the level of acetylcholine in brain circuits devastated by a lack of this neurotransmitter. Donepezil reduces the rate of cognitive deterioration in about 40 per cent of cases, but has no effect on dementias caused by failure of cerebral circulation. These drugs can induce unwanted dose-related cholinergic side-effects that include nausea, vomiting, diarrhoea, dizziness, insomnia and rarely **syncopy** (fainting). Acetylcholinesterase inhibitors should be prescribed only by consultants specialising in the treatment of dementia. Prescribing a drug treatment is based on careful assessment of the patient's cognitive abilities and behaviour, including their abilities in providing for themselves a suitable level of self-care. Assessments should be repeated every six months. The patient's carer should be included in the assessment process and in any decision to prescribe a drug, with administration routine, dosage and side-effects fully explained to them. This is because cognitive decline in the patient may lead to poor drug compliance, and therefore supervision of medication by a responsible carer can become essential. After initial specialist assessment, drugs may continue to be prescribed by the patient's own doctor under a shared-care protocol.

These drugs are well absorbed from the gut so they are suitable for oral use. They are metabolised in the liver and are excreted via the kidneys. Donepezil has a 100 per cent oral bioavailability and a long-half-life (70 hours), and is usually given at night. Galantamine also has 100 per cent oral bioavailability, but a much shorter half-life (5 to 7 hours). Rivastigmine has a 40 per cent oral bioavailability due to first pass metabolism, and a very short half-life (1 hour).

Memantine is an NMDA glutamate receptor antagonist which reduces the damaging overactivity of glutamate within nerve cells. It also has antagonistic activity at the serotonin 5-HT3 and nicotinic acetylcholine receptors, and an agonistic effect on dopamine D2 receptors. It has become a treatment for moderate to severe dementia although its high cost has limited its use in the UK.

Future drugs for dementia

There are about 675 clinical trials going on testing new treatments and diagnostic procedures for AD. A large number of these are new drug treatments for dementia in various stages of development. Some could be in clinical use within a few years. Amongst these new drug studies there are:

1. Inhibitors of the enzymes that produce beta-amyloid.
2. Blockers of beta-amyloid aggregation.
3. Drugs which combat hyperphosphorylated tau production and accumulation.
4. Agents which protect neurons against death and promote brain cell health.
5. Vaccines or antibodies which clear away accumulated beta-amyloid.

Ampakines are a class of drugs that improve memory by a different mechanism (Figure 14.6). They prolong the memory by stimulating glutamate binding to

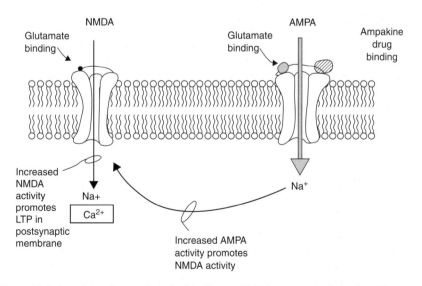

Figure 14.6 Ampakine drug action. By binding to AMPA receptors, these drugs increase glutamate activity at that receptor. The increased sodium entry here promotes NMDA receptor activity in the same cell membrane, resulting in a large calcium influx, which boosts memory.

AMPA receptors. Increased AMPA receptor activity then promotes the function of NMDA receptors and thereby establishes improved LTP in the postsynaptic membrane. When they come into clinical practice, ampakines may be the next generation of memory-enhancing drugs to replace the acetylcholinesterase inhibitors (Concar 1997). However, there is a downside to memory-boosting drugs. Growing evidence indicates that memory is closely associated with pain, both the memory of and the sensation of pain (Day 2002). Boosting memory with drugs may have the adverse effect of increasing pain sensitivity, so everything that hurts normally would hurt even more with these drugs. It is a stark choice for the elderly with dementia: improve your memory but suffer more pain, or live in comfort and memory loss. It may be possible, however, to target the drugs to different areas of the brain, i.e. to the areas that process memory and not to the areas that process pain. In addition, other drugs that block pain-related enzymes in the spine may reduce the sensation of pain in persons taking these drugs (Day 2002).

Also in late trials is a Russian developed drug called **Dimebon (Dimebolin)**. This agent slows down brain cell death by improving mitochodrial function. However, it is controversial because many believe the early success rate observed is based on unreliable data.

Rember is another trial drug that could be in clinical use by 2012. This drug contains a form of **methylene blue**, which is an inhibitor of Tau protein aggregation, i.e. it prevents the formation of tangles in AD. The 2008 trials showed an 81 per cent improvement in patient cognitive ability for those taking 60mg three times a day for nearly a year. Rember also increases specific mitochondrial biochemical pathways which are in decline in both AD and Parkinson's disease (PD). For this reason, and because Rember also acts on the **synuclein** fibres in the brain, it is also *See page 264*   being considered as a treatment for Parkinson's Disease.

New cells for old!

Speculation is growing about the possibility that new neurons can be grown to replace cells lost from dementia. **Stem cells** are undifferentiated cells, i.e. they are cells at a very early stage of development, and have not yet been designated as any particular cell type. The hope is that stem cells can be artificially manipulated to form specialised brain cells. These could then be used to replace missing cells in dementia, and maybe restore brain function. It amounts to rebuilding a damaged mind, but the research is at an early stage, and it is therefore a potential treatment for the future.

Key points

The ageing brain

- Naturally occurring neuron loss can begin as early as 23 years of age, but is insignificant during these early years. It is likely to increase after 60.
- Neuron losses may be attributed to reduced blood flow to the brain caused by age-related changes in the arteries that supply the head.
- Neurons are oxygen and glucose-sensitive and will not function when faced with a decline in the oxygen and glucose supply.
- Synapses are vital for memory and learning.

The hippocampus and memory

- The hippocampal complex consists of the dentate gyrus and Ammon's horn, which is further divided into areas CA1, CA2, CA3 and CA4.
- The subiculum, the entorhinal cortex, the perirhinal cortex and the parahippocampal cortex are all areas of the temporal lobe linked to the hippocampus.
- Memory is based on the formation of long-term potentiation (LTP) at the synapse.
- Damage to Ammon's horn CA1 and CA3 areas, the fornix, the mammillary bodies and the anterior thalamic nucleus can cause memory loss.

Alzheimer's disease

- Alzheimer's disease is a dementia with the presence of extracellular plaques and intracellular neurofibrillary tangles.
- The early-age onset of AD is more genetically based than the late-age onset.
- The plaques have a central core of abnormal beta-amyloid protein (Aβ42).
- Familial Alzheimer's disease (FAD) usually has mutations of the *APP* (chromosome 21), *PSEN-1* (chromosome 14), *PSEN-2* (chromosome 1) and *HSD17B10* (chromosome X) genes.
- The tangles inside the neurons are made from an abnormal form of tau protein.
- The over-65 age group have an increased risk of dementia if they have the *ApoE$_\varepsilon$-4* (apolipoprotein E) gene variation on chromosome 19.
- AD may be inflammatory in nature and is possibly caused by infections in some cases.
- AD is linked with Down syndrome through chromosome 21.

The drugs used in dementia

- Donepezil, Galantamine and Rivastigmine are reversible acetylcholinesterase inhibitors.
- Ampakines are future drugs which are being investigated for improvement of memory.
- They increase activity of the AMPA receptors that boost NMDA receptor function in memory and learning.
- Rember is a possible future drug that improves cognitive abilities in AD.
- It reverses tangle formation and improves mitochondrial activity.
- AD patients often require supervision by nurses and carers during drug administration to ensure patient safety and compliance.
- Nurses and carers should also be alert to drug side-effects.

References

Beardsley T. (1997) The machinery of thought. *Scientific American*, Aug: 58–63.

Bentley P. (1999) Dementia demystified. *Nursing Times*, **10** (95): 47–49.

Biernacki C. and Barratt J. (2001) Improving the nutritional status of people with dementia. *British Journal of Nursing*, **10** (17): 1104–1114.

Blows W. T. (2000) The nervous system, part 2. *Nursing Times*, **96** (40): 45–48.

Concar D. (1997) Brain boosters. *New Scientist*, 8 Feb.: 32–36.

Day S. (2002) Painful memories. *New Scientist*, **173** (2332; 2 March): 29–31.

Kang J. E., Lim M. M., Bateman R. J., Lee J. J., Smyth L. P., Cirrito J. R., Fujiki N., Nishino S. and Holtzman D. M. (2009). Amyloid–beta dynamics are regulated by orexin and the sleep-wake cycle. *Science* **326** (5955): 1005–1007.

Katzman R. and Kawas C. (1998) Risk factors for Alzheimer's disease. *Neuroscience News*, **1** (4): 27–34.

Maier-Lorentz M. M. (2000a) Neurobiological basis for Alzheimer's disease. *Journal of Neuroscience Nursing*, **32** (2): 117–125.

Maier-Lorentz M. M. (2000b) Effective nursing interventions for the management of Alzheimer's disease. *Journal of Neuroscience Nursing*, **32** (3): 153–157.

Smith D., Clark R., Jobst K. A., Sutton L., Ueland P. M. and Refsum H. (1998) Hyperhomocysteinemia: an independent risk factor for histopathologically-confirmed Alzheimer's disease, in *Homocysteine: A Possible Risk Factor for Alzheimer's Disease*. Available online: http://www.sciencedaily.com/releases/1998/05/980504125421.htm.

15 Learning, behavioural and developmental disorders

- Introduction
- Learning disorders
- Communication disorders
- Behavioural disorders
- Developmental disorders
- Mental retardation
- Tic disorders
- Key points

Introduction

The learning and developmental disorders generally begin during childhood and have a combination of causes. Some have a genetic basis interacting with social, psychological and environmental factors. These are referred to as having a **polygenic** aetiology.

A classification of such disorders includes the following:

- Learning disorders (dyslexia, dysgraphia and dyspraxia).
- Communication disorders (expressive language disorder, stuttering).
- Behavioural disorders (attention deficit hyperactivity disorder).
- Developmental disorders (autism, Asperger's syndrome, Rett syndrome).
- Mental retardation (phenylketonuria, Tay-Sachs disease, fetal alcohol syndrome).
- Tic disorders (Tourette syndrome).

Learning disorders

Dyslexia

Dyslexia is a reading/writing disorder in which any three of the following symptoms may be present:

1 Words or letters being reversed during reading after the age of eight years;
2 Deterioration of writing;

3   Difficulty with hearing;
4   Difficulty with learning by rote.

Between 5 and 10 per cent of school children have significant deficits in their reading skills. Reading begins with the understanding of the phonics (or sounds) of words, or different parts of words, learnt first from the spoken language. After this, the child must learn to associate the phonic sounds with the written symbols of the language as printed on the page, so reading becomes a translation of the written symbols into spoken sounds. Sufferers of dyslexia appear to find this very difficult, although in all other respects they are usually intellectually well developed. Developmental dyslexia appears to be familial, suggesting a genetic basis to the disorder.

Multiple genes have been identified as associated with dyslexia:

- **DYX1** (dyslexia specific 1) found at 15q21, a gene linked to single-word reading and spelling. Disorder of this gene results in both spelling and reading difficulties, providing a biological basis that accounts for the linkage between these two skills.
- **DYX2** (dyslexia specific 2) found at 6p21.3, a gene linked to the awareness of phonics in the spoken word.
- **DYX3** found at 2p15–16, **DYX4** found at 6q13–16, **DYX5** found at 3p12-q13, **DYX6** found at 18p11.2, **DYX7** found at 11p15.5, **DYX8** found at 1p36-p34 and **DYX9** found at Xq27.3 are all susceptibility genes, meaning that if mutations of these are inherited they increase the risk of this disorder.

Disorganised cell layers in a part of the thalamus known as the **lateral geniculate nucleus (LGN)** have been found in dyslexia. This area of the thalamus is the relay point for visual stimuli from the retina of the eye to the visual cortex within the occipital lobe of the cerebrum. The thalamic cells that are disrupted are those of the **magnocellular layers** (Figure 15.1), large cells that convey sensory impulses relating to visual depth of field and the visual perception of movement to the visual cortex. Other thalamic cells within the LGN, the **parvocellular layers**, which

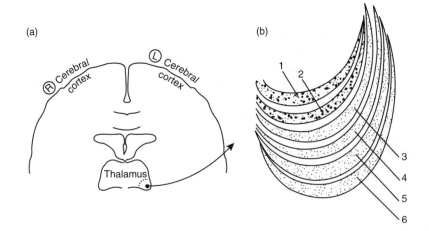

Figure 15.1 The magnocellular layer (layers 1 and 2) of the lateral geniculate nucleus of the thalamus, which are disrupted in dyslexia. Layers 3 to 6, the parvonuclear layers, are unaffected.

convey colour and fine detail impulses to the cortex, are unaffected by the disorder. Pathways from the magnocellular layers of the LGN activate the part of the visual cortex called V5, which functions in the event of movement within the visual field. In dyslexia, V5 activation by the sensory input from the LGN magnocellular layers appears not to happen. Reading is affected, possibly because words appear to the reader to move around on the page and become jumbled, and this is a common complaint made by those with dyslexia. They transpose letters within a word and this causes them to misread words; for example, the written word *dog* may be read as *god*. Perhaps the magnocellular layers are distorting the visual image of words and may be adding unnecessary movement, possibly in relation to the movement of the eyes themselves. Movement involves space, and other symptoms associated with dyslexia show disturbance to movement and space-related skills including poor handwriting, difficulties with balance (e.g. when riding a bicycle), delayed walking skills and slowness in learning how to tell the time. These skills require visual input and the difficulties found in dyslexia suggest problems associated with the development of the posterior parietal lobe, i.e. the primary visual cortex, or its input from the visual pathways via the LGN (Carlson 2010).

Dyslexic people also seem to have part of their upper temporal lobe, the **planum temporale**, equal in size on both sides. Normally, the left planum temporale is larger than the right (Figure 15.2). Only 11 per cent of the population have a

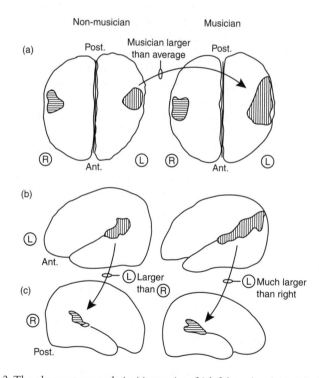

Figure 15.2 The planum temporale in (a) superior, (b) left lateral and (c) right lateral views. Normally, the left planum temporale is larger than the right in most people. In musicians, especially those with perfect pitch, the left planum temporale is considerably larger than the right. In those with dyslexia the planum temporale tends to be of equal size on both sides.

right planum temporale larger than the left. The fact that they are more or less symmetrical in dyslexia is significant. This region contains **Wernicke's area,** the language area, and this has led to speculation that the planum temporale is normally larger and more dominant on the left because it is involved in language and speech perception. Whether this is true or not is a debate that continues.

Dysgraphia and dyspraxia

Dysgraphia is a disorder of writing, causing problems with spelling, in two main forms:

- **Phonological dysgraphia**, the inability to write words phonetically, or according to the sounds of words. This disorder is thought to be caused by neuronal damage to the superior temporal lobe. The ability to write whole words is retained.
- **Orthographic dysgraphia**, the inability to write and spell visually based irregular words. Here the ability to write whole words is poor, whilst phonetic writing is preserved. This disorder is thought to be caused by neuronal damage to the inferior parietal lobe.

Writing is a function primarily of that half of the brain dominant for speech, the left hemisphere of the cerebral cortex in most people. It is here that the twin speech areas are located, **Wernicke's area** for language construction and **Broca's area** for the motor organisation of the muscles for speech.

Dyspraxia is a disorder of movement (**praxis** means *to do* or *to act*) in which specific motor skills cannot be carried out despite there being no evidence of paralysis. It is the speed of movements that appears to be impeded. Speech is affected in some cases (**verbal dyspraxia**) because speech involves rapid, skilled movements of the jaw and tongue. In normal speech we are capable of producing as many as 15 sounds every second. Sufferers of dyspraxia may also have some degree of difficulty with reading (an overlap with dyslexia) or with purposeful movements, thus appearing clumsy (sometimes called **motor dyspraxia**). Swallowing and sucking movements remain normal. The term **developmental dyspraxia** is used frequently since the disorder appears to be a failure to correctly organise the motor (or movement) pathways in the brain during brain development.

Communication disorders

Children with **expressive language disorder** find problems in expressing themselves verbally, due to limited vocabulary and difficulties in learning new words. They may also have problems retrieving words from memory and find it hard to apply correct grammar. Two main forms of this disorder are recognised: 1. the *developmental* form, where symptoms start sometime after birth as the child grows, the cause is unknown; 2. the *acquired* version that occurs after a stroke or head injury later in life. The child's ability to understand others' spoken language is unimpaired. Those children who do fail to understand language that is spoken to them have a variation of the disorder call **receptive-expressive language disorder**.

Stuttering (or **persistent developmental stuttering, PDS**), is the interruption to normal fluent speech by the reiteration of single sounds or word syllables, or by prolonged delays. It affects about one million adults worldwide. The cause is now becoming clearer. Excess dopamine in circuits of the brain, especially the basal ganglia, have been indicated because dopamine antagonist drugs help to prevent stuttering, but they do cause side-effects which prevent them from being a first-line treatment. Normally the left hemisphere of the brain is used in fluent speech. Brain scans reveal a dysfunction in the left hemisphere during stuttering, with a compensatory overactivity of the same areas in the right hemisphere. Also, in normal speech, the left frontal lobe (involved in language planning) is activated moments before the central cortex (involved in speech execution). The frontal lobe activity was absent, or even came after the central cortex activity, in those who stutter. This was a timing error between the left frontal lobe and the central cortex. Further studies revealed a structural defect in the pathways that link the frontal lobe with the central cortex, and it appears that the right hemisphere activation may be trying to bypass this defect. Females lateralise their speech skills less than males (see Chapter 2 for lateralisation). This is possibly the reason why boys that stutter have four times less chance of recovery than girls.

The genetic basis of this disorder is now better understood. Several gene mutations have been linked to stuttering. The **GNPTAB** gene, the **GNPTG** gene and the **NAGPA** gene are all involved in lysosomal activity (**lysosomes** contain digestive enzymes which break down unwanted cellular components). The *GNPTAB* gene, at 12q23.3, codes for a protein which helps in the breakdown and recycling of cell components inside the lysosomes of the cell. The *GNPTG* (16p) and *NAGPA* (16p13.3) genes code for proteins which are also important for enzyme activity related to lysosomal metabolism. The link between these proteins and the problem of stuttering is not yet clear. **STUT1** at 18p11.3–11.4 and **STUT2** at 12q24.1 are two further genes associated with stuttering.

Behavioural disorders

Attention deficit hyperactivity disorder

The two related conditions, **attention deficit disorder** (**ADD**) and **attention deficit hyperactivity disorder** (**ADHD**), affect learning by disrupting the child's ability to raise attention and concentrate on any specific subject. The difference between these two disorders is solely the degree of additional hyperactive disruptive behaviour, which becomes a dominant feature of the condition in ADHD, although many authors consider them to be different degrees of the same disorder.

The symptoms of ADHD include severe impulsive, disruptive and aggressive behaviour, restlessness and inability to concentrate on a subject. Approximately 3 per cent of the population suffer from this condition, mostly children. The cause and the associated pathology are not fully understood, but recently there have been some interesting test results suggesting that these children lack some of the systems in the brain that inhibit impulsive and aggressive behaviour (Taylor 1999). Such an inability to block disruptive behaviour would result in acting without thinking or realising the consequences.

Genes are a key factor in about 75 per cent of ADHD patients, and an autosomal dominant inheritance pattern can be found in families with this disorder. The mutations involved are mostly centred around dopamine and serotonin receptor genes. The D4 receptor gene (**DRD4** at 11p15.5) mutation may account for about 30 per cent of the genetic risk of this disorder. ADHD is often inherited along with other conditions which further complicate the picture. ADHD is regularly associated with substance abuse, for example alcoholism, and with depression. One gene in particular, found at locus 5p15.3, is strongly implicated in the condition. Called **DAT1**, this gene codes for a protein that transports the neurotransmitter dopamine across the cell membrane, but it not clear how this is involved in the condition.

The brains of sufferers show little gross difference from normal brains. There is a small reduction in brain volume, in particular the prefrontal cortex. The lateral prefrontal cortex, dorsal anterior cingulate cortex, caudate nucleus and putamen all appear to be involved in this disorder, but the changes are not obvious. The most important differences are disturbances in the biochemistry of the brain in ADHA. There appears to be an overall reduction in dopamine, and an 8 per cent reduction in glucose metabolism in the premotor cortex and prefrontal cortex (both parts of the frontal lobe of the cerebrum).

The treatment of ADHD may include prescription of the drug **methylphenidate hydrochloride** (**Ritalin**). Related to amphetamines, it stimulates the central nervous system with increasing levels of dopamine, improving alertness and concentration. The drug remains controversial because it can produce side-effects such as nervousness, loss of appetite, insomnia, headaches, dizziness and, rarely, hallucinations. The controversy is also fuelled by the growing debate centred on whether society should be medicating children. The concern is about what possible long-term harm this may be doing to our children at a time of important brain development. Methylphenidate can also affect the rest of the body, causing possible growth failure, damage to heart muscles and low blood-cell counts. Some parents of affected children taking Ritalin have claimed remarkable transformations in their children in terms of better behaviour and concentration. However, other parents have said that this drug has not been beneficial, causing additional behavioural problems. In either case, there is clearly a need for a comprehensive treatment plan for all sufferers from ADHD, in which dugs such as Ritalin may or may not form part of the therapy, based on a joint decision between medical staff and the parents (Scott 2000).

Developmental disorders

Autism

Autism is so called because affected children appear to withdraw from normal social interactions, including parental relations, and prefer their own company in isolation (auto = self). They also show restricted, stereotypical and ritualised patterns of interests and behavior. They fail to develop the skills necessary for normal human interactions; notably, communication skills are lacking to varying degrees or even absent. The social isolationism is akin to that seen in schizophrenia, a disorder to which autism is linked. Autism is also sometimes associated with other conditions, notably epilepsy, Rett's syndrome, Down syndrome, various single-gene defects, infections (e.g. congenital **rubella**, or German measles), some temporal lobe tumours and **hydrocephalus** (Rapin 1998). Hydrocephalus is excessive water around the brain due to a build-up of **cerebrospinal fluid** (**CSF**), which can cause extensive brain damage. The term **autistic spectral disorder** (**ASD**) is used to indicate that this disorder occurs at various degrees of severity, from mild at one end of the spectrum through to severe at the other end. The cause of autism appears to be multifactorial, not purely genetic. The condition affects about 1 in 250,000 infants (0.0004 per cent), with boys being more often affected than girls.

At least some forms of autism are genetically inherited. Twin studies offer the best evidence of this. If one **monozygotic** (**identical**) **twin** has autism, the other twin has up to 96 per cent chance of having autism; that is, there is a **concordance rate** of 96 per cent. In a case of concordance, both twins will develop the disorder, while in a case of **discordance**, one will but the other will not develop the disorder. In **dizygotic** (**nonidentical**) **twins** the concordance rate is about the same as for ordinary siblings with the disorder (i.e. 2–3 per cent). Even 2 per cent is a very much higher chance of developing the disorder than the 0.0004 per cent recorded for the population as a whole, indicating that the figures for twins and sibling relationships are strongly influenced by inherited genetic factors. Understanding of the genes themselves has grown, with 133 genes now linked to autism. The important genes (and their gene loci) are *AUTS1A* (7q36), *AUTS1B* (7q31), *AUTS2* (3q25-q27), *AUTS3* (13q14), *AUTS4* (15q11–13), *AUTS5* (2q), *AUTS6* (17q21), *GLO1* (6p21.3), *AUTSX1* (Xq13), *AUTSX2* (Xp22.33), *AUTSX3* (Xq28) and *SPCH1* (7q31), a gene involved in speech.

Another important factor in autism is damage to the central nervous system of the fetus during or shortly after pregnancy. The highest incidence of autism occurs if fetal brain development is disturbed during the early stages of pregnancy. One type of autism is called the **regressive form** because the child starts developing normally after birth but then mentally regresses. Investigations have shown that mothers of children with autism, particularly of the regressive type, have **IgG** (**Immunoglobulin G**) **antibodies** in their blood which are specific to fetal brain cells. By crossing the placenta, these antibodies get into the fetal circulation and brain where they can disrupt brain development. IgG and complement proteins are also found in the digestive system of autistic children. These are normally blood plasma immune proteins, and are not expected to be found inside the bowel. Their presence outside the blood is similar to conditions seen in autoimmune disorders.

In autism there appears to be an abnormal acceleration of brain growth in early life (before two and up to five years old), both in grey and white matter, so the brain is larger than non-autistic peers of the same age. Later in childhood (from five to nine years old) this accelerated brain growth slows down dramatically, so non-autistic children have a chance to catch up. By adolescence there is little difference between the sizes of autistic and non-autistic brains. This abnormal brain growth in autism varies across the brain, with the prefrontal cortex and the amygdala showing the biggest growth, whilst the motor cortex shows the least growth.

Studies involving the biochemistry of the **prefrontal cortex** in males suffering from autism indicate disordered levels of the energy-related molecules, including reduced levels of **phosphocreatinine** (**PCr**), suggesting that a hypermetabolic state exists in neurons of the frontal lobes with a lack of synthesis of cell membranes (Maier 1998). The **cerebellum** in autistic sufferers is also affected, showing a poorly developed **vermis** (Figure 15.3). The cerebellar vermis is a median lobe

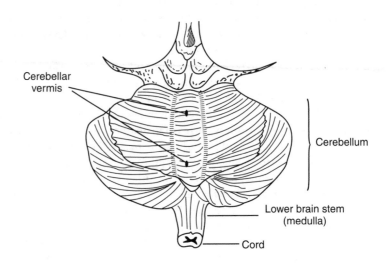

Figure 15.3 The cerebellum, dorsal view showing the vermis (the central ridge), malformation of which is becoming important in mental health.

(that is, it runs along the midline) that appears worm-like (vermis = worm). The cerebellar vermis is also poorly developed, and sometimes missing, in an autosomal recessive disorder called **Joubert syndrome**. Children with this condition also show symptoms of autism, suggesting cerebellar involvement in the cause of some aspects of autism.

Other brain changes that have been identified are as follows:

- The visual cortex of the occipital lobe processes impulses from the eyes concerning facial recognition by assigning this task mainly to part of the **fusiform gyrus** and a few other areas nearby. In autism, the fusiform gyrus has fewer and smaller neurons than normal, and as a result the area is hypoactive. This would account for autistic children having difficulties with social interactions with other people, since these interactions are dependent on identification of people, and that, in turn, relies on facial recognition (van Kooten 2008).
- **Mirror neurons** occur in the premotor cortex, part of the frontal lobe, and their purpose is to allow individuals to copy the actions of others. Copying is a vital component of learning, and these neurons not only perform this task but are apparently involved in higher cognitive functions related to copying, including language and understanding others' intentions. These mirror circuits were first found in monkeys, and were called '*monkey-see, monkey-do neurons*'. In autism, these neurons appear only to respond to what they do, not to what they see others do. This is thought to be partly responsible for the lack of social skills related to learning and people interactions that are seen in autism.

Autism in both children and adults often presents great challenges for nurses, parents and other carers at home. The principal problems centre on communication difficulties, and specialist advice and support are often required (Aylott 2000a, b). Part of the management of autism may be diet-based. Some affected children have been found to benefit from the exclusion from the diet of both **gluten** (a wheat-based protein) and **casein** (a milk-based protein) (Miller 1995). The theory suggests that when these peptides (small proteins) are absorbed they inhibit brain activity to some extent. Their removal from the diet is thought to give the brain greater potential to interact with the environment, improving the ability to talk and reducing the autistic traits. Dietary management is not a cure but it may help to improve the child's communication skills and increase interaction with the family.

Some individuals are considered to have a milder form of autism called **Asperger's disorder** (or **Asperger's syndrome**), named after Hans Asperger, an Austrian physician. They demonstrate varying degrees of the following symptoms:

- an inability to respond to normal social interactions with other people;
- restricted interests and behavioural patterns;
- inability to form peer relationships;
- poor reciprocal emotional abilities;
- abnormal nonverbal gestures.

This behaviour tends towards the isolationism also seen in autism, but in Asperger's verbal communication and cognitive development are normal (Sadock et al. 2009).

Linked with autism is the contradictory and puzzling phenomenon known as **savantism**. About 30 per cent of autistic people have an extraordinary talent in one particular skill, usually centred on music, mathematics, art or memory. These people are known as **savants**. There is some debate as to how or why a selection of people with a disability such as autism can excel to such an advanced degree in one specialised subject. Their particular skill does involve exceptional practice, especially in music, but the question remains: are these talents 'built in' to the brain from birth, and does practice serve to sharpen these skills to a very high level? The attention to detail demonstrated by savants is amazing, and it is this that sets them apart from others in the same field of talent. Some brain differences have been found in savants, e.g. they may show an increase in brain size in those areas involved in their particular talents, but they equally show thinner than normal areas in other parts of their brains. However, this brain thickening could result from the large amounts of practice they carry out for their skill. The notion of brain thickening as a result of persistent practice is getter better understood as part of **plasticity**, i.e. the brain's ability to adapt to changes in circumstances. So savantism may therefore be a question of motivation, i.e. it may be that some autistic children become highly motivated to develop one particular skill which they then develop to an amazingly high standard. Perhaps if this level of motivation was found more often in non-autistic children they could equally develop similarly amazing talents and skills.

Rett syndrome

Rett syndrome is another condition that involves the clinical symptoms of autism. The sufferers, almost entirely girls, develop normally for about the first few months of life, then further development is arrested at about 12–18 months, followed by a serious decline in growth and development. This rapid decline includes autistic symptoms with dementia, and these may be the first clinical signs of this disorder. The symptoms progress to include motor problems such as abnormal hand movements and failure to walk, failure of head growth leading to **micro-cephaly** (a smaller head) and in some cases a slight increase in the level of ammonia in the blood (**hyperammonaemia**). Rett syndrome is caused by mutations of the gene **MECP2 (methyl CpG binding protein 2)** on the X chromosome (Xq28). Such mutations result in loss of noradrenaline from the locus coeruleus, and low levels of noradrenaline in the brain generally, which is a pathological feature of this disorder. Mutations of another gene called **SYN1** (found at Xp11.23) may be involved in Rett syndrome. The normal gene codes for the protein **synapsin I** which is one of several proteins called **synapsins** which are critically involved in **synaptogenesis** (the formation of synapses) and in the modulation of neu-rotransmitter release at the synapse. Exactly how this gene mutation causes the symptoms is not yet clear, but neuronal developmental problems have been found on brain examination. Brain cells show membrane-bound **inclusions** (abnormal structures within the cell body) in both neurons and oligodendrocytes, and a loss of dendrites from neurons extending from the motor and limbic cortex has also been identified.

Mental retardation

Mental retardation is characterised by a seriously below-average intellectual abil-ity involving cognitive deficits over a wide range of skills. These skill deficits in-clude those related to the standard skills required for normal daily living, such as communication, self-care, interpersonal sills and academic ability. Mental retarda-tion can be regarded as a spectral phenomenon, i.e. being very mild at one end of the spectrum to very severe (or profound) retardation at the other end of the spectrum. This varying degree of severity determines the level and types of support these children will require. Mental retardation may cause varying degrees of lan-guage development problems, various motor deficits causing movement problems, weak academic performance and poor social skills.

The biological causes of mental retardation are numerous, ranging from genetic through to environmental factors. Chapter 6 identifies a number of mental retarda-tion syndromes of genetic and chromosomal origin, specifically of the X chromo-some (see Figure 6.13 and Table 6.3). Other causes include toxins, infections, brain trauma, metabolic and nutritional disorders.

Some genetic causes of mental retardation

Phenylketonuria (PKU) is an autosomal recessive gene disorder which affects about 1 in 20,000 children worldwide. In this disorder the *essential* dietary amino acid phenylalanine cannot be metabolised fully due to a recessive gene error found at 12q22-q24.1, the gene coding for the enzyme **phenylalanine hydroxylase** (Figure 15.4). This enzyme converts phenylalanine to tyrosine which is the precur-sor to dopamine and noradrenaline.

See page 60

As a result of the failure of the enzyme, phenylalanine builds up in the blood and the brain. Phenylalanine has to be transported across the blood–brain barrier by a protein, the **large neutral amino acid (LNAA) transporter**. This transporter protein is also essential for carrying other LNAAs across the blood–brain barrier.

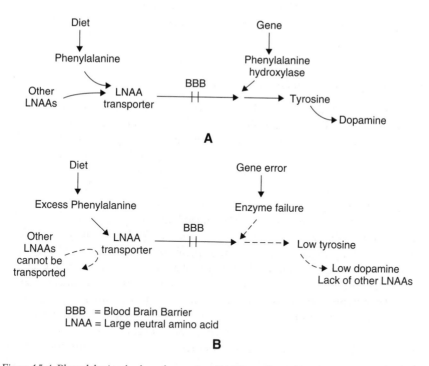

Figure 15.4 Phenylalanine hydroxylase action (A) Normally and in (B) Phenylketonuria.

In the event of excessive phenylalanine in the blood, the transporter is swamped and working only on phenylalanine. Therefore, a shortage of the other LNAAs in the brain causes brain damage leading to mental retardation (Figure 15.4). The severity of the mental retardation varies from mild to profound, sometimes with microcephaly, mood disorders and behavioural problems. A simple test can detect the problem early, and this can allow sufferers to reduce the complications with a low phenylalanine diet (allowing just enough for tissue growth and repair) and sometimes medication with **saproterin**. This drug is a synthetic form of the dietary nutrient **tetrahydrobiopterin**, which acts as a co-factor necessary for the function of phenylalanine hydroxylase. Occasionally, it is an absence of this co-factor that is the reason phenylalanine hydroxylase fails, and phenylalanine builds up causing PKU.

Tay-Sachs disease is a recessive inherited disease more common in the Jewish population. Children with this disorder initially develop normally from birth, but between three and six months old they suffer a progressive degeneration of the nervous system. The CNS degeneration causes blindness, fits, paralysis, mental retardation and usually death between two and six years old. The gene, found at 15q23-q24, codes for a sub-unit of the enzyme **beta-hexosaminidase A (*HEXA* gene)**. The gene can have any of the 120 or more mutations that have been found in Tay-Sachs disease. Beta-hexosaminidase A is an enzyme found in the lysosomes of neurons. It breaks down a fatty waste called **GM2 ganglioside**, which is then normally excreted from the cell. Failure of this sub-unit, due to one of the many gene errors, results in this waste accumulating within the neuron, which then subsequently dies. Although every generation carries the faulty gene, being recessive the disease does not appear in every generation, but skips one or more generations.

Some teratogenic causes of mental retardation

Fetal alcohol syndrome (FAS) occurs when women drink too much alcohol during pregnancy (Figure 15.5). The alcohol acts as a **teratogen**, which is an agent that crosses the placenta and harms the developing fetus. A teratogenic agent may be living (e.g. a virus) or non-living (e.g. a chemical or drug, such as alcohol). As a result of excessive alcohol consumption during pregnancy, the child may show signs of mental retardation along with multiple physical abnormalities, such as low birth weight, facial and skeletal abnormalities and nervous system damage. They have low to average intellectual abilities, including poor judgement skills and difficulties in learning from experience. As an older child they are unlikely to demonstrate anything higher than an average performance at school, and they have problems following directions. The worst problems occur when drinking alcohol during the earliest stages of pregnancy when the embryonic development is taking place. There is probably no safe level of alcohol to be drunk during pregnancy since even low prenatal consumption is shown to cause learning, memory and growth problems in the child at school. A similar problem occurs with illicit drugs taken by mothers during pregnancy. **'Crack babies'** are born to cocaine abuse mothers who took the drug during pregnancy. These children are less alert than normal, with poor emotional and cognitive responses. They also have disturbed sleep

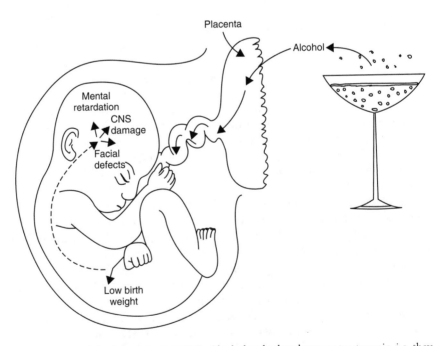

Figure 15.5 Fetal alcohol syndrome (FAS). Alcohol and other drugs are teratogenic, i.e. they cross the placenta and have serious adverse effects on the child.

patterns, irritability and possible mental retardation. Cocaine causes constriction of blood vessels supplying the fetus, resulting in less oxygen supply, which in turn restricts growth and development.

Nicotine is another teratogen which will affect the fetus if the mother smokes during pregnancy. Nicotine has the effect of narrowing blood vessels (much like cocaine) and this reduces the blood supply to the fetus. In addition, the **carbon monoxide** in cigarette smoke binds tightly to the haemoglobin, preventing oxygen from binding, so the maternal and fetal blood both carry less oxygen. Embryonic and fetal growth requires a good oxygen supply, and this is exactly what is lacking when nicotine and carbon monoxide are introduced into the maternal blood by smoking. Fetal mental retardation is due to the reduced oxygen supply to the fetal nervous system. In addition, most of the other 4,000 or more toxic chemicals found in cigarette smoke, such as the poison **cyanide** and the neurotoxic metal **lead**, will enter the maternal blood and cross as teratogens into the fetal blood. The results of this chemical assault on the fetus are catastrophic, including more than doubling the risk of loosing the baby through stillbirth. Babies born live to mothers who smoked during pregnancy are of low birth weight and may be born premature. Low birth weight usually means than the vital organs are underdeveloped and therefore do not perform as well as they should for a newborn child. The brain is chief amongst these organ deficits. The fetal neural damage caused by maternal smoking has a life-long effect on the child's brain, causing poor intellectual development, learning difficulties and behavioural problems (e.g. increased risk of ADHD). Motor and sensory deficits are more common in babies born to smoking mothers (Figure 15.6).

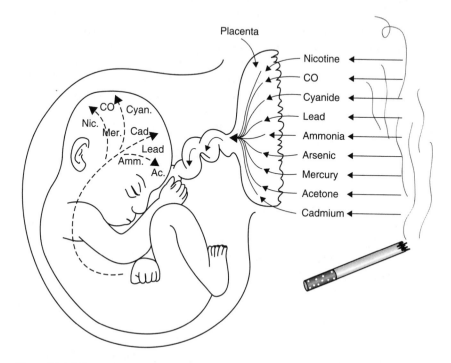

Figure 15.6 Effects of smoking during pregnancy on the fetal brain.

Tic disorders

Gilles de la Tourette syndrome (or **Tourette's syndrome**) is characterised by motor and vocal **tics**, i.e. uncontrollable and repetitive muscle twitches of the head and shoulders particularly, and involuntary abnormal vocal sounds (e.g. grunts, barks, whistles). These tics are associated with abnormal behaviour, such as pulling hair and self-mutilation, and especially the compulsion to utter obscene words (**coprolalia**) and to repeat words many times (**echolalia**). The symptoms of the condition begin between the ages of 2 and 15 years and about 75 per cent of the patients are male. The mutation involved in the aetiology of this disorder is of the gene ***BTBD9*** at 6p21 (a mutation of this gene is also linked to another neurological condition called **restless leg syndrome**). This gene error appears to be responsible for the 'pure' form of the disorder, i.e. without any additional signs of the other conditions which sometimes accompany it, notably **obsessive compulsive disorder** (**OCD**) and **attention deficit disorder** (**ADD**). ***BTBD9*** normally codes for a protein in the amygdala, caudate nucleus, cerebellum and the hippocampus, although the function of this protein is unknown. Other genes linked to this disorder have been located to 11q23 and 13.q31. However, the genes themselves are still under investigation.

The pathology of the brain in Tourette's syndrome appears to be centred on the dopaminergic systems of the basal ganglia. Dopamine receptor antagonists, particularly D_2 antagonists such as haloperidol, have reduced symptoms significantly, while drugs with a dopamimetic action (i.e. mimicking dopamine) make the symptoms worse. The basal ganglia is implicated in the disease because of its motor function and because some discrepancy in the symmetry of both the putamen and the lentiform nucleus have been identified in some sufferers (Breedlove et al. 2010). In addition, the caudate nucleus shows some reduction in a particular cell type known as the '**parvalbumin positive**' cells (Kalanithi et al. 2005). These cells have a regulatory control function on the basal ganglia circuits routed through the caudate nucleus. A new treatment, **deep brain stimulation**, appears to improve the symptoms in the few cases where the treatment was tried. It consists of electrodes implanted deep into the brain to stimulate brain activity. It is still in the trial stages and the long-term consequences of this approach are unknown.

Key points

Dyslexia

- Nine genes have been identified associated with dyslexia, *DYX1* (dyslexia specific 1) through to *DYX9* (dyslexia specific 9).
- The brains of dyslexia sufferers show disorganised cell layers within part of the thalamus, called the lateral geniculate nucleus (LGN), part of the visual pathway.

Dysgraphia and dyspraxia

- Dysgraphia is a disorder of writing and spelling, in two forms: phonological dysgraphia and orthographic dysgraphia.

Attention deficit hyperactivity disorder

- A gene called *DAT1*, found at locus 5p15.3, may be one factor causing attention deficit hyperactivity disorder (ADHD). It codes for a protein that transports dopamine across the cell membrane.

Autism

- Autistic children appear to withdraw from social interactions, including parental relations, and become isolated (auto = self).
- Autism is caused or influenced by multiple genes.
- Autistic spectral disorder (ASD) is used to indicate that this disorder occurs at various degrees of severity.
- The prefrontal cortex in autism indicates disordered levels of the energy-related molecules, especially reduced levels of phosphocreatinine (PCr), suggesting that a hypermetabolic state exists in neurons of the frontal lobes.
- The cerebellum in autistic sufferers is also affected, showing a poorly developed vermis.
- A milder form of autism is called Asperger's syndrome.

Rett syndrome

- Rett syndrome also involves the clinical picture of autism, the sufferers being almost always girls.
- The gene causing Rett syndrome is *MECP2* (methyl CpG binding protein 2) at Xq28, and a second gene at locus Xp11.4–11.2, a gene called *SYN1*, is likely to be involved.

Phenylketonuria

- Metabolism of the essential dietary amino acid phenylalanine fails due to a recessive gene mutation.
- The gene codes for the enzyme phenylalanine hydroxylase.
- As a result of the failure of the enzyme, phenylalanine builds up in the blood and in the brain causing mental retardation.
- A phenylalanine-free diet can allow normal mental development.

Tay-Sachs disease

- The gene for Tay-Sachs disease normally codes for a sub-unit of the enzyme beta-hexosaminidase A (*HEXA* gene).
- Beta-hexosaminidase A is an enzyme involved in the normal break down the fatty waste GM2 ganglioside in neuronal lysosomes.
- In Tay-Sachs disease this waste accumulates causes neuronal death.

Fetal alcohol syndrome

- Too much alcohol consumed during pregnancy acts as a teratogen and affects the fetus.

- The result is a mix of both physical and mental abnormalities.
- There is no safe level of alcohol consumption during pregnancy.

Tourette's syndrome

- Tourette's syndrome is characterised by motor and vocal tics, i.e. uncontrollable and repetitive muscle twitches of the head and shoulders particularly, and involuntary abnormal vocal sounds (e.g. grunts, barks, whistles).
- The main gene involved in Tourette's syndrome is *BTBD9* at 6p21.

References

Aylott J. (2000a) Understanding children with autism: exploding the myths. *British Journal of Nursing*, **9** (12): 779–784.

Aylott J. (2000b) Autism in adulthood: the concepts of identity and difference. *British Journal of Nursing*, **9** (13): 851–858.

Breedlove S. M., Watson N. V. and Rosenzweig M. R. (2010) *Biological Psychology: An Introduction to Behavioral, Cognitive and Clinical Neuroscience* (6th edition). Sinauer Associates, Massachusetts.

Carlson N. R. (2010) *Physiology of Behavior* (10th edition). Allyn and Bacon, Boston.

Folstein S. E., Haines J. and Santangelo S. L. (1998) The genetics of autism. *Neuroscience News* **1** (4): 14–17.

Kalanithi P. S. A., Zheng W., Kataoka Y., DiFiglia M., Grantz H., Saper C. B., Schwartz M., Leckman J. F. and Vaccarino F. M. (2005) Altered parvalbumin-positive neuron distribution in basal ganglia of individuals with Tourette syndrome. *Proceedings of the National Academy of Sciences of the United States of America*. Online at: http://www.pnas.org/content/102/37/13307.full-aff-1

Maier M. (1998) Magnetic resonance spectroscopy in neuropsychiatry, in Ron M. A. and David A. S. (eds), *Disorders of Brain and Mind*, pp. 303–335. Cambridge University Press, Cambridge.

Miller K. (1995) Psychoneurological aspects of food allergy, in Leonard B. E. and Miller K. (eds), *Stress, the Immune System and Psychiatry*. Wiley, Chichester.

Rapin I. (1998) What a neurologist would like to know about autism and doesn't. *Neuroscience News*, **1** (4): 6–13.

Sadock B. J., Sadock V. A. and Ruiz P. (2009) *Kaplin and Sadock's Comprehensive Textbook of Psychiatry* (9th edition). Lippincott, Williams and Wilkins, Baltimore.

Scott S. (2000) Bad behaviour. *New Scientist*, **166** (2239): 44–45.

Taylor E. (1999) Early disorders and later schizophrenia: a developmental neuropsychiatric perspective, in Ron M. A. and David A. S. (eds) *Disorders of Brain and Mind*. Cambridge University Press, Cambridge.

van Kooten I. A. J., Palmem S. J. M. C., Cappeln P., Steinbusch H. W. M., Korr H., Heinsen H., Hof P.R., van Engeland H. and Schmitz C. (2008) Neurons in the fusiform gyrus are fewer and smaller in autism. *Brain*, **131** (4): 987–999.

Index